Ward-Based Critical Care
A Guide for Health Professionals

OTHER CLINICAL CARE BOOKS FROM M&K:

The ECG Workbook
ISBN: 978-1-905539-14-7 2008

Routine Blood Results Explained 2/e
ISBN: 978-1-905539-38-3 2007

Arterial Blood Gas Analysis: an easy learning guide
ISBN: 978-1-905539-04-8 2008

Haemodynamic Monitoring & Manipulation: an easy learning guide
ISBN: 978-1-905539-46-8 2009

Deep Vein Thrombosis and Pulmonary Embolism: a guide for practitioners
ISBN: 978-1-905539-51-2 2008

Self-assessment in Axial Skeleton Musculoskeletal Trauma X-rays
ISBN: 978-1-905539-47-5 2009

Perspectives on Death & Dying
ISBN: 978-1-905539-21-5 2009

Research Issues in Health & Social Care
ISBN: 978-1-905539-20-8 2009

Nurses and Their Patients: informing practice through psychodynamic insights
ISBN: 978-1-905539-31-4 2009

Ward-Based Critical Care
A Guide for Health Professionals

Edited by

Sally A. Smith MSc DipHE Nursing ENB100 998 RN

Nurse Consultant in Critical Care Outreach, Maidstone and Tunbridge Wells
NHS Trust, Tunbridge Wells, Kent, UK

Ann M. Price MSc PGCE BSc (Hons) ENB100 RN

Senior Lecturer, Canterbury Christ Church University, Canterbury, Kent, UK

Alistair Challiner FRCA FIMCRCSEd EDIC DCH

Consultant Intensivist, Maidstone and Tunbridge Wells NHS Trust, Maidstone
Hospital, Intensive Care Unit, Maidstone, Kent, UK

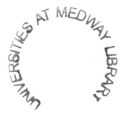

Ward-Based Critical Care: a guide for health professionals
Edited by Sally A. Smith, Ann M. Price and Dr Alistair Challiner
ISBN: 978-1-905539-03-1
First published 2009

British Library Catalogue in Publication Data
A catalogue record for this book is available from the British Library

Notice
Clinical practice and medical knowledge constantly evolve. Standard safety precautions must be followed, but, as knowledge is broadened by research, changes in practice, treatment and drug therapy may become necessary or appropriate. Readers must check the most current product information provided by the manufacturer of each drug to be administered and verify the dosages and correct administration, as well as contraindications. It is the responsibility of the practitioner, utilising the experience and knowledge of the patient, to determine dosages and the best treatment for each individual patient. Any brands mentioned in this book are as examples only and are not endorsed by the Publisher. Neither the Publisher nor the author(s) assume any liability for any injury and/or damage to persons or property arising from this publication.

The Publisher
To contact M&K Publishing write to:
M&K Update Ltd · The Old Bakery · St. John's Street
Keswick · Cumbria CA12 5AS
Tel: 01768 773030 · Fax: 01768 781099
publishing@mkupdate.co.uk
www.mkupdate.co.uk

Designed and typeset in 11/13 Candara by S. Maria Hampshire.
Cover and graphics by Luke Kelsey.
Printed in England by Ferguson Print (Keswick) Ltd.

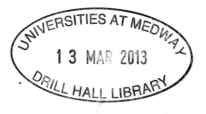

Contents

Introduction

Airway Management   A

Breathing   B

Circulation   Ⓒ

Disability   Ⓓ

Exposure and Environment · E

Practical Skills

Contents

Acknowledgements

This book has been the result of collaboration between many contributors. The Editors thank each of them individually.

Thanks are also extended to The Practice Development Group of the Kent and Medway Critical Care Network for the use of the Tracheostomy Wall Chart; East Kent Hospitals NHS Trust and Philips Respironics for their advice and use of guidance with non-invasive ventilation information; The Kent and Medway Critical Care Network for their input into the book; and Dr Ron Daniels of Survive Sepsis at Good Hope Hospital for his specialist advice.

We would also like to thank Mike Roberts at M&K Publishing and Maria Hampshire at Shoreline BioMedical for their support and help with this book.

Finally, we extend our gratitude to the many clients and patients we have worked with over the years.

Sally A. Smith, Ann M. Price and Alistair Challiner
November 2009

List of contributors

Gaurav AGARWAL *Specialist Registrar in Acute Medicine, Maidstone Hospital, Maidstone and Tunbridge Wells NHS Trust, Kent, UK*

Dr Kuno BUDACK *Cardiology Staff Grade, Kent and Sussex Hospital, Maidstone and Tunbridge Wells NHS Trust, Kent, UK*

Dr Russell E. M. CANAVAN *Consultant Gastroenterologist and General Internal Medicine, Bronglais Hospital, Caradog Road, Aberystwyth, Ceredigion, Wales, UK*

Dr Alistair CHALLINER *Consultant Intensivist, Maidstone and Tunbridge Wells NHS Trust, Maidstone Hospital, Intensive Care Unit, Maidstone, Kent, UK*

Tim COLLINS *Clinical Nurse Educator, Intensive Care Unit, Maidstone Hospital, Maidstone, Kent, UK*

Julie COOK *Acute Pain Nurse Specialist, Kent and Sussex Hospital, Maidstone and Tunbridge Wells NHS Trust, Kent, UK*

Jane DONN *Acute Pain Nurse Specialist, Maidstone and Tunbridge Wells NHS Trust, Maidstone Hospital, Maidstone, Kent, UK*

Sarah ELLIOT *Physiotherapy Practitioner in Respiratory Care, Medway Maritime Hospital, Medway NHS Foundation Trust, UK*

Jayne FRASER *Senior Outreach Sister, Kent and Sussex Hospital, Maidstone and Tunbridge Wells NHS Trust, Kent, UK*

Deborah HIGGS *Consultant Nurse in Critical Care, East Kent Hospitals University NHS Foundation Trust, Margate, Kent, UK*

Dr Simon MERRITT *Consultant, Respiratory and Sleep Medicine, Conquest Hospital, Hastings, UK*

Victor NEBBIOLO *Resuscitation Consultant, Victor Nebbiolo Ltd, East Sussex, UK*

Catherine PLOWRIGHT *Consultant Nurse Critical Care, Medway NHS Foundation Trust, Medway Maritime Hospital, Gillingham, Kent, UK*

Ann M. PRICE *Senior Lecturer, Canterbury Christ Church University, Canterbury, Kent, UK*

Sally A. SMITH *Nurse Consultant in Critical Care Outreach, Maidstone and Tunbridge Wells NHS Trust, Tunbridge Wells, Kent, UK*

Amanda SUDAN *Senior Sister, Critical Care Outreach, Kent and Sussex Hospital, Maidstone and Tunbridge Wells NHS Trust, Kent, UK*

Dr Angus TURNER *Consultant in Anaesthesia and Intensive Care, Maidstone and Tunbridge Wells NHS Trust, Maidstone Hospital, Kent, UK*

Philip WOODROW *Practice Development Nurse, Critical Care, East Kent Hospitals University NHS Foundation Trust, Kent, UK*

Preface

Sally A. Smith, Ann M. Price and Alistair Challiner

This book is designed to guide a variety of healthcare professionals in the management of critically ill patients within the ward setting. It is particularly relevant for medical students, nursing and physiotherapy students and newly qualified staff in these areas. Its purpose is to be a handy reference for both studying and updating knowledge and skills as part of one's job. Healthcare professionals should find it useful for consolidating what they learn in lectures or clinical placements, as well as for understanding the rationale of care and practical help in acute care wards.

The book utilises the ABCDE approach for assessing and managing patients who are deteriorating in the ward so that a systematic approach is adopted and so that prompt, appropriate management is instigated. It aims to help healthcare professionals to prevent further deterioration, where possible, and take relevant action.

The Department of Health recognised in their publication Comprehensive Critical Care (Department of Health, 2000) that critically ill patients were frequently cared for within the ward setting. At this time it was acknowledged that care in the ward for critically ill adults was sometimes suboptimal (McQuillan *et al.*, 1998), due to lack of knowledge, training and skills. Consequently a huge programme of training for acute care staff in high-dependency skills was implemented and 'critical care outreach' teams were initiated in an attempt to address the issues and improve patient care. In 2005 the National Confidential Enquiry into Patient Outcome and Death (NCEPOD, 2005) noted that suboptimal care was still a problem for a variety of reasons including staff knowledge and support and lack of staff, and because there were more acutely ill patients in the general wards. Indeed, NCEPOD data highlights that some deteriorating patients are still not being adequately monitored or treated on the ward prior to an intensive care admission.

In 2007, the National Institute for Health and Clinical Excellence (NICE) and the National Patient Safety Agency (NPSA) issued guidelines for the assessment and management of acutely ill patients in hospital in an attempt to ensure that consistent practice is achieved. The main priorities of these documents are:

- carrying out initial physiological observations at admission and/or assessment
- implementing a clear treatment plan based on diagnosis and past medical history and stating frequency of physiological observations
- using 'track and trigger' systems (see Chapter 1)
- developing staff competency to respond to and care for critically ill patients
- applying a graded response strategy (low, medium and high) so that the most appropriate personnel for dealing with the situation are mobilised swiftly
- ensuring comprehensive handover when a patient is transferred to a critical care area, addressing both physiological and psychosocial needs.

With these issues in mind, this book attempts to give the reader a structure on which to base an initial assessment and treatment and highlights when urgent or emergency action and referral is needed.

There is also reference made to recent NICE guidance on the rehabilitation of patients following a spell on the critical care unit. This enables ward staff to learn and follow current evidence after a person has been critically ill.

With infection control being a top priority, some chapters refer to the high-impact interventions when looking after unwell patients in the ward setting, such as caring for a central venous cattheter (Department of Health, 2007).

The book is divided into eight sections, and these follow a logical sequence that is routinely used and taught in critical care and resuscitation training, namely the ABCDE assessment (Resuscitation Council 2006a; 2006b). There are many cross-references between chapters and sections to help illuminate a discussion point or provide practical advice on a linked topic. Pictures and diagrams are used liberally to aid understanding.

Each chapter addresses only the most important points to ensure the best outcome for patients in the initial treatment phase. Readers should refer to other works to address more complex issues and may need to discuss specialist needs with appropriately qualified staff or referral centres. Our aim is to make initial patient care – when deterioration in condition is recognised – as swift and appropriate as possible.

The chapters generally follow a standard format, comprising background and definitions used, the pathophysiology, aetiology and mechanism of each condition and its therapy, and monitoring and management based on current evidence (references are included but not extensive to make the book easy to use). Most contain a short case history or clinical scenario that relates to the chapter subject; these features are used to explain or explore the topic further within the clinical setting. Practical tips and 'Hot Tips' are given whenever possible, to remind readers of key points, as well as useful internet resources and published references.

As the editors, we hope that you find this book informative and useful in the practical setting. We hope it will clarify the initial assessment and management of your patients with a view to improving their long-term mortality and morbidity and preventing admission to a critical care unit. All the contributors and editors of this book are critical care and acute care clinicians from a variety of professions, and all have over 10 years' experience in their field.

References and further reading

Department of Health (2000). *Comprehensive Critical Care: A Review of Adult Critical Care Services*. London, Department of Health.

Department of Health (2007). *Saving Lives Campaign: High-Impact Interventions No. 1: Central Venous Catheter Care Bundle*. London, Department of Health.

McQuillan, P., Pilkington, S., Allan, A. *et al.* (1998). Confidential enquiry into quality of care before admission to intensive care. *British Medical Journal*, **316**, 1853–58.

National Confidential Enquiry into Patient Outcome and Death (2005). *NCE into Patient Outcome and Death: An acute problem?* London, NCEPOD.

National Institute for Health and Clinical Excellence (2007). *NICE Guideline 50: Acutely ill patients in hospital: Recognition and response to acute illness in adults in hospital*. London, NICE.

National Patient Safety Agency (2007). *Safer care for the acutely ill patient: Learning from serious incidents.* 5th Report from the Patient Safety Observatory. London, NPSA.

Resuscitation Council (2006a). *Advanced Life Support*, 5th edn. London, UK Resuscitation Council.

Resuscitation Council (2006b). *Intermediate Life Support*, 2nd edn. London, UK Resuscitation Council.

Introduction

1 Critical care outreach

Deborah Higgs

In recent years, the term 'critical care outreach' has become synonymous with the management and care of acutely ill patients on general wards within acute trusts across the UK. Outreach teams have become a popular choice for organisations managing an increasingly complex group of patients with higher acuity of illness. This chapter explores the role of outreach teams in the context of today's healthcare system.

Background

Access to critical care facilities is crucial for effectively managing sick patients. However, there are capacity issues in the provision of these services. The increased complexity of medical and surgical interventions, an ageing inpatient population, and a continuing reduction in the number of hospital beds has led to an increased acuity of hospital inpatients. The situation is compounded further by the continuing debate over the management of acutely ill patients outside designated critical care areas.

There is an increasing body of evidence to show that patients who become, or who are at risk of becoming acutely unwell on general wards may have received suboptimal care (McQuillan et al., 1998). Significantly earlier recognition and management of the premonitory symptoms of serious deterioration, including cardiac arrest, might improve outcomes for these patients (Franklin and Mathew, 1999; McQuillan et al., 1999; Buist et al., 1999; Goldhill et al., 1999; McGloin et al., 1999). Concurrent work in Australia focused around the development of the medical emergency team, or the MET (Lee et al., 1995); this group of multidisciplinary staff responded to predefined physiological criteria in order to detect early clinical deterioration. The UK National Health Service (NHS) devised clinical services for recognising and managing the onset of deteriorating health; these took the form of critical care outreach teams, and were based on the foundation of the MET initiative.

This early work influenced the recommendations made in the Department of Health report entitled Comprehensive Critical Care (2000). This reviewed adult critical care services and recognised the need to modernise them. It promoted a hospital-wide approach with services that extended beyond the physical boundaries of the intensive care unit (ICU). Critical care was to be driven by patient need – not by location or specialty. The deployment of outreach services was therefore a key recommendation of the report.

Critical care outreach teams

Critical care and acute trusts enthusiastically embraced the concept of outreach. In a survey of NHS acute hospitals in England that routinely provide level 1 care, 73% (139) had a formal outreach team (McDonnell et al., 2007). Level 1 care is the level of care a patient requires that can be delivered on the ward, although they may need extra help from critical care teams. The main aims of the service were:

- to prevent admission to critical care or ensure admission is appropriate
- to enable discharges from critical care
- to share skills with ward and community staff.

Since then, the outreach services have continued to evolve, primarily to meet local trust requirements. While the rapid devolvement of teams across the NHS led to a wide variability of service models – from a single nurse-led service to a multidisciplinary team with allied health professionals and medical input – the common aim to improve care for acutely ill patients remained a key priority. Working collaboratively, the National Outreach Forum and the Critical Care Stakeholders Forum joined together to produce a document that described the role of outreach in supporting patient care (The National Outreach Forum and the Critical Care Stakeholders Forum, 2007). It provided indicators of effectiveness for outreach services, and noted that the objectives of any service should be:

- to improve the quality of acute patient care, patient experience and reduce adverse clinical events
- to enhance clinical staff confidence, competence and experience through training and the sharing of skills
- to improve organisational agility and resilience by delivering comprehensive care across organisational and professional boundaries, directorates or locations.

The pathway of care can conveniently be divided into three phases:

- The recognition and management of the acutely unwell patient on the general wards.
- Clinical involvement on the general wards in the care of patients after a period of critical illness.
- Outpatient support to the patient following discharge from hospital.

Due to the variability of service provision, teams may deliver some or all of the above. However, what remains pivotal to the success of such interventions is the ability of staff to recognise critical illness. Clinical deterioration can happen at any point in a patient's illness, or care pathway, but patients are particularly vulnerable following an emergency admission to hospital, after surgery, and during recovery from a critical illness. It is important for nursing and medical staff to be competent in recognising and responding to signs of critical illness.

Unfortunately, for a variety of reasons – many poorly understood – ward-based teams often do not recognise patients who deteriorate. Articulating the reasons for substandard care is difficult because many factors may contribute – organisational problems, inadequate supervision, failure to seek advice from senior staff and poor communication, among others. The National Confidential Enquiry into Patient Outcomes and Death (NCEPOD, 2005) found that delayed recognition of acutely unwell patients, poor communication between teams, and the institution of inappropriate therapy all lead to poor outcome. The National Patient Safety Agency issued a report entitled Safer Care for the Acutely Ill Patient: Learning from Serious Incidents (2007). They identified deterioration as a key theme. Over a period of a year it was found that 11% of reports relate to the subject of deterioration that is not recognised or acted upon. This was attributed to three key themes:

1. No observations were made for a prolonged period, therefore changes in the patients' condition and vital signs were not detected.

2. There was no recognition of the importance of the deterioration and/or no action was taken other than recording of observations.

3. There were delays in the patients receiving medical attention, even when that deterioration had been detected and recognised.

The aim is to develop strategies that equip healthcare providers with the right skills and knowledge to begin treatment of acutely ill patients at the earliest stage of their deterioration. Outreach plays an important role in supporting ward staff to identify sick patients. A key aspect of the work is about sharing critical care skills, by being clinically available at the bedside. Nursing staff often claim that they know intuitively when the patient 'is not right'; although intuition is a useful aid, it is important to use a systematic physiology-based approach when assessing critically ill patients (Subbe, 2006). Outreach services are aware that effective assessment of patients at risk is a prerequisite for early recognition of critical illness, and they use a variety of strategies to educate ward teams.

HOT TIPS

Early recognition of critical illness improves outcomes.

Physiological track and trigger systems

Physiological 'track and trigger' systems are designed to help ward staff quickly identify patients who are at risk of developing critical illness. Scores are allocated to each abnormal vital sign parameter, resulting in a total score, and this score may or may not indicate a need to call for assistance.

The majority of acute trusts in the UK have adopted such a system in an effort to reduce serious adverse events relating to the deteriorating patient. Vital sign measurement is an important aspect of inpatient care. Efficient and thorough recording can reveal vital trends about the patient's progress. NICE has produced guidance on the recognition of and response to acute illness in adults in hospital. This clinical guideline makes evidence-based recommendations on the recognition and management of acute illness in acute hospitals and provides key priorities for implementation by acute trusts (NICE, 2007). They place much emphasis on the importance of physiological observations.

A key recommendation was that track and trigger systems should be used to monitor all adult patients in acute hospital settings. As with the varying outreach models, there are many different track and trigger systems. Local needs dictate the specific system that is employed. NICE do not recommend one particular system; instead they recommend a multiparameter or aggregated weighted score that allows a graded response and includes monitoring the patient's heart rate, respiratory rate, systolic blood pressure, level of consciousness, oxygen saturation and temperature. For more detail, see *http://www.nice.org.uk*.

Box 1.1 summarises some important points about physiological track and trigger systems.

Box 1.1   Physiological track and trigger systems (based on NICE, 2007)

Physiological track and trigger systems should be used to monitor all adult patients in acute hospital settings.

Physiological observations should be monitored *at least* every 12 hours, unless a decision has been made at a senior level to increase or decrease this frequency for an individual patient.

The frequency of monitoring should increase if abnormal physiology is detected, as outlined in the recommendation on graded-response strategy.

An example of a track and trigger scoring system is shown in Table 1.1. An effective and thorough assessment is crucial, and staff caring for patients in the acute setting should have the skills to identify patients who are at risk of deterioration, and intervene in a timely and appropriate manner.

Many clinicians will use a systematic physiology-based approach when assessing patients. The problems found by McQuillan and colleagues (1998) as mentioned earlier in the chapter led to the development of the Acute Life-threatening Events Recognition and Treatment course, otherwise known as ALERT™. The ALERT™ course is based on other life-support training programmes, such as the ALS, ATLS, and BLS, and uses a structured and prioritised system of patient assessment and management. This approach assists healthcare professionals because it uses Airway, Breathing, Circulation, Disability and Exposure (ABCDE) as the fundamental assessment, therefore ensuring they perform to a safe and consistent standard.

Many outreach services use this approach in conjunction with their local resuscitation team. Once the initial ABC assessment is completed, a more thorough assessment should be undertaken, including a review of the patient's past medical history and drug history. Many outreach personnel, via extended roles, have the ability to take arterial blood gases, order x-rays and prescribe drugs. Such extensions in practice enable a timely response to any deterioration in a patient's clinical condition.

Sharing skills

Effective sharing of critical care skills is crucial, and outreach teams play a key role in the planning and delivery of trust-wide education in critical care (NHS Modernisation Agency, 2003). Provision of education and training courses on acute clinical interventions (such as non-invasive ventilation, care of the tracheotomy and chest auscultation) have been delivered both in local hospitals and nationally. The ultimate goal is that ward-based teams will need less support from outside organisations.

The success in terms of improved patient outcomes of any system that promotes the early recognition of critical illness depends on the effectiveness of the response strategy (Subbe, 2006). The support of critically ill ward patients via outreach services is achieved through the knowledge, expertise and experience of the staff that make up the team. Outreach nurses appear to develop clear and focused action plans and contribute to clinical decision making by co-coordinating medical and nursing care and facilitating communication (Coad *et al.*, 2002; Chellel *et al.*, 2006).

The follow-up of patients who have had a critical care stay ensures that one of the most vulnerable groups receives seamless care; work continues to develop around the rehabilitation of patients who have experienced profound critical illness.

Table 1.1 **A track and trigger scoring system. If the patient scores 5 or more or scores 3 in any one area, get help from outreach, the site practitioner and the patient's team**

	3	2	1	0	1	2	3
Breaths per minute	–	<9	–	9–19	20–29	30–39	>40
Oxygen saturation	<85%	85–89%	90–94%	>95%	–	–	On 0% oxygen
Heart rate (b.p.m)	–	<40	40–50	51–100	101–110	111–129	≥130
Systolic blood pressure	<70	71–80	81–100	101–199	–	200 or more	–
Urine output (mL/h in last 2 hours)	<30	31–40	–	–	–	–	>250
Temperature	–	Up to 35.0	–	35.1 to 37.4	37.5 to 38.4	38.5 or more	–
Conscious level	Unresp-onsive	Responds to pain stimulus	Responds to voice	Alert	–	–	–
Pain	–	Unrelieved by analgesia	Severe or (7–10)	–	–	–	–

Conclusions

It appears that critical care outreach services remain a key resource for ward-based teams. Concerns about the endorsement of a service not introduced on the back of clear evidence, but on set objectives, have meant that outreach continues to attract attention in the literature.

The variation among service models makes it difficult for researchers to evaluate the impact teams have in practice (McDonnell *et al.*, 2007).

The complexities were illustrated in the MERIT (Medical Early Response Intervention and Therapy) study – the only multicentre cluster randomised-controlled trial of a similar service with wide variability in models of provision. Outcomes were cardiac arrest, unexpected death and unplanned admission to intensive care; they were not significantly reduced (MERIT, 2005). However, outreach provision still exists across the country and is still at the forefront of improvement initiatives related to patient safety and reducing adverse clinical incidents. Outreach teams support junior medical and inexperienced nursing staff in complex clinical situations using their skill and knowledge to improve the care that acutely ill patients receive. Outreach teams can provide a valuable support to ward staff, facilitate the early recognition of deteriorating patients and trigger early intervention (Coad *et al.*, 2002; Chellel *et al.*, 2006).

Any change in service provision requires organisations to evaluate and review the impact of the intervention. Critical care provision is continually evolving, responding to the ever-changing environment of the NHS. It is important for the service to use audit and research to shape the future of critical care outreach.

References and further reading

Buist, M.D., Jarmolowski, E., Burton, P.R., Bernard, S.A., Waxman, B.P. and Anderson, J. (1999). Recognising clinical instability in hospital patients before cardiac arrest or unplanned admission to intensive care. A pilot study in a tertiary-care hospital. *Medical Journal of Australia*, **171**, 22–25.

Chellel, A., Higgs, D. and Scholes, J. (2006). An evaluation of the contribution of critical care outreach to the clinical management of the critically ill ward patient in two acute NHS trusts. *Nursing in Critical Care*, **11**(1), 42–51.

Coad, S. and Haines, S. (2002). Supporting staff caring for critically ill patients in acute areas. *Nursing in Critical Care*, **4**, 24–48.

Critical Care Stakeholders Forum, National Outreach Forum (2007). *Clinical Indicators for Critical Care Outreach Services: Clinical Document*. London, Department of Health.

Department of Health (2000). *Comprehensive Critical Care – A Review of Adult Critical Care Services*. London, Department of Health.

Department of Health, NHS Modernisation Agency (2003). *Critical Care Outreach: Progress in Developing Services*. London, DH and NHS Modernisation Agency.

Franklin, C. and Mathew, J. (1994). Developing strategies to prevent in hospital cardiac arrest, analyzing responses of physicians and nurses in the hours before the event. *Critical Care Medicine*, **22**, 244–47.

Goldhill, D.R., White, S.A. and Sumner, A. (1999). Physiological values and procedures in the 24 hours before intensive care unit admission from the ward. *Anaesthesia*, **54**, 529–34.

Lee, A., Bishop, G., Hilman, K. and Daffurn, K. (1995). The medical emergency team. *Anesthetic Intensive Care*, **23**, 183.

McDonnell, A., Esmonde, L., Morgan, R., *et al.* (2007). The provision of critical care outreach services in England: Findings from a national survey. *Journal of Critical Care*, **22**, 212–18.

McGloin, H., Adam, S. and Singer, M. (1999). Unexpected deaths and referrals to intensive care of patients on general wards. Are some cases potentially avoidable? *Journal of the Royal College of Physicians of London*, **33**, 255–59.

McQuillan, P., Pilkington, S., Allan, A., *et al.* (1998). Confidential inquiry into quality of care before admission to intensive care. *British Medical Journal*, **316**, 1853–58.

MERIT Study Investigators (2005). Introduction of the medical emergency team (MET) system: A cluster-randomised controlled trial. *Lancet*, **365**, 2091–97.

National Confidential Enquiry into Patient Outcome and Death (2005). *An Acute Problem?* London, NCEPOD.

National Patient Safety Agency (2007). *Safer Care for the Acutely Ill Patient: Learning from Serious Incidents*. London, NPSA.

Subbe, C. (2006). Recognition and assessment of critical illness. *Anaesthesia and Intensive Care Medicine*, **8**(1), 21–23.

The National Institute for Health and Clinical Excellence (2007). *Clinical Guideline 50: Acutely Ill Patients in Hospital: Recognition of and Response to Acute Illness in Adults in Hospital*. London, NICE.

Useful websites

National Institute for Health and Clinical Excellence (NICE)
www.nice.org.uk

National Outreach Forum
www.norf.org.uk

National Patient Safety Agency
www.npsa.nhs.uk

Patient Safety First Campaign
www.patientsafetyfirst.nhs.uk

2 Assessing and monitoring the acutely ill ward patient

Alistair Challiner and Sally A. Smith

I t is well recognised that the acuity of ward patients is increasing (Audit Commission, 1999; Department of Health, 2000; National Institute of Health and Clinical Excellence (NICE), 2007). The patient population is ageing, with greater dependency and higher coexisting morbidity (NICE, 2007). Technology is becoming more complex with regard to the management and monitoring of acutely ill ward patients.

It is now more common to be caring for patients with tracheostomies, non-invasive ventilation and continuous positive airway pressure (CPAP) in the ward setting; these are perceived as advanced therapies (Ball, 2005) that sometimes enable ward staff to prevent patients requiring admission to the intensive care unit (ICU). Due to the pressure on beds in the high-dependency and intensive care units, it is becoming inevitable that acutely ill patients residing in ward beds require close assessment, observation and monitoring. This increasing complexity is placing more pressure on ward staff and many staff caring for these patients feel they do not possess adequate critical care knowledge and expertise.

This chapter will outline how to assess a sick patient effectively and quickly, and then describes in more detail how to assess a patient at each point. At the end of this chapter you will be able to: outline a systematic way of assessing an acutely ill patient and describe the required monitoring and observation.

The detailed assessment of an acutely ill patient is essential. Attention to detail is also imperative. A systematic and simple assessment protocol will ensure a thorough assessment is undertaken. Always using the same systematic approach ensures the whole team works towards the same therapeutic goals (Smith, 2003). Many systems have been designed to aid appropriate examination and assessment of a patient, and many of them use the ABC system, which prioritises the airway before breathing before circulation and before neurological aspects. The systems may be applied to trauma, impending cardiac arrest or paediatrics.

How to examine an acutely unwell patient

The first assessment performed by experienced clinicians is to look at the patient and gauge how sick the patient is. This is achieved by experience, but the three key observations (according to the paediatric assessment triage PEPP course manual; The Resuscitation Council, 2005) to make are:

- the apparent level of consciousness
- the colour of the patient
- the breathing pattern and approximate rate.

Case Scenario

A 58-year-old woman is admitted to a surgical ward with pancreatitis. Previously fit and well, she says she smokes 40 cigarettes per day, has a minimal alcohol intake, but reports having felt lethargic and in pain for the previous 5 days. She is admitted to a surgical ward. An intravenous infusion is commenced at 125 mL per hour, and she is made nil by mouth. Antibiotics are commenced. Overnight her blood pressure remains low for several hours with a systolic of 70–90 mmHg, and a urine output of 15–20 mL per hour. Other observations are stable, although at 8 A.M. her respiratory rate is 20 breaths per minute, her SpO_2 is 92%, her heart rate is 120 beats per minute and her blood pressure is 90/40 mmHg. The nursing staff called the surgical team to review. Her track and trigger score is 6, requiring an urgent review.

If you were the nurse caring for this patient, or the house officer asked to review, what assessment, observations and monitoring would you undertake or request?

A patient who is deteriorating (like the woman in the scenario above) will require an immediate 'triage-type' assessment, to identify the immediate resuscitation or interventions required in the short term, while a more detailed examination will follow once he or she is stabilised. This will largely be a physical assessment commencing with the Airway, then Breathing, Circulation and Disability (neurological assessment) then Exposure/Examination/Everything Else – namely, the ABCDE approach.

The principle of this method is to deal with each aspect before moving on to the next. For example, if a patient's airway is compromised, this needs to be managed before breathing can be assessed.

Level of consciousness

The level of consciousness must be assessed quickly:

- Is the patient awake?
- Does he or she look at you and follow you with their eyes?
- If they look like they are asleep, do they respond to speech, or are they unresponsive even to touch?

Answers to these questions give a rapid indication of how ill a patient is. Any decrease in consciousness indicates a very sick patient.

Think of the causes as:

1. Hypoxaemia.
2. Hypercapnia from ventilatory failure.
3. Shock or circulatory failure.
4. Neurological impairment from metabolic, or non traumatic cerebral injury.
5. Drug or alcohol intoxication.

This pattern follows the ABCDE system.

Colour

The colour of the patient gives a rapid indication of sickness and underlying problems. For example:

- A blue patient is hypoxaemic until proved otherwise.
- A pale patient may have acute blood loss or shock.
- Skin mottling may indicate sepsis.
- The patient may be sweaty or dry-skinned.

Respiratory rate

The rate and pattern (particularly the depth of the breaths) are important.

- A *very rapid* respiratory rate, particularly if it is over 30 breaths per minute (with 2 seconds between breaths) may be due to severe compromise of the respiratory system or circulatory system.
- A *very slow* rate, of less than 10 breaths per minute, implies respiratory depression from exhaustion, carbon dioxide narcosis, or respiratory depressant drugs.
- Deep, rapid breaths are typical of the effects of metabolic acidosis or lung diseases such as acute pneumonia.

Does the patient look like he or she has just run a marathon despite lying in a bed? If so, then there are severe respiratory or circulatory problems. The patient will not keep breathing like this forever because they will get tired and develop respiratory failure. Also look at whether the respiratory pattern implies obstruction of the airway. What position have they placed themselves in? Partial upper airway obstruction usually causes a patient to sit up, drool and look very frightened. This rapid assessment takes just a few seconds with experience, but it tells the observer a great deal and reflects the real-life clinical situation.

HOT TIPS

The ABCDE system is very good for teaching and using as a prioritised assessment and treatment algorithm, but do *not* wait until Step D of ABCDE to decide whether the patient is unconscious or not! Assess for this quickly then get appropriate help and undertake appropriate treatment.

Following the initial quick look, the ABCDE system should be run through to exclude acute life-threatening risks.

Assessing an acutely ill patient using the ABCDE system

The **ABCDE** system (**A**irway, **B**reathing, **C**irculation, **D**isability, **E**xposure/**E**nvironment/**E**verything **E**lse) will identify:

1. Whether the airway is clear, obstructed or potentially obstructed.

2. Whether air is going in and out of each lung (exclude clinical pneumothorax and examine clinically the unventilated lung and the nature of breath sounds, particularly wheeze and crackles).

3. Respiratory rate and pulse oximetry.

4. Heart rate, pulse volume (central and peripheral), skin temperature and blood pressure (it gives the observer an overall an idea of circulatory impairment or shock, and checks for any obvious blood loss).

5. Level of consciousness, Glasgow Coma Scale (see Chapter 45) or AVPU (see Box 2.1), pupils and posture.

6. Any relevant factors in the environment and everything else, depending on the clinical situation (e.g. trauma or medical). As part of Step E also look at (7) below.

7. Look at what has been done (e.g. oxygen mask and percentage of oxygen, intravenous lines and fluids, urinary catheterisation) and what is coming out (e.g. surgical drains or central venous catheters, if present).

Box 2.1   AVPU assessment

A—Patient is **Alert**
V—Patient responds to **Verbal** stimulation or command
P—Patient responds to **Painful** stimuli
U—Patient is **Unresponsive**

Each section of the system will now be discussed in more detail.

A—Airway

The goal is to ensure a patent airway. A simple question to the patient may be enough to assess it. If the patient is able to speak clearly, then they have a patent airway.

Look (inspect)

Look for chest and abdominal movements. A patient with an obstructed airway who is making respiratory effort will have paradoxical chest and abdominal movements. Tracheal tug may be noted, along with use of their accessory muscles (tracheal tug is a rhythmic downward pull; Jarvis, 2000). The patient may also be cyanosed or dusky in colour (remember that skin tone may mask these signs). The patient will clearly be distressed unless the obstruction has led to unconsciousness with possible respiratory arrest.

Feel (palpate)

If there is doubt at this stage regarding the airway, feel for airflow at the mouth and nose. An effective way is to moisten your cheek and feel for airflow against your cheek.

Listen (auscultation)

In partial airway obstruction, the entry of air is reduced, although breathing is noisy. Box 2.2 describes commonplace sounds.

Box 2.2   Sounds of partial airway obstruction

Expiratory wheeze—obstruction of lower airways which tend to collapse and obstruct during expiration.

Gurgling—suggests presence of liquid or semi-solid material in upper airways.

Snoring—pharynx partially occluded by tongue or palate.

Crowing—laryngeal obstruction or spasm.

Stridor—obstruction above or at the level of the larynx.

If you have any doubt regarding the patency of a patient's airway, summon urgent help and commence basic life support manoeuvres. Please see the section on Airway Management. The patient in this scenario had a patent airway and was able to answer questions from the surgical team.

B—Breathing

The assessment of breathing is an essential aspect of the monitoring and observation of the acutely ill ward patient. According to the National Confidential Enquiry into Patient Outcome and Death, changes in respiratory function are sensitive indicators of deterioration (NCEPOD, 2005; NICE, 2007). A change of 5 respirations per minute in a resting patient is very significant, but we know that respiratory rates are frequently not recorded on vital sign charts (National Patient Safety Agency, 2007; NICE, 2007). Using the 'look, listen, feel, measure' approach, breathing can be accurately assessed, with the goal of ensuring adequate oxygenation of vital organs.

Look (inspect)

When assessing an acutely ill deteriorating patient, the way he or she looks will give many clues as to their wellbeing. Observation and assessment of the following are necessary:

- The patient's colour – if there is evidence of central cyanosis (bluish tinge on the lips and tongue) they are very seriously ill because this is a late sign of poor oxygenation.

- Does the patient look distressed? Are they sweating? Are they using accessory muscles to breathe? Routinely assess their respiratory rate (count for a full minute), the depth of each breath and whether the chest is moving equally on both sides. Any abnormalities need to be addressed immediately.

Feel (palpate)

Place your hands on the patient's chest wall to enable you to assess the bilateral chest movement, feel surgical emphysema, and possibly crepitus (crackling due to presence of secretions). Assessing the position of the trachea is vital because any deviation may indicate a pneumothorax or fluid in the chest (i.e. mediastinal shift requiring immediate treatment). If you are concerned about your findings, get senior help from a medical registrar or anaesthetist. See Chapter 46 on making a physical examination of the chest.

Feel (percuss)

Examination of the chest also involves percussing the lung fields. If trained to undertake it, this assessment will enable you to validate your palpation examination.

Listen (auscultate)

You will have already noted airway sounds when assessing the airway. Before using the stethoscope, listen to the patient's breathing and note what you can hear. You may hear rattling of secretions or wheeze. The stethoscope will allow you to evaluate the quality of breathing, and whether there is bilateral air entry throughout, or any fluid, secretions and wheeze. Note any abnormality and treat it.

Measure (monitoring and intervention)

You may at this stage consider it necessary to undertake an arterial blood gas, while monitoring is being established. Observation and monitoring of respiratory function can be via continuous pulse oximetry, increasing the vital sign observations to hourly or more frequently if required. In our case scenario, oxygen was administered in order to maintain the patient's SpO_2 above 95%. She required 60% oxygen to meet this goal. A respiratory rate of 20 breaths per minute was high for her at rest, and her arterial blood gas showed a metabolic acidosis with a pH of 7.1 (see Chapters 40 and 41). She was clearly attempting to compensate by increasing her respiratory rate. Her chest sounded quiet, with crackles at the bases. She required close observation to monitor for any further deterioration in her condition. Continuous monitoring of her oxygen saturations was commenced. All critically ill patients should receive oxygen in order to prevent further organ damage or sudden deterioration. The use of high-flow oxygen (15 litres/ minute) via a reservoir oxygen mask will provide a high percentage of supplementary oxygen to a patient with low saturations and respiratory problems. If the rate or depth of breathing is deemed to be inadequate, artificial ventilation via a bag–valve mask should be commenced and urgent assistance sought.

C–Circulation

Assessment of this patient's airway shows that it is patent. Her breathing requires supplementary oxygen, and hourly respiratory rate and continuous monitoring of her oxygen saturations is in progress. Relevant tests have been undertaken and noted (these will vary with the suspected cause of the acute illness). Assessment of circulation is usually determined by taking the pulse and blood pressure. Temperature monitoring is also useful for obtaining supplementary information. Assessment of circulation can now take place; the goal is to ensure the patient is well perfused.

Look (inspect)

A patient who is compromised cardiovascularly will look pale and sometimes sweaty; observe for this. These patients may also look drowsy. Look also for any evidence of external bleeding, but consider whether internal bleeding or fluid loss could be present. Assess the capillary refill time (Box 2.3), which is a quick and easy way of assessing perfusion.

Box 2.3   Capillary refill

Take the patient's hand and press firmly on the nail bed of one finger (ideally on the first digit) for 5 seconds.

Then release the pressure and observe the nail bed. The nail will look pale but should return to a pink colour within seconds.

If there is a slow response, it may indicate poor perfusion.

Observe the heart rhythm of the patient. Either undertake a 12-lead ECG or place the patient on a cardiac monitor for continuous monitoring. A knowledgeable person will need to assess any ECG findings, but consider if the rhythm is regular, fast or slow (over 100 or below 60 beats per minute). If a heart rhythm changes, first check how the patient feels and ensure it is not due to artefact. If the patient feels worse, call for assistance. If the patient does not respond, follow cardiac arrest procedures. If competent to do so, assess for jugular venous distension. Many hypotensive patients are also hypovolaemic. If their instability is cardiac, this will also help you make a clinical judgement in the absence of advanced monitoring techniques in ward areas.

Look at the patient's fluid chart, if they have one (if not, commence one). This particular patient had received 6 litres of crystalloid and colloid overnight. The fluid had no impact on her blood pressure or her urine output. Her daughter described her as boggy and swollen looking. Assessment of how dry the patient's mouth is will give some indication of hydration needs.

Feel (palpate)

More and more observations are being taken by non-registered personnel in the ward areas. It is common practice for medical devices to be used to take pulse and blood pressure recordings. The negative aspect of this is that it has now become less routine practice to feel a pulse on a patient, which means that vital information can be missed. Palpating peripheral and central pulses will give you an idea of perfusion. The pulse needs to be assessed for strength, rate, regularity and equality at each point. Thready pulses suggest a poor cardiac output and bounding pulses suggest sepsis. See Chapters 13, 14 and 15 on shock, hypovolaemia and sepsis, respectively. Feeling limb temperature is also required, and will give a good idea about how well perfused the patient is. A warm limb usually means well perfused, and a cold limb usually means not. Note at which point the limbs become cool.

Listen (auscultate)

Listening to the patient's blood pressure is the most common way of checking perfusion. If the blood pressure machine is unable to record a blood pressure, palpate one manually using a stethoscope and a manual blood pressure manometer. Remember to follow the manufacturer's instructions about frequency of observations when using monitoring devices as they can be inaccurate in certain situations.

Shocked, poorly perfused patients will have low blood pressures. However some patients may maintain an adequate blood pressure due to compensatory mechanisms, but will have other signs of compensation such as high heart rate or poor urine output. Consider this in the light of your other cardiovascular assessment findings.

Auscultation of the heart may also reveal valvular abnormalities, although it has limited value in the immediate assessment of an acutely unwell patient. Observe for the Portsmouth Sign (Smith, 2003) whereby the heart rate is higher than the systolic blood pressure. This is a late sign of a seriously ill patient and needs urgent action.

Measure (monitoring and intervention)

The patient in our scenario presented with a low blood pressure that had not responded to fluid resuscitation. She was oliguric and looked puffy. We already know that she had a metabolic acidosis. A patient like this requires very close monitoring and observation. Many hypotensive patients are hypovolaemic and the administration of a fluid challenge may well reduce heart rate and increase blood pressure, enabling them to pass urine and perfuse vital organs more effectively. A mean arterial blood pressure of 70 mmHg and urine output of at least 0.5 mL/kg per hour (use a urometer to measure hourly urine) are acceptable goals; they can be easily measured and monitored in the ward area. If the patient does not improve, consider the use of vasopressors (drugs that improve blood pressure). For this, the advice of critical care personnel and senior members of the multidisciplinary team will be required, and transfer to a specialist area is usually required.

In acutely ill patients who have not responded to initial resuscitative treatment, and whose cardiovascular system remains a concern, monitoring the central venous pressure via a central venous catheter will be necessary (see Chapter 38 on setting up and transducing a central venous catheter). This can be continuously monitored via a transduced line and monitor, and is becoming more commonplace in ward areas.

The observation and monitoring of this patient includes continuous monitoring of respiratory rate, oxygen saturations, heart rate and rhythm, blood pressure, central venous pressure, and hourly recording of vital signs, urine output and fluid input, with four-hourly fluid balance measurements. Bloods for urea and electrolytes and other tests need to be considered at this point.

D—Disability

Assessment of the patient's conscious level is undertaken once airway, breathing and are stabilised. With the acutely ill patient this can be undertaken swiftly and crudely AVPU system (Alert, Verbal, Pain, Unconscious; see Box 2.1). Measurement of blood use should be made and treated, if low, with 50% glucose intravenously (according to local hospital policy). In the meantime, position the patient with altered conscious level in the lateral recovery position to maintain their safety while the cause of the change is investigated, and more in-depth neurological examination is carried out. The patient in our scenario was alert and orientated, and able to cooperate with the care she was receiving. See Chapter 45 on how to undertake a Glasgow Coma Score properly.

E—Exposure, Environment, Examination and Everything Else

Once the initial assessment of vital signs and interventions to stabilise the patient have been carried out, a closer examination of the patient should be undertaken. This will ensure no detail is missed and will involve careful and systematic exposure of the patient. This is where you can check drips and drains, observe abdominal distension, check patency of lines and tubes, observe fluid loss or bowel actions and not anything else of relevance.

At this point you should have a good idea of how sick the patient is: are they getting worse or stabilised, and what are you going to do next? Now is a good time to look at the patient's chart to look at the temperature, and any trends in blood pressure and heart rate, respiratory rate, GCS, if recorded, blood glucose and fluid balance.

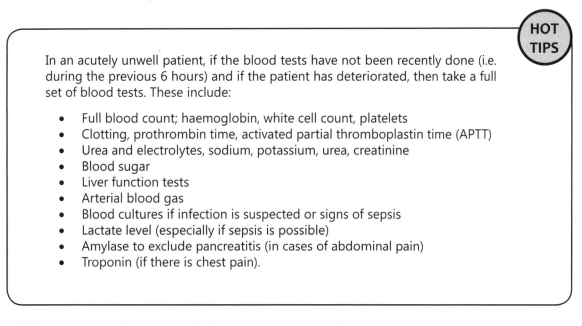

HOT TIPS

In an acutely unwell patient, if the blood tests have not been recently done (i.e. during the previous 6 hours) and if the patient has deteriorated, then take a full set of blood tests. These include:

- Full blood count; haemoglobin, white cell count, platelets
- Clotting, prothrombin time, activated partial thromboplastin time (APTT)
- Urea and electrolytes, sodium, potassium, urea, creatinine
- Blood sugar
- Liver function tests
- Arterial blood gas
- Blood cultures if infection is suspected or signs of sepsis
- Lactate level (especially if sepsis is possible)
- Amylase to exclude pancreatitis (in cases of abdominal pain)
- Troponin (if there is chest pain).

This is an appropriate time to look at the notes if the patient is new to you. Look at existing blood tests, ECGs and radiology. Look at the latest blood results, ideally noting the trends. Check the potassium; is it dangerously high or low? Compare a low potassium with the magnesium, as this is usually concurrently low. The sodium value is commonly related to intravenous fluid infusions. The urea and creatinine may be increased due to renal impairment. Ideally compare with an earlier result to identify chronic renal failure. The haemoglobin level not only identifies blood loss or anaemia but is also related to the fluid status. Excess intravenous fluids can cause an apparent anaemia, and dehydration can haemoconcentrate and make the haemoglobin look higher.

The white blood count (WBC) is usually raised due to infection or other cause of stress. A very low WBC or high WBC can be caused by sepsis. The platelet count may be decreased due to disseminated intravascular coagulation (DIC). If so, look at the clotting results. A prolonged prothrombin time (PT) or INR (international normalised ratio) and a prolonged activated partial thromboplastin time (APTT) give a good indication of this in a very sick patient. The INR may be deranged due to warfarin treatment or liver impairment which can be confirmed by review of the liver function tests.

A blood gas is very valuable for assessing lung function with respect to ventilation and oxygenation. The base excess and bicarbonate identify acid–base abnormalities the commonest of which in acutely ill patients will be a metabolic acidosis. Take the blood samples at the same time that a cannula is sited, except for the blood gas and blood culture.

An ECG is essential in any patient with chest pain, any arrhythmia or hypotension. Previous ECGs are useful for comparison to identify acute changes. Look at the most recent chest x-rays and obtain one if the patient is acutely unwell because the chest is commonly involved as a primary cause or complication.

When reviewing the notes, look at the last entries to see what the last clinician was thinking about, diagnosed and treating. Then look at the original admission notes to get a full history. Also look at the letters section of the notes. Previous admissions or specialist consultations should have a letter with important information on pre-existing diseases. It is also very important to review the nursing notes. Their documentation of events is usually very detailed and may tell what happened during the gaps that may exist in the medical notes. At this point you should have:

- identified how sick the patient is, with the intention of knowing what to do next or who to call
- initiated life saving treatment based on the ABC principles
- have a good idea why the patient is in hospital, their past medical history and what has happened to them.

With acutely ill patients the priority is to keep them alive and stable by correcting the physiology as much as possible. A precise diagnosis may not be possible; for example, a patient may be identified as being in septic shock.

Life-saving treatment includes oxygen, intravenous access and fluids and broad-spectrum antibiotics. The patient should have a central line inserted and a urinary catheter, and one-to-one nursing. The blood pressure may not respond to fluids, therefore urgent referral to intensive care is required for invasive, intensive monitoring, for vasopressor therapy and possibly for ventilation. The source of sepsis may not be a priority compared to urgent treatment and referral; the C-reactive protein and CT scan can wait.

Continuing assessment

It is very difficult for ward staff to provide the level of care that is available in high dependency units (HDU) and intensive care units (ICU). However, patients who are unstable and acutely unwell must not be left unattended for long periods. From a nursing perspective they will require continuous input. From a medical perspective they must be reviewed (at the very least) twice during the day and again by the hospital-at-night team.

The use of a track and trigger scoring system may help staff detect trends and changes in the patient's condition. Handover to other teams at the end of the shift must be succinct and clear, with the management plan agreed and documented to maintain continuity (NICE, 2007; NPSA, 2007).

Many Trusts now have a critical care outreach team, who need to be made aware of patients such as this, and can support ward staff with monitoring and management.

Conclusions

The patient in this scenario was successfully managed by the ward teams with support and input from the critical care outreach team. She required physiotherapy for her chest, and humidified oxygen. Her acidosis and renal failure improved as her blood pressure increased. She was treated for fluid overload with diuretics and began to pass urine. Her pancreatitis slowly resolved. She did not require inotropic support or high-dependency facilities.

The full monitoring of this patient with the use of a central line made it possible to manage her fluids, respiratory and cardiovascular systems effectively. Eventually she was discharged home.

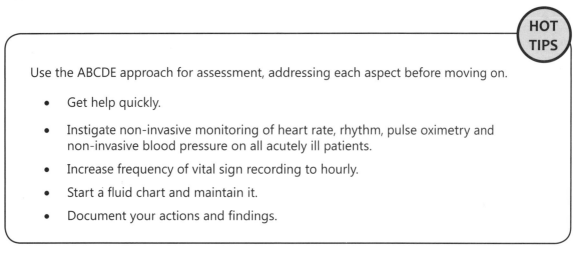

HOT TIPS

Use the ABCDE approach for assessment, addressing each aspect before moving on.

- Get help quickly.

- Instigate non-invasive monitoring of heart rate, rhythm, pulse oximetry and non-invasive blood pressure on all acutely ill patients.

- Increase frequency of vital sign recording to hourly.

- Start a fluid chart and maintain it.

- Document your actions and findings.

References and further reading

Audit Commission (1999). *Critical to Success: The Place of Efficient and Effective Critical Care Services within the Acute Hospital.* London, The Audit Commission.

Ball, C. (2005). Ensuring a successful discharge from intensive care. *Intensive and Critical Care Nursing*, 21, 1–4.

Department of Health (2000). *Comprehensive Critical Care: A Review of Adult Critical Care Services.* London, The Stationery Office.

Jarvis, C. (2000). *Physical Examination and Health Assessment*, 3rd edn. Philadelphia, WB Saunders.

National Confidential Enquiry into Patient Outcome and Death (2005). *An Acute Problem?* London, NCEPOD.

National Institute for Health and Clinical Excellence (2007). *Acutely Ill Patients in Hospital: Recognition of and Response to Acute Illness in Adults in Hospital*. Available at http://guidance.nice.org.uk/page.aspx?o=421416 (last accessed November 2009).

National Patient Safety Agency (2007). *Safer Care for the Acutely Ill Patient: Learning from Serious Incidents. Fifth Report from the Patient Safety Observatory*. London, NPSA.

Resuscitation Council (2005). *European Paediatric Life Support (EPLS) for Use in the UK*, 2nd edn. London, Resuscitation Council.

Smith, G. (2003). *Acute Life-Threatening Events Recognition and Treatment: A Multiprofessional Course in the Care of the Acutely Ill Patient*. Portsmouth, University of Portsmouth.

Useful websites

National Outreach Forum
www.norf.org.uk

Resuscitation Council
www.resus.org.uk

The Deteriorating Hospital Patient
www.thedeterioratinghospitalpatient.co.uk

A B C D E

Airway Management

3

Assessing and managing the airway

Alistair Challiner and Sally A. Smith

This chapter will cover the assessment of a patient's airway and how to intervene using basic life support techniques. It will also describe how to use simple airway manoeuvres to maintain the airway, and how to use simple airway adjuncts.

Assessing the airway

It is imperative that patients are able to maintain their airway in order to breathe properly, and in order to protect themselves from aspirating secretions (possibly leading to aspiration pneumonia) or from blocking their airway with their tongue. The goal is to ensure a patent airway. Assessing the airway is the first step in any assessment of an acutely unwell patient. Recognition of airway obstruction can be made using the 'look, listen, feel' technique.

Look (inspect)

Look for the presence of cyanosis, a 'seesaw' breathing pattern, use of accessory muscles, tracheal tug (as the patient breathes in you will see the tracheal area move up and down as if being pulled), alteration of conscious level, any obvious obstruction (e.g. a foreign body or vomit), and whether the patient is in any form of distress (Anderson, 2003).

Listen (auscultate)

Listen for sounds such as gurgling, snoring, crowing, stridor or wheeze (see Box 2.4 in the previous chapter).

Feel (palpate)

Feel for airflow on inspiration and expiration with the back of your hand or your cheek that has been moistened. If the airway is totally blocked the patient will require emergency resuscitation. A totally blocked airway can be recognised by a cyanosed patient, who is in deep distress and who may have no breath sounds. In this situation, summon urgent help (put out a cardiac arrest call) and commence basic life support.

Simple manoeuvres

Immediate measures must be undertaken if a patient's airway is compromised in order to clear it. These include the head tilt, chin lift and jaw thrust (Fig. 3.1). Turn the patient onto their back and then open the airway using the head tilt and chin lift:

- Place your hand on the forehead and gently tilt the head back.
- Place your fingertips under the point of the chin, lift the chin to open the airway.

The administration of high-flow oxygen (at 15 L/min) and the monitoring of saturations via pulse oximetry (SpO₂) will be required if there is any compromise to the airway. It is also imperative to get help quickly from someone who is skilled in advanced airway techniques (such as the on-call anaesthetist).

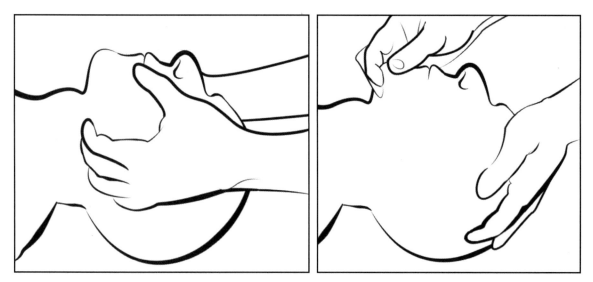

Figure 3.1 Jaw thrust (left) and head tilt and chin lift (right).

Using airway adjuncts to maintain the airway

Sometimes patients require their airway to be maintained using an airway adjunct. This enables easy suctioning of secretions and administration of oxygen.

Inserting an oropharyngeal airway

Oropharyngeal airways such as the Guedel (Fig. 3.2) are used for patients who have obstruction due to reduced consciousness, usually because the tongue falls backwards in the mouth. An oropharyngeal airway ensures that the tongue is moved forwards and reduces obstruction so enabling the patient to breath. The size of the adjunct to be used is determined by lining up the airway against the side of the patient's cheek and ensuring the flange is level with the front teeth and the end is at the angle of the jaw line.

Insert the airway upside down – in other words curling upwards – so its concavity is directly upward, until the soft palate is reached. Then rotate the airway by 180°, so that the concavity is directed inferiorly and the airway is slipped into place over the tongue. This ensures the tongue cannot block the airway as the device is being inserted.

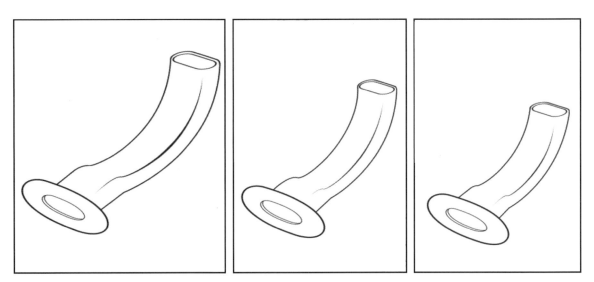

Figure 3.2 Oropharyngeal airways.

Oropharyngeal airways are coughed out by patients when they begin to be able to manage their own airway. If a patient tolerates the oropharyngeal airway, it means they have no protective gag reflex, and they are, therefore, at risk of aspiration of their gastric contents. Skilled help is required if the patient needs intubation. Get help immediately using your own hospital's procedures such as dialling 2222 for the resuscitation team. If the patient is breathing, then they would be safer lying on their side so that any secretions or regurgitation drains from the mouth.

Inserting a nasopharyngeal airway

Nasopharyngeal airways are useful for patients who are not necessarily unconscious, but do have a compromised airway, or have difficulty in expectorating secretions, as occurs in patients with myasthenia gravis or Guillain–Barré syndrome, or someone with a decreased conscious level. The choice of airway is generally a size 3 for a female and a size 4 for a male.

Lubricate the tube and then pass it into the right nostril, as if aiming it in a straight line from the front to the back of the head, directing it posteriorly and toward the ear (not up and over as you may feel inclined to do, parallel to the palate). Gently pass the nasopharyngeal airway through the nostril into the oropharynx with a slight rotatory motion, until the flange rests against the nostril.

This procedure can cause some trauma to the nasal passages, so a gentle smooth movement is best. Try the other nostril if you have difficulty on insertion.

Suctioning the airway using a Yankauer sucker

This technique is useful for removing oral secretions from the mouth. The sucker is bent in the middle so that as you pass it into the oral cavity your hand does not occlude your view. Attach the sucker to the suction tubing and pass the catheter into the mouth, removing secretions gently. Always make sure you can see the tip of the catheter – never pass it beyond direct vision.

Giving oxygen via a bag-valve mask

Administering oxygen via a bag-valve mask is an advanced technique which is usually taught on advanced life support courses. Ward staff members may be able to assist by either holding the mask securely to the patient's face with both hands, or squeezing the bag gently. For training and competence in this manoeuvre, refer to your own Resuscitation Training teams.

Indications for the insertion of a laryngeal mask or an endotracheal tube

Laryngeal masks (LMAs) are more frequently used to maintain an airway in an unconscious patient, such as during anaesthesia or at a cardiac arrest situation. Certainly in the ward emergency situation they are helpful because they can be inserted by practitioners who have received training but are not necessarily an anaesthetist.

The laryngeal mask is a device that acts as a mask over the larynx and thus is easier to maintain than holding a face mask. It is inserted into the mouth and the cuff is inflated. It can only be used in patients with no airway reflexes, as in a cardiac arrest, and is used to administer ventilation via a bag device. Aspiration is still a risk, but no more so than with a face mask.

Endotracheal tubes are the preferred device for maintaining the airway in a patient who may go on to require ventilation in an intensive care environment. The technique requires hands-on training and should be performed by a skilled practitioner.

Placing a patient in the recovery position

There are several ways of undertaking this manoeuvre, each with its own advantages. No single position is perfect for all patients. The position should be stable, near to a true lateral position, with the head dependent (lower) and with no pressure on the chest to impair breathing (The Resuscitation Council (UK), 2005).

Training is required, usually from the resuscitation team, in order to undertake this manoeuvre competently. In brief, it involves positioning of the person on their side, protecting their airway and ensuring their limbs are safely positioned. One person can undertake this, although in a hospital setting two or more people can safely position the patient.

Conclusions

Assessing the airway is the first step in assessing an acutely unwell patient. The goal is to ensure a patent airway at all times. There are several airway adjuncts and maneouvres that can be used to achieve this goal.

Practitioners can learn these skills through basic and advanced resuscitation training in their own hospitals. However, with any patient whose airway is compromised it is essential to call for expert help as soon as possible.

References and further reading

Anderson, I.D. (2003). *Care of the Critically Ill Surgical Patient*, 2nd edn. London, Royal College of Surgeons.

The Resuscitation Council (UK) (2005). *Adult Basic Life Support*. Available at: www.resus.org.uk (last accessed November 2009).

Useful websites

The Resuscitation Council
www.resus.org.uk

4 Temporary tracheostomies

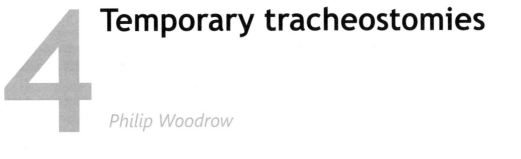

Philip Woodrow

Tracheostomies are a medical intervention to alleviate a medical problem. This chapter discusses care for adult patients with existing temporary tracheostomies. Most Trusts, or their Critical Care Networks, publish care bundles for tracheostomy care; readers should follow care bundles approved for use within their own Trust.

After reading this chapter you should be able to describe what tracheostomies are, why they are used, and the nursing care required by a patient with one. Paediatric care, although not specifically described, is generally similar but the equipment is smaller. Figure 4.1 shows a typical tracheostomy tube. A *tracheotomy* is the operation that creates a *tracheostomy* – a stoma in the trachea. There are three types of tracheostomy:

- a permanent tracheostomy
- a temporary tracheostomy
- a mini-tracheostomy.

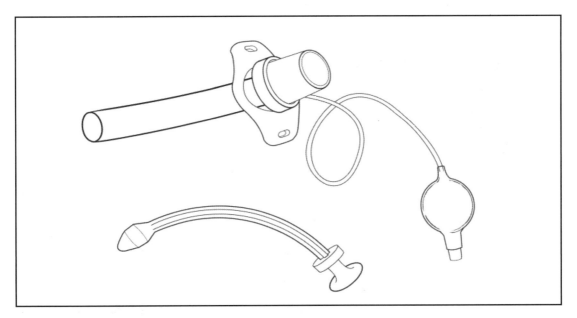

Figure 4.1 Tracheostomy tube.

Temporary tracheostomies are most frequently encountered in acute hospitals. Permanent tracheostomies are often similar, but part of the upper airway may have been removed, usually because of cancer. Well-formed permanent stomas do not always need tubes, but if tubes are present they will not have cuffs. Mini-tracheostomies are not an airway but a means of access for tracheal suction; they are rarely used and will not be discussed here.

Because no gas exchange occurs until air reaches alveoli, the space between where air enters the body (normally the nose and/or mouth) and the alveoli is called dead space. Normal adult dead space is about 150 mL. During expiration, this space is filled with the oxygen-poor and carbon-dioxide-rich air from the lungs. Therefore during inspiration, about the first 150 mL of air to reach alveoli is this same oxygen-poor and carbon-dioxide-rich air. Normal (healthy) resting adult tidal volumes (breath sizes) of 300–500 mL leave sufficient good-quality (21% oxygen, 0.04% carbon dioxide) air for the volume of dead space not to cause problems, but shallow breathing (which commonly occurs with respiratory failure) increases the proportion of poor-quality air reaching lungs, resulting in hypoxia, and often hypercapnia. Creating a tracheostomy approximately halves the volume of dead space, so with severe respiratory failure it significantly increases the quality of air – and the quantity of oxygen – reaching alveoli, while reducing the quantity of re-breathed carbon dioxide, thus improving carbon dioxide clearance.

Case Scenario

A man with a 7-year history of chronic obstructive pulmonary disease was admitted 3 weeks ago with an acute exacerbation, which necessitated admission to intensive care, where he was ventilated for 18 days. On day 5 he had a percutaneous tracheostomy formed and is now making a slow but steady recovery. He is transferred to a medical ward, where you admit him. His tracheostomy is size 7.5 mm. The cuff remains inflated.

After reading this chapter, plan this patient's nursing care for the next few days.

Percutaneous tracheostomies

Most tracheostomies are now formed percutaneously (Walz *et al.*, 1999; Freeman *et al.*, 2000), a needle hole into the trachea is dilated until the tube can be inserted. Percutaneous is quicker and safer than surgical formation, and it can be performed at the bedside (although is often safer when performed in an operating theatre) and it causes less scarring (Eggert and Jarwood, 2003).

Tube size

To maintain patency, a tube is inserted into a temporary stoma. Most adult tubes are internal diameter (ID) sizes 7.0, 7.5, 8.0 or 8.5 mm, although smaller and larger sizes are available. The size is stated on the plastic flange at the side of the tube, and printed on the bladder.

Cuffs

Temporary tracheostomies have a cuff around the outside which can be inflated with air to protect the patient's airway. Most cuffs usually hold about 5 mL (this varies mainly according to tracheostomy size). If cuff pressures exceed capillary pressure, ulcers (pressure sores) may develop in the trachea. Tracheal ulcers can cause permanent tracheal stenosis. So the pressure inside an inflated cuff should be checked, ideally with a cuff pressure manometer (see Fig. 4.2). Like tyre pressure gauges, cuff pressure manometers attach to the air inlet.

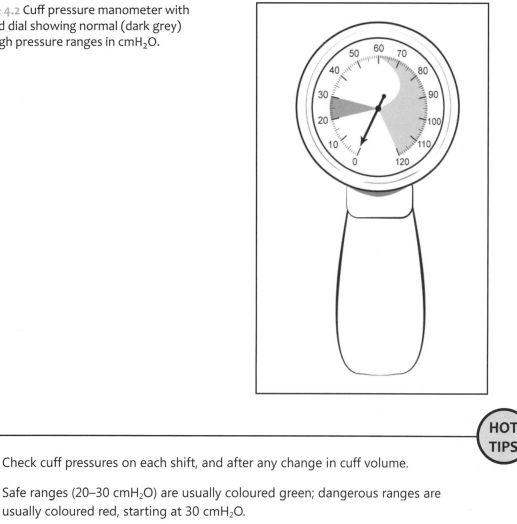

Figure 4.2 Cuff pressure manometer with shaded dial showing normal (dark grey) and high pressure ranges in cmH_2O.

HOT TIPS

- Check cuff pressures on each shift, and after any change in cuff volume.

- Safe ranges (20–30 cmH_2O) are usually coloured green; dangerous ranges are usually coloured red, starting at 30 cmH_2O.

- The lowest pressure that prevents an air leak (so that no air can be felt through the mouth or nose, and no bubbling is heard from the throat) should be used.

- If a pressure above 25 cmH_2O is needed to prevent a leak, the tube may be too small, so further advice should be sought from an anaesthetist or from the critical care outreach team.

If cuff pressure manometers are not available, the external bladder gives an approximate indication of pressure. Significant resistance to squeezing the external bladder probably indicates cuff over-inflation. However, this is not a fully reliable assessment so most critical care outreach teams carry (or have access to) cuff pressure manometers.

Acute respiratory diseases, including exacerbations of chronic obstructive pulmonary disease (COPD), often cause tracheal oedema and inflammation. With recovery, especially with steroid therapy, oedema and inflammation subside, increasing the diameter of the trachea to its normal size. Large cuff leaks may enable patients to 'speak past' cuffs, and may indicate that the tracheostomy is no longer needed, or that it needs to be replaced by a larger tube.

Problems associated with tracheostomies

Cuffs do not form a perfect seal. Saliva and other fluids often accumulate above the cuff, and usually trickle past into the lungs. Excessive secretions usually necessitate removal with oral or nasopharyngeal suction.

Tracheostomies cause various potential problems to patients. Nursing care should, therefore, minimise the risks and problems to patients. Problems discussed here are:

- communication
- nutrition
- weak cough
- wound care.

Communication

Tracheostomy tubes are sited below the vocal cords. If cuffs are inflated, no air passes through the cords, so the patient's voice is lost. Loss of speech is frightening and isolating. Nurses should explain to patients, and their families, that loss of their voice is caused by the tube, and that when the tube is removed, or the cuff deflated, their speech should return.

HOT TIPS

Discourage patients from placing a finger over the tracheostomy to speak. Each square centimetre of skin may harbour 3 million organisms (Hinchliff, 1996) so this can place three million bacteria 75 mL away from the alveoli that are recovering from pneumonia.

While patients are unable to speak, nurses should optimise other means of communication. These will vary between individual patients, nurses, and depend on which aids are available, but may include:

- lip reading
- sign language
- writing

- picture, letter and word boards
- laptop-style computer aids.

When acute disease subsides, the voice may be restored by:

- one-way speaking valves
- fenestrated tubes.

Speaking valves allow air to enter the tracheostomy, retaining benefits from the reduced airway dead space, but they prevent exhalation through the tube. It is therefore essential that cuffs are fully deflated before placing speaking valves on the tubes. With the tracheostomy blocked, exhalation is forced around the tube and so through the vocal cords. Alternatively, 'fenestrated' tubes, with small holes on the curve of the tube, allow sufficient air to escape to create a voice. Fenestrated tubes are seldom used in acute care.

> **HOT TIPS**
>
> Various artificial 'voice boxes' are available for people with permanent tracheostomies, but these are only likely to be seen in acute (non-ENT) wards if patients already have them when admitted.

Nutrition

Because the oesophagus is adjacent to the trachea, tracheostomy tubes make swallowing difficult, especially if the cuff is inflated. This creates a risk of aspiration. So most Trusts' policies state that patients should not eat or drink when the cuff is inflated; once the cuff is deflated, swallowing should be assessed by a speech and language therapist, or another specialist, before commencing with an oral fluid diet. Nutrition is fundamental to health, so malnourishment delays recovery. Until the patient is able to eat orally, alternative means of nutrition should be supplied (such as nasogastric feeding). Dieticians should be actively involved, and the diet closely monitored, especially when oral intake is resumed.

Weak cough

Although cough and gag reflexes may be present, many patients with tracheostomies have weak coughs. Patients should be individually assessed, but may need staff to remove secretions with suction. Suction can cause trauma, so if patients are able to clear their airways effectively, they should be allowed to do so. Some patients may be able to cough secretions to the end of the tracheostomy, requiring a nurse to remove secretions from the tip of the tube – often a clean Yankauer catheter is best for this. But if coughs are too weak to achieve this, a soft suction catheter should be used to remove secretions from just above the carina. Safe suction requires skill, so it should only be performed by someone who is competent to do so. Suction pressures should be low, and many practitioners limit pressure to 20 kPa. Suction is either performed with a clean (glove) or sterile (glove) technique and the practice varies between Trusts. Normal adult suction catheter sizes are Fg10, FG12 and (sometimes) FG14, usually colour-coded black (FG10), white (FG12) and green (FG14); use the smallest size that will be effective. The suction catheter should be inserted into the trachea, to reach below the tube but above the carina. Most patients will cough once the catheter touches the trachea. Further advice on suctioning is included in Chapter 37.

Wound care

Before routine re-dressing of a tracheostomy site, staff should check for the following:

- specific medical instructions (e.g. a new tracheostomy may remain undisturbed for 4–2 hours)
- wound care product instructions (many dressings are designed for daily replacement, but some may remain in place longer if not soiled).

Re-dressing can only safely be undertaken with two people. The assistant is required to hold the tube in place once the tube-holder has been removed, so it may be anyone who is competent to undertake this task. Once the assistant is holding the tube, the tube-holder and old dressing are discarded. Excessive secretions around the stoma may be removed with a sterile suction catheter (soft catheters are easiest). The wound is then cleaned using standard sterile wound-cleaning procedures. The underneath of the plastic flange should also be cleaned and dried. Tracheostomy tubes are now seldom stitched to the skin, but if there are stitches then sterile cotton buds are often easiest for cleaning.

Most tracheostomy wound dressing pads have two distinct sides. Check which side should be placed against the skin – some dressings can be visually deceptive. Tube-holders are often custom-made, with two different lengths. Both lengths usually have Velcro™ fastenings, which are placed through the holes in the flange. The longer length is then passed behind the patient's neck, and attached to the shorter length with a further Velcro™ fastening (Fig. 4.3).

Figure 4.3 Tracheostomy in situ with dressing, fastener and 'Swedish nose'.

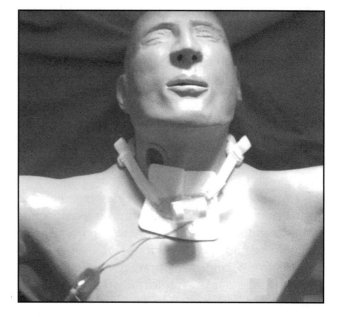

The tube-holder should be just tight enough to place two fingers between it and the patient's neck (Docherty and Bench, 2002). If it is any slacker, it may fail to hold the tube in place; if tighter, it may cause discomfort.

Replacing normal respiratory functions

The upper airways have the following effects on inspired air:

- warming
- moistening
- filtering.

These functions must be achieved to prevent drying and encrustation of the lower airways. One option is a 'Swedish Nose' – a heat- and moisture-exchanging filter (Fig. 4.3). Alternatively, supplementary oxygen should be humidified.

Tube occlusion

Usage of (and frequent changing of) inner tubes significantly reduces problems from occlusion. Inner tubes should initially be changed at least 2-hourly and cleaned according to manufacturer's instructions. As patients recover, specialist staff (e.g. critical care outreach teams or respiratory physiotherapists) may advise less frequent changes. If partial occlusion is suspected, the inner tubes should be changed more frequently. Any occlusion causes respiratory arrest. Like any arrest situation, help should be summoned urgently. Encrusted secretions usually cause occlusion, so removal of the inner tube often resolves the problem.

A patent inner tube can then be inserted. If removing the inner tube fails to establish a patent airway, suction is usually attempted; if it fails, the old tube should be removed and replaced, ideally with a tube of the same size. If a similar size tube cannot be inserted, either the stoma may be dilated with tracheal dilators or a tube that is a half-size smaller should be inserted (see more about changing tracheostomies in Chapter 36).

Nurses caring for patients with a temporary tracheostomy should check the emergency equipment at each shift, checking that the suction equipment works. They should also check the size of tube in the patient (the internal diameter size is usually printed on the bladder).

Changing and removing tubes

An anaesthetist or suitably qualified person usually changes or removes tracheostomy tubes; many Trusts have specific policies about who can change tubes (see Chapter 36 on changing a tracheostomy). Decannulation increases the *work of breathing* (muscular work and energy 'cost', especially of oxygen) by 30% (Cheddar *et al.*, 2002) so respiratory function should be closely monitored following decannulation.

Conclusions

Caring for patients with tracheostomies requires skill and knowledge. Their care is summarised in Fig. 4.4 (overpage). Where tracheostomies are rarely seen, staff have few opportunities to develop these skills and are likely to forget knowledge because it is not frequently needed.

The tracheostomy is the patient's airway, so maintaining patency is of fundamental importance. Staff should seek advice about any aspect of care that they are unsure about and take opportunities to develop skills under competent supervision. Unless other ward staff are

TRACHEAL SUCTIONING

Carry out every hour (or, if in doubt, no less than every 2 hours). Use the correct size of catheter (i.e. tube size minus 2 x 2). Use a suction pressure of no more than 13.5 to 20 kPa per 150 mmHg. For patients who have copious secretions, consider a closed-suction system for infection control.

Enter the size of tube here: _____

HUMIDIFICATION

Inspired air and oxygen must always be humidified using either a heat–moisture exchange humidifier (also known as a 'Swedish nose') or a Respi-Flo™ system and wide-bore tubing.

INNER CANNULA

Use a plain non-fenestrated inner cannula in the ward setting. Inspect it every 4 hours and clean it, if necessary. Do not use brushes or swabs. Rinse with water. Replace it if it is difficult to clean. Store in a dry container.

THIS TRACHEOSTOMY WAS INSERTED BY THE ANAESTHETISTS/ENT TEAM
(delete as necessary)

Any problems,
please contact the team

Date inserted: _____

Tube size: _____

Due for change on: _____

EXPERIENCED PERSONNEL
Outreach Bleep _____
Site practitioners Bleep _____
Physiotherapist Bleep _____
ENT wards Ext. _____
ICU Ext. _____

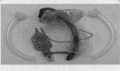

Non-fenestrated cuffed
double cannula
(e.g. BLUELINE ULTRA™)

TAPES

Change the tapes regularly when soiled, at least every 24 hours. This is a two-person procedure.

STOMA

Clean stoma with normal saline as required and apply a foam dressing at least every 24 hours. This procedure is for a two-person procedure.

TUBES

Change at 28 days unless indicated otherwise. The procedure should only be undertaken by an experienced person.

CUFF (if inflated)

If an audible leak is heard or cuff is over-inflated or under-inflated, pressures need to be checked either with a cuff pressure gauge or minimal occlusive technique. Contact an experienced person.

EATING AND DRINKING

Refer to speech and language therapist before allowing a patient to eat or drink. Patients should not eat and drink with an inflated cuff.

COMMUNICATION

Please remember to consider other means of communication (e.g. pens, paper, spelling board) and consider using a speaking valve.

IN THE EVENT OF THE TUBE FALLING OUT

**Give oxygen via stoma and face mask.
Use tracheal dilators if necessary to maintain airway.
Call Resuscitation Team on 2222.**

IN THE EVENT OF RESPIRATORY DISTRESS

Call for medical help as usual. Remove inner cannula if used. Apply oxygen and sit patient up. If suction catheter *can* be passed, apply oxygen and sit patient up. Proceed to respiratory or cardiac arrest action if necessary. If suction catheter *cannot* be passed, patient is in severe distress—call the Resuscitation Team on 2222.

IN THE EVENT OF CARDIAC ARREST

**Call Resuscitation Team on 2222.
Inflate cuff.
Bag via tracheostomy using high-flow oxygen.
Check chest is rising.**

Figure 4.4 **Sample of a tracheostomy care wall chart based on the one used by Kent and Medway Critical Care Network.**

experienced in tracheostomy care, the critical care outreach team should be included in the multidisciplinary team. Tracheostomies are increasingly being used in various clinical areas, so many Trusts provide or purchase study days about tracheostomy care, which staff should attend.

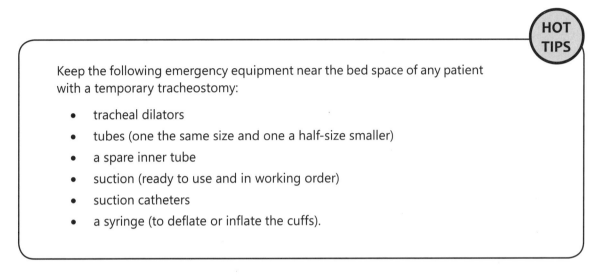

HOT TIPS

Keep the following emergency equipment near the bed space of any patient with a temporary tracheostomy:

- tracheal dilators
- tubes (one the same size and one a half-size smaller)
- a spare inner tube
- suction (ready to use and in working order)
- suction catheters
- a syringe (to deflate or inflate the cuffs).

References and further reading

Cheddar, K., Louis, B., Beanies, L., *et al.* (2002). Physiological effects of decannulation in tracheostomised patients. *Intensive Care Medicine*, **28**(12), 1761–67.

Docherty, B. and Bench, S. (2002). Tracheostomy management for patients in general ward settings. *Professional Nurse*, **18**(2), 100–04.

Eggert, S.M. and Jarwood, C.J. (2003). Percutaneous tracheostomy. *BJA CEPD Reviews*, **3**(5), 139–42.

Freeman, B.D., Isabella, K., Lin, N. and Buchman, T.G. (2000). A meta-analysis of prospective trials comparing percutaneous and surgical tracheostomy in critically ill patients. *Chest*, **118**(5), 1412–18.

Hinchliff, S.M. (1996). Innate defences. In: S.M. Hinchliff, S.E. Montague, R. Watson (eds) *Physiology for Nursing Practice*, 2nd edn. London, Baillière Tindall, pp. 623–53.

Walz, M.K., Peitgen, K., Thürauf, N., *et al.* (1998). Percutaneous dilational tracheostomy – early results and long-term outcome of 326 critically ill patients. *Intensive Care Medicine*, **24**(7), 68–90.

Useful websites

St George's Healthcare NHS Trust Guidelines
www.smiths-medical.com

NHS Quality Improvement Scotland
www.nhshealthquality.org

• A B C D E •

B

Breathing

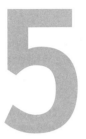

5 Asthma

Simon Merritt

Asthma is the commonest chronic respiratory disease in the UK, so all health professionals working in an acute medical environment should have a good working knowledge of its signs, symptoms and treatment.

Around 5.2 million people in the UK are currently believed to suffer from asthma (Asthma UK, 2004) and in 2002 there were 4.1 million GP consultations, 69,000 admissions to hospital and 14,000 deaths due to asthma (Asthma UK, 2004). At the end of this chapter you should be able to:

- understand the pathophysiology of asthma
- assess the severity of an attack
- institute emergency treatment.

Asthma has been defined by an international consensus report as 'a chronic inflammatory disorder of the airways'. In susceptible individuals, inflammatory symptoms are usually associated with widespread, but variable, airflow obstruction and an increase in airway response to a variety of stimuli. Obstruction is often reversible, either spontaneously or with treatment (National Heart, Lung and Blood Institute, National Institutes of Health, 1992). The diagnosis of asthma is not always straightforward since not all that wheezes is asthma. For example, a middle-aged or old smoker who tells you that they have asthma may actually have a history more suggestive of chronic obstructive pulmonary disease (COPD). (See Chapter 7.)

Wheeze is associated with a number of medical conditions (see Table 5.1). Whatever the cause, however, the principles of assessment and treatment of the acutely unwell wheezing patient follow the same ABCDE format. Some clinicians still use the term asthma rather than explaining to their patient that actually they have COPD, which is a smoking-related lung disease.

Causes of wheeze include:

- viral or bacterial respiratory tract infection
- COPD
- congestive cardiac failure
- bronchiectasis
- localised airway obstruction (e.g. tumour or foreign body)
- vocal cord dysfunction
- cystic fibrosis.

Diagnosis

The diagnosis of asthma depends upon the presence of suggestive symptoms such as wheeze, shortness of breath, atopy (allergy), cough and chest tightness. Characteristically the wheeze and shortness of breath are worse during the night and first thing in the morning. These symptoms may also be triggered by exercise, pollens, dust and animals (British Thoracic Society, 2007). Several objective tests are used to assist in the diagnosis of asthma, the most common of which is the completion of a peak flow diary whereby the patient performs a peak flow each morning and evening.

Asthma is suggested by the presence of more than a 20% diurnal variation in peak expiratory flow rate (PEFR) in three or more days in a week for two weeks (British Thoracic Society, 2007). See Box 5.1.

Box 5.1   Peak expiratory flow rate (PEFR)

The normal PEFR values for a particular person depend upon their height, age, sex and, to a lesser extent, their ethnicity.

Tables of normal values are available from a number of sources. There are also simple programs that can be downloaded to a desk-top computer or PDA which will calculate the values.

One such program can be found at: www.peakflow.com/top_nav/normal_values/index.html.

Asthma fatalities

A significant number of patients with asthma die each year. Most of those who die have chronically severe asthma; only in a minority will the fatal attack occur suddenly in a patient who has mild to moderate asthma.

Beta-blockers and non-steroidal anti-inflammatory drugs (NSAIDs) (see Box 5.2) are known to potentially exacerbate asthma and should be avoided (British Thoracic Society, 2007).

Examples of commonly used NSAIDs include, aspirin, ibuprofen (same as Neurofen™) and diclofenac (Voltarol™).

Box 5.2   Non-steroidal anti-inflammatory drugs (NSAIDs) and asthma

NSAIDs, especially aspirin, will precipitate an asthma attack in about 5% of asthmatic patients. Exactly why these patients are particularly susceptible is not completely understood. However this phenomenon occurs almost exclusively in patients who have both nasal polyps and asthma.

It is known that NSAIDs interfere with the cyclo-oxygenase (COX) pathway, eventually leading to the metabolism of a substance called arachidonic acid to produce leukotrienes.

These are known to induce bronchospasm in susceptible patients.

Asthma severity

It is crucial to judge the severity of an asthma attack; the PEFR, pulse, blood pressure (BP), oxygen saturations and the patient's ability to complete a sentence in one breath, all give very important prognostic information, and indeed guide both the treatment and the need for critical care, as illustrated in Table 5.1.

Table 5.1 Levels of severity of acute asthma exacerbations (adapted from the British Thoracic Society, 2007)	
Near-fatal asthma	Raised $PaCO_2$ and/or requiring mechanical ventilation with raised inflation pressures
Life-threatening asthma	Any *one* of the following in a patient with severe asthma: PEFR < 33% best or predicted SpO_2 < 92% PaO_2 < 8 kPa Normal $PaCO_2$ (4.6–6.0 kPa) Silent chest Cyanosis Feeble respiratory effort Bradycardia Dysrhythmia Hypotension Exhaustion Confusion Coma
Acute severe asthma	Any *one* of: PEFR 33–50% best or predicted Respiratory rate ≥ 25/min Heart rate ≥ 110/min Inability to complete sentences in one breath
Moderate asthma exacerbation	Increasing symptoms PEFR > 50–75% best or predicted No features of acute severe asthma
Brittle asthma	*Type 1*: wide PEFR variability (> 40% diurnal variation for > 50% of the time over a period > 150 days) despite intense therapy *Type 2*: sudden severe attacks on a background of apparently well-controlled asthma

Pathophysiology

The pathophysiology of asthma is not completely understood. It is likely that asthma, a term that is used widely, is in fact composed of a number of different disease entities, as illustrated by different ages of onset, different triggers for an attack, and (most importantly) different levels of responsiveness to inhaled steroids, which form the mainstay of asthma treatment. The common factor – that is the primary abnormality in asthma – is variable obstruction (narrowing) of the medium and small-calibre airways. This is thought to be due to inflammation and airway wall infiltration.

Case Scenario

You are concerned about a 19-year-old asthma patient who was admitted 2 days prior with a severe asthma attack, but was due to go home the next day having recovered quickly. She has become increasingly wheezy throughout the morning and has used three nebulisers in the last 4 hours. This happened within 10 minutes of taking her morning medication and your colleague thinks that maybe one of the tablets is at fault. You study the drug chart and at once spot that she has been given a dose of Ibuprofen 400 mg (a non-steroidal anti-inflammatory drug), which you remember can cause asthma attacks in some asthmatic people.

You go at once to see the patient. She appears very short of breath and you can hear her wheezing from the end of the bed. Oxygen therapy has been commenced. Her observations are as follows: respiratory rate 40 b.p.m., oxygen saturation (SpO_2) 91% on 40% oxygen via mask, pulse 115 b.p.m., blood pressure 150/96 mmHg.

What would you do to stabilise and treat her? What investigations would you perform?

Airway inflammation

Asthma is a chronic inflammatory disease of the airways, characterised by airway epithelial damage, increased numbers of mucus-secreting cells and an inflammatory reaction due to infiltration by activated eosinophils, lymphocytes and mast cells (different types of white blood cells). The lymphocytes release a number of cytokines (see Box 5.3) which recruit and upregulate inflammatory cells in the airways.

Box 5.3 Cytokines

These are proteins released by cells of the immune system, after exposure to an antigen, which act as intercellular signals in the generation of an immune response. They can have either pro-inflammatory or anti-inflammatory effects.

Activated eosinophils release a variety of proteins that are toxic to airway cells, such as leukotrienes. There is a direct correlation between the number of eosinophils in the airway walls and the severity of airways obstruction. Mast cells, which are naturally present in the normal airway wall, are upregulated and sensitised by immunoglobulin E (IgE, a type of antibody) which is directed against a specific antigen (e.g. house dust mite excreta). When these mast cells are exposed to the antigen to which they are sensitised, they synthesise and release a number of inflammatory mediators, such as histamine and leukotrienes. These mediators, and others, can cause smooth muscle contraction, increased mucus secretion and secondary stimulation of airway nerves, therefore causing airway narrowing (obstruction) which sometimes requires treatment (see Box 5.4). There is also airway smooth-muscle hyperplasia and hypertrophy and collagen deposition below the basement membrane (termed airways remodelling). Over a long period of time, in a subgroup of asthmatic patients, this can lead to fixed (i.e. irreversible) airways obstruction.

Box 5.4   Inhaled and oral steroids in asthma

Steroids form the mainstay of the management of both acute and chronic asthma. They downregulate the troublesome inflammatory pathways, and also decrease the expression of some of the more harmful cytokines. Typically, inhaled steroids are used over a long period to reduce inflammation and prevent asthma attacks (e.g. budesonide, beclomethasone and fluticasone). During an acute attack of asthma short courses of oral steroids are used (e.g. prednisolone). Occasionally, in cases of very severe asthma, intravenous hydrocortisone can be used, until the patient is well enough to take tablets.

Physiology of airway obstruction

Asthma is characterised by airflow obstruction, which is for the most part reversible with bronchodilators. Obstruction of the airways leading to a variable reduction in airflow, can be caused by contraction of airway smooth muscle, by the presence of an increased volume of thick sticky sputum and also by thickening of the airway wall. These changes are variably found throughout the bronchial tree during an asthma attack.

> **HOT TIPS**
>
> Refer to the BTS NICE guidelines for a thorough review of asthma and its evidence-based acute and chronic management. They are provided on the following website: www.brit-thoracic.org.uk

On arrival at the patient's bedside, a full set of vital signs needs to be obtained, and a monitor should be attached to the patient to measure continuous pulse oximetry (SpO_2), heart rate and non-invasive blood pressure at regular intervals (see Chapter 3).

> **HOT TIPS**
>
> It is helpful to perform your examination by first inspecting the patient and their surroundings, then palpating, percussing and finally auscultating. The assessment of the patient from the above case history will be detailed here, but note that in an emergency situation assessment and treatment are occuring simultaneously rather than one after the other as described below.

You can immediately hear the patient in our scenario wheezing. She is sitting bolt upright and gripping on to the sides of the bed with her hands, thus enabling the use of her accessory muscles of respiration. She is able to talk, but can only manage a few words at a time before taking another breath. She tells you that she is frightened and asks you to help her. You also establish that she has been ventilated on the intensive care unit in the past, so this immediately worries you and indicates the severity of her asthma.

A—Airway
Since she is alert and talking to you, her airway is fine at present. However you appreciate that the principle problem in asthma is bronchoconstriction (narrowing of the airways) and realise that this must be addressed as soon as possible.

B—Breathing
Her respiratory rate is 40 breaths per minute and her oxygen saturation is 91% on 40% oxygen via a Venturi mask. Inspection of her chest reveals equal but mildly reduced chest expansion and the use of accessory muscles already described. Palpation of her trachea reveals it to be central. Percussion of her chest is normal. Auscultation reveals a diffuse polyphonic wheeze (see Box 5.5) throughout the chest anteriorly and posteriorly. Breath sounds are normal in volume. At this stage you measure her peak flow. She has great difficulty performing the manoeuvre but after three attempts she manages 200 L/min, which you calculate to be about 40% of her best peak flow.

> **Box 5.5 Wheeze**
>
> A wheeze is a musical sound that results from the passage of air through narrowed airways. It principally occurs on expiration. It is a prominent feature of both asthma and chronic obstructive pulmonary disease (COPD).

C—Circulation

Assessment of this patient's circulation reveals a tachycardia of 115 beats per minute and an elevated blood pressure of 15460/96 mmHg. Her jugular venous pressure (JVP) is difficult to see due to the contraction of the sternocleidomastoid muscle (one of the accessory muscles) but it does not appear unduly elevated. Her heart sounds are also difficult to elicit due to the loud wheezes.

D—Disability

Since she is alert and orientated, formal assessment of her alertness and mental disability gives a Glasgow Coma Score (GCS) of 15/15 or 'A' on the AVPU (Alert, Verbal, Pain, Unconscious; see Box 2.1) score (see Chapter 44 on how to do a GCS properly).

E—Exposure, Environment and Everything Else

The last part of your assessment comprises full exposure of the patient to ensure that there are no other physical signs that have been missed thus far. You find a red band around her right ankle revealing an allergy to ibuprofen (you learn later that it was getting in the way when it was around her wrist and so was moved yesterday). You move it back to her wrist. Her temperature is 36.8°C.

Investigations

The British Thoracic Society guidelines on asthma (British Thoracic Society, 2008) state that a chest x-ray is not routinely recommended in acute asthma, unless the patient has life-threatening asthma with atypical symptoms, or is not responding to treatment, or is suspected to have either pneumonia or a pneumothorax. A chest x-ray is therefore not indicated at this moment.

As a rule arterial blood gases (ABGs) are only required in acute asthma if there are features of life-threatening asthma or if the patient's saturations are less than 92%, which they are in this case (see Chapters 48 and 49).

Box 5.6 **Arterial blood gas results**	
Oxygen	40%
PaO$_2$	8.9 kPa
PaCO$_2$	4.0 kPa
pH	7.45
Saturations	91%B
Base excess	+2

The ABG reveals hypoxia and hypocapnoea (a low PaCO$_2$). If the PaCO$_2$ was normal this would be extremely worrying and the asthma attack would be classified as life threatening (Table 5.1).

Severity of attack

Worrying features specific to this case would include any of the features of life-threatening or near-fatal asthma. It is worth noting that this patient has been ventilated on the intensive care unit before, which usually indicates severe longstanding asthma. This patient has a peak flow of 40% predicted, a respiratory rate of 40 per minute, a heart rate of 115 beats per minute, and is unable to complete sentences in one breath, indicating that she has acute severe asthma.

HOT TIPS

Remember that assessment is an ongoing process and it is important to continually re-assess the patient, especially if his or her condition changes (for better or worse) and to assess response to any treatment.

Management

A—Airway

It has already been established that this patient's airway is intact, however any patient who is short of breath will derive considerable improvement if sat up at 90°. It aids them in the use of their accessory muscles of respiration.

B—Breathing

'Breathing' will be the principle therapeutic target in the treatment of any acute asthma attack. The use of high-flow oxygen is encouraged in asthma; the aim should be to keep the oxygen saturations above 92%. It is important to remember that although oxygen can help to correct any hypoxia it will not significantly bronchodilate on its own and, therefore, is an adjunct to treatment of an acute asthma attack, rather than the main treatment. It is important to monitor ABGs in critically ill patients, especially if changes have been made to their treatment or inspired oxygen concentration.

Nebulisers

The mainstay of acute asthma management is nebulised bronchodilators and oxygen therapy (British Thoracic Society, 2007). High-dose nebulised beta-2 agonists (5 mg of salbutamol or terbutaline) should be given as soon as possible. Ideally the nebuliser should be driven with oxygen, not air, but this should not prevent administration of nebulised beta-2 agonists in a timely fashion. During administration of the nebuliser, the patient should be encouraged to take slow, deep breaths through the mouth where possible and discouraged from talking, to ensure maximal drug deposition. A single dose of 5 mg of salbutamol may not completely resolve the bronchospasm, therefore it is advised in the BTS guidelines either to give nebulisers at 15–30 minute intervals or to provide continuous nebulisation at a rate of 5–10 mg per hour (British Thoracic Society, 2007). This author prefers the latter approach, sometimes even giving four or five 'back-to-back' nebulisers over a 60-minute period for severe attacks. At these high doses, tremor and tachycardia are common but only rarely interfere with the treatment.

After this period of stabilisation, salbutamol is commonly given 1-hourly to 4-hourly, with a provision on the drug chart for extra doses as and when necessary. Ipratropium bromide (Atrovent™) has a lesser role to play in the treatment of acute asthma than in COPD. However, research has shown that in acute severe asthma or life-threatening asthma it can produce significantly more bronchodilation than salbutamol alone. Ipratropium should initially be given at a dose of 500 µg every 4 to 6 hours. The most recent addition to the BTS asthma guidelines is the administration of intravenous magnesium sulphate (1.2 g to 2 g) in either acute severe asthma that has responded poorly to bronchodilators or immediately in a patient diagnosed with life-threatening or near-fatal asthma. It should be given only once and slowly over a 20-minute period (British Thoracic Society, 2007). See Chapter 8 for more details on drug therapy in COPD.

Steroids and antibiotics

The administration of steroids is a very important part of the treatment of an acute asthma attack and – if given early – reduces mortality in an acute attack (British Thoracic Society, 2007). An initial dose of 40 mg of oral prednisolone is usually sufficient (a course of 7–14 days would be normal). If the patient is too unwell to take oral medication then 100 mg hydrocortisone intravenously, four times daily, is a good substitute. Bacterial infections are not a particularly common trigger for an acute asthma attack, however in the presence of green sputum, consolidation (shadowing caused by infection) on the chest x-ray, a temperature above 37.5°C, and/or elevated white blood cells and C-reactive protein (CRP; an acute-phase protein which is almost always elevated when there is significant infection or inflammation), it would be wise to commence antibiotic treatment. A thorough review of community-acquired pneumonia and its antibiotic treatment has been produced by the BTS (2007); reference to it is recommended.

HOT TIPS

It is imperative to re-assess the patient at this stage, ideally noting their PEF, pulse, BP, oxygen saturations and ability to complete a sentence in one breath (i.e. their asthma severity).

If all are improving, then continue as above; however if your patient is still deteriorating then it is advisable to perform an ABG and seek senior help as soon as possible.

C—Circulation

The circulatory system in asthma is not usually a major problem, apart from the sinus tachycardia commonly caused by salbutamol. However, some patients are particularly susceptible, and can develop arrhythmias. The best treatment for these is to ensure the electrolytes (sodium, potassium, magnesium, calcium and phosphate) are normal and to reduce the dose and/or frequency of salbutamol nebules, if clinically possible. If that fails then, depending on the nature of the rhythm and the blood pressure, amiodarone, digoxin, verapamil or DC cardioversion can be used, as per the Resuscitation Council's *Advanced Life Support Guidelines* (Resuscitation Council, 2005). It is good practise to establish intravenous access and take routine bloods (full blood count, urea and electrolytes, CRP and blood cultures) in all acutely unwell patients. Patients with an acute asthma attack are liable to develop hypokalaemia, mainly due to the high doses of salbutamol being administered. They are also prone to becoming dehydrated and, therefore, usually need maintenance intravenous fluids with added potassium, until they are able to eat and drink normally (see Chapter 21 for more on electrolytes).

The role of intravenous aminophylline and salbutamol

The majority of patients will respond to the treatment outlined above, but one of the commoner reasons for an apparent lack of response is undertreatment with nebulisers. In the past it has been advocated that patients with severe asthma that does not improve with nebulised bronchodilators should be treated with intravenous aminophylline and/or salbutamol. There are, however, very few circumstances in which this treatment can be advocated, mainly because extensive research has failed to show significant clinical benefits with either, in addition to nebulised salbutamol, compared to just nebulised salbutamol alone (Parameswaran *et al.*, 2001). Even in ventilated patients on the intensive care unit it is preferable to add salbutamol to the ventilator circuit and, therefore, deliver it to the lungs, rather than intravenously; however, if there is any doubt regarding adequate drug delivery to the lungs, intravenous salbutamol or aminophylline can be initiated on the intensive care unit. If aminophylline is used, then care must be taken to ensure that the loading dose is omitted if the patient already takes oral aminophylline, and that levels are performed on a daily basis (see more about intravenous dosing regimens in the *British National Formulary*; BNF, 2009).

Referral to the intensive care unit

There should be a low threshold for seeking advice from a critical-care physician or a chest specialist when it is felt that a patient requires ventilation, or for patients who have severe acute or life-threatening asthma who are not responding to appropriate therapy. Worrying features to look out for are described in Box 5.6.

Box 5.6   Signs of deterioration

- Deteriorating PEFR
- Worsening hypoxia
- Elevated pCO_2
- Acidosis on ABG
- Exhaustion/poor respiratory effort
- Drowsiness or confusion
- Respiratory arrest

Monitoring the patient

Monitoring in the patient with acute asthma is very similar to the close monitoring involved with any critically ill patient, as described in Chapter 3. The level and frequency of monitoring depends on the severity of the attack, but the minimum in an acutely unwell asthmatic would be to nurse them in an area on the ward that is easily visible, to measure their respiratory rate, oxygen saturation, heart rhythm, pulse and blood pressure continuously and formally record it at least hourly. Bloods (specifically potassium) should be monitored daily (more often if very low < 3.0 mmols/L) and fluid balance recorded regularly. The only additional monitoring required is the PEFR, which should ideally be done pre- and post-nebuliser. However, it is unlikely that more than four recordings (pre- and post-nebuliser) per day would be of further benefit. A slow but steady improvement should be seen both acutely and also day-to-day. Once the patient is stable, usually after 24 hours, the frequency of monitoring can be reduced, along with the frequency of the nebulisers.

Conclusions

This patient in our case scenario was given back-to-back salbutamol nebulisers (5 mg), with the first also containing 500 µg of ipratropium. Her oxygen was humidified and increased to 60% via

Venturi mask and her saturations increased to 96%. A repeat ABG 20 minutes later revealed a PaO_2 of 14 kPa, with a low $PaCO_2$ and normal pH. She was also given a dose of 40 mg prednisolone. In this case antibiotics were not felt to be necessary. Her PEFR improved to 250 litres per minute after four back-to-back nebulisers and her respiratory rate dropped to 25 breaths per minute. She was then able to complete sentences in a single breath and was understandably very flattering about the expert management she received !

HOT TIPS

- Immediately work out the severity of the attack.
- Patients with life-threatening or near-fatal asthma must be moved to a critical care environment as soon as possible.
- Administer enough oxygen to maintain the saturation above 94%.
- If your patient is requiring high-flow oxygen to maintain this saturation (or if saturations are below 92%) then perform an arterial gas and call for senior help immediately.
- Administer salbutamol (5 mg) via a nebuliser on a continuous basis (i.e. one after the other) until there is a clinical improvement with better saturations, reduced respiratory rate and the patient is able to talk in full sentences.
- Administer intravenous magnesium sulphate for acute severe asthma or worse.
- Never administer Bi-PAP on the general ward for an asthmatic patient who is acidotic – there is little evidence for this outside of the intensive care unit (for more on Bi-PAP see Chapter 8).
- Intravenous aminophylline has no place in the management of the average asthmatic patient.

References and further reading

Asthma UK (2004). *Where Do We Stand?: Asthma in the UK Today*. Available at: www.asthma.org.uk/health_professionals/ordering_materials/where_do_we.html (last accessed November 2009).

British National Formulary (2009). *British National Formulary: Number 54*. London, BMJ Publishing Group.

British Thoracic Society and Scottish Intercollegiate Guidelines Network (2008). *British Guideline on the Management of Asthma: a National Clinical Guideline*. Available at: www.brit-thoracic.org.uk/ClinicalInformation/Asthma/AsthmaGuidelines/tabid/83/Default.aspx (last accessed November 2009).

National Heart, Lung and Blood Institute, National Institutes of Health (1992). International Consensus Report on the Diagnosis And Treatment of Asthma. *European Respiratory Journal*, **5**, 601–41.

Lanes, S.F., Garrett, J.E., Wentworth, C.E., *et al.* (1998). The effect of adding ipratropium bromide to salbutamol in the treatment of acute asthma: a pooled analysis of three trials. *Chest*, **114**, 365–72.

Parameswaran, K., Belda, J. and Rowe, B.H. (2001). *Addition of intravenous aminophylline to beta 2-agonists in adults with acute asthma. Cochrane Review. The Cochrane Library. Issue 3.* Oxford, Update Software.

Resuscitation Council (2005). *Advanced Life Support Course*, *Provider Manual*, 4th edn. London, Resuscitation Council.

Useful websites

Asthma UK
www.asthma.org.uk

British Thoracic Society
www.brit-thoracic.org.uk

Lung and Asthma Information Agency
www.laia.ac.uk

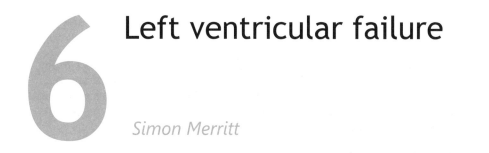

Left ventricular failure

Simon Merritt

Left ventricular failure is a common and potentially life-threatening cause of acute respiratory distress. In an ageing population with an increasing prevalence of ischaemic heart disease, a patient with acute left ventricular failure is not an uncommon sight either in the emergency department or on the ward.

Rapid treatment, which involves optimising oxygenation and reducing cardiac preload and afterload, is essential. Despite recent advances in drug therapy the prognosis of patients admitted to hospital with heart failure is relatively poor with only 48.4% alive after 5 years (Varela-Roman *et al.*, 2002). By the end of this chapter you should be able to:

- define left ventricular failure
- understand its causes
- make a rapid assessment of a patient with left ventricular failure
- understand its immediate management.

Acute left ventricular failure occurs when there is a sudden reduction in the ability of the left ventricle to pump blood effectively to the vital organs. This directly causes an increase in the pulmonary capillary pressure and, therefore, an accumulation of fluid in the alveoli. The presence of fluid in the alveoli impairs gas exchange, and this results in hypoxia (Box 6.1).

Box 6.1   Hypoxia

Hypoxia is a lack of sufficient oxygen in both the blood and tissues. The lower level of normal in terms of partial pressure of oxygen in the blood stream is 11 kPa; anything below this is termed hypoxia. If the pO_2 is < 8 kPa, then the patient is said to be in respiratory failure.

There are two distinct groups of patients who suffer from acute left ventricular failure: those whose left ventricle fails as a result of a myocardial infarction or as a result of an arrhythmia, and those who already have chronic heart failure (usually oedematous) who require a much smaller insult for their heart failure to worsen. Essentially the first is a reflection of an acute deterioration in the heart's pumping capability and the second is a combination of chronic impairment of pumping capability and fluid overload, which may be acute (e.g. too much intravenous fluid postoperatively) or chronic. The distinction is important because the presenting history and prioritisation of the various treatments differs between the groups.

You are worried about a 65-year-old woman on the medical ward who was transferred from the coronary care unit after a recent myocardial infarction. You are concerned because she has suddenly become short of breath, pale and sweaty. She requires urgent help. Her observations are as follows: respiratory rate 30 b.p.m., oxygen saturations 89% on 35% oxygen, pulse 130 b.p.m. and blood pressure 180/110 mmHg.

What would you do to stabilise and treat her?

What investigations may she require?

Pathophysiology and aetiology

Acute left ventricular failure may be secondary to severe myocardial ischaemia or infarction, to valvular heart disease (aortic or mitral) or to an arrhythymia (bradycardia or tachycardia). See Chapter 17 for more on the management of tachyarrhythmias). Other causes include fluid overload (e.g. over-enthusiastic postoperative fluid replacement), a hypertensive crisis, acute myocarditis (infection of the heart muscle), or secondary to drug toxicity (beta-blockers, tricyclic antidepressants and calcium channel blockers). All these put a further strain on a compromised heart muscle and compound the failure.

Coronary heart disease is the most common cause of left ventricular dysfunction (Varela-Roman, 2002). A more thorough review of the mechanisms of acute left ventricular failure following myocardial infarction is provided by Struthers *et al.* (2005). Box 6.2 gives a brief explanation of preload and afterload, as illustrated in Fig. 6.1.

For further information about cardiac ischaemia and infarction, refer to Chapter 18 on cardiac chest pain.

Box 6.2   Preload and afterload

Preload is the amount of tension on the heart before it begins to contract. The preload is determined by the end diastolic volume (the amount of blood in the heart after it has completely relaxed).

Afterload is the amount of tension the heart must build up before it can start to contract. This depends on the aortic pressure; before the ventricle can start to move blood through the aortic valve the pressure in the ventricle must equal that in the aorta.

Assessment

Assessment, as well as management, of a patient with acute left ventricular failure should be performed using the ABCDE method (see Chapter 2 for an overview of assessing and monitoring the acutely ill patient).

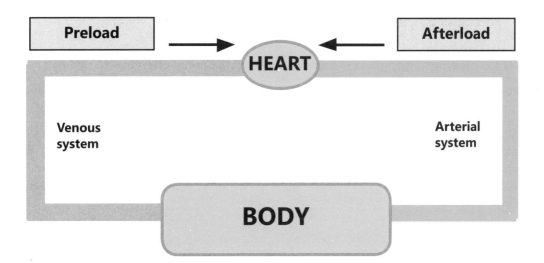

Figure 6.1 Preload and afterload.

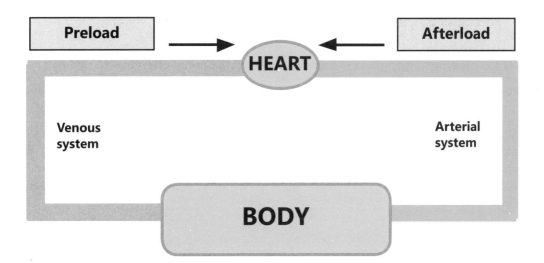

HOT TIPS

It is helpful, but not imperative, to perform your examination by first inspecting the patient and their surroundings, then palpating, percussing and finally auscultating.

The assessment of the patient from the above case scenario will be detailed here, but it is important to note that in an emergency situation, assessment and treatment occur simultaneously rather than one after the other as described below.

A—Airway

On assessment the patient is so short of breath that she is unable to talk in full sentences. However she can indicate that she has no chest pain. You notice that she is sitting bolt upright in bed and is agitated, but not confused. The very fact that she is talking to you, albeit in single words, and is alert, indicates that her airway is fine for now and not the major problem.

B—Breathing

While assessing her breathing you observe both sides of her chest are moving equally. Her respiratory rate is now 40 breaths per minute and her trachea is central. Percussion of her chest is equal and resonant throughout both lung fields.

Auscultation reveals crackles audible during inspiration, when listening posteriorly (see Box 6.3 on recognising added sounds). Her oxygen saturation has been measured at 89% (on 35% oxygen via a Venturi mask).

> **Box 6.3 Recognising added sounds (based on Munro and Edwards, 1995)**
>
> **Crackles (crepitations):** Non-musical sounds mainly heard during inspiration caused by:
>
> - re-opening of occluded small airways such as in fibrosing alveolitis, pulmonary oedema
> - air bubbling through secretions such as in bronchiectasis.
>
> They may be described as fine or coarse but this serves little clinically useful purpose. Asking the patient to cough to note whether the sounds change may assist in defining their cause (e.g. there may be secretions in the major bronchi and/or dilated bronchi and pulmonary cavities). To hear what crackles sound like, pull Velcro™ apart (fine crackles) or crunch up a supermarket plastic bag (coarse crackles).
>
> **Rhonchi (wheezes):** Musical sounds produced by air passing through narrowed airways such as in asthma.
>
> **Pleural friction rub:** Leathery or creaking sounds produced by movement of roughened pleural surfaces (e.g. in pleurisy). Usually associated with pleural pain.

C—Circulation

Assessment of this patient's circulation starts with the general observation that she is pale which suggests she is either anaemic or (as is more likely in this situation) her cardiac output is low. Feeling the temperature of her hands and fingers is very important and provides useful information regarding her cardiac output. In this case you notice that her hands are cool but sweaty. Her pulse is 130 beats per minute (regular) and feels weak. Her blood pressure was measured at 180/110 mmHg several minutes ago. Even though she is sitting bolt upright you can still see her jugular venous pressure (JVP) visible up to the level of her ear lobe (see Box 6.4 on examining jugular venous height). She has mild ankle oedema.

Auscultation of her heart reveals what sounds like three separate heart sounds: the first two are close together and the third follows after a short gap. Together they sound like a horse galloping. This is a third heart sound producing a so-called 'gallop' rhythm, which is characteristically heard just before the first heart sound. It is pathognomic of heart failure.

It is important to view a 12-lead ECG at this point because she may be suffering from another myocardial infarction or may have an arrhythmia that has precipitated her left ventricular failure. Attach her to a cardiac monitor to monitor her heart rate and oxygen saturations.

D—Disability

Next, consider an assessment of the patient's level of alertness and any mental disability. This can be done using the 15-point Glasgow Coma Scale, or more simply the AVPU scale, both of which are described elsewhere (see Chapters 2 and 44). This patient is agitated but alert and orientated, with a GCS of 15 and 'A' on the AVPU scale. In very severe or pre-terminal acute left ventricular failure, patients may become confused and drowsy or even unconscious.

Box 6.4 Examining the height of the jugular venous pressure

1. Ensure the patient is positioned on his or her back at an angle of 45° with their head resting on a pillow and their neck relaxed (note that patients who are breathless may find it difficult to lie in this position).

2. Ask the patient to turn their head just a little left of centre. By looking across their neck, identify the pulsation of the internal jugular vein (it is normally visible just above the level of the clavicle).

3. You will see the internal jugular vein (JVP) pulsate twice for every one heart beat (except if there is atrial fibrillation). This is one way to distinguish it from the carotid pulse (another is that venous pulsations are impalpable).

4. Estimate the height of the JVP using the sternal angle as 0 cm; the height of the top of the pulsation is the JVP. It should not be much higher than 4 cm above the sternal angle.

5. Run your fingers along one of the clavicles to the midline – this point is the sternal notch. By running your fingers down the sternum at this point for a few centimetres the *sternal angle* is felt as a palpable 'lump'.

E—Exposure, environment and everything else

The last stage of assessment would be to fully expose the patient to check that there are no physical signs that you have missed. There are none in this case. An arterial blood gas (ABG) provides invaluable information and must be performed; it should not, however, delay appropriate treatment.

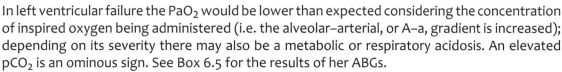

It is a common misconception that arterial blood gases (ABG) need to be performed whilst breathing air. This is not true and can be detrimental to the patient. The oxygen concentration, however, must be recorded on the ABG result.

In left ventricular failure the PaO_2 would be lower than expected considering the concentration of inspired oxygen being administered (i.e. the alveolar–arterial, or A–a, gradient is increased); depending on its severity there may also be a metabolic or respiratory acidosis. An elevated pCO_2 is an ominous sign. See Box 6.5 for the results of her ABGs.

A chest x-ray can be useful in confirming the diagnosis. Portable x-rays obtained on the ward are frequently of poor quality, but treatment certainly cannot wait until the x-ray is taken and returned to the ward. Provided it is of adequate quality a chest x-ray would classically reveal the presence of bilateral perihilar alveolar oedema giving a typical 'butterfly' appearance. It is important to realise that assessment is an ongoing process and it is vital to continually re-assess the patient, especially if his or her condition changes (for better or for worse) or if he or she receives any treatment.

Box 6.5	Arterial blood gas results at 35% oxygen
Oxygen	40%
PaO_2	7.5 kPa
$PaCO_2$	4.2 kPa
pH	7.44
Saturations	85%
Base excess	− 1
Bicarbonate	21 mmol/L

Worrying features generally include those at either end of the scale on most 'patient at risk' scoring systems, such as a very fast or very slow pulse, a very high blood pressure or, of more concern, a very low blood pressure and of course low oxygen saturations. Chapter 2 discusses track and trigger systems in greater depth.

Management

As mentioned previously the priority of the various treatments differs depending on whether it is truly acute left ventricular failure, for which vasodilator treatment is most important, or whether it is acute on chronic left ventricular failure (mainly fluid overload), in which diuretics are as important, if not more so, than vasodilators. The patient in our case scenario was previously reasonably fit and well and had recently suffered a myocardial infarction. There were no signs of chronic fluid overload, so it is reasonable to suppose that this is true acute left ventricular failure.

A—Airway

The first priority is to ensure her airway is adequate. If she is talking to you and is alert then it is fine for the moment.

B—Breathing

Increasing her oxygen concentration to bring her saturation to above 92% will help her breathing, as will sitting her at 90°. If increasing the oxygen concentration to maximum (using a mask and non-rebreath bag with 15 litres oxygen) does not increase the oxygen saturation, consider using continuous positive airways pressure (CPAP), which will provide a higher oxygen concentration and will also 'force' some of the pulmonary oedema out of the alveoli and back into the circulation. In this sort of situation CPAP, if used correctly, can be literally life saving; its application is discussed in more detail in Chapter 8.

Since the remainder of the treatment involves the administration of intravenous drugs, the insertion of one (or preferably two) cannulae at this point is vital. At this time blood should be taken for full blood count, urea and electrolytes and cardiac enzymes. Intravenous glyceryl trinitrate (GTN; see Box 6.6) is the most important treatment for this woman and this should be commenced immediately through one of the cannulas.

Box 6.6   Glyceryl trinitrate (GTN)

GTN works by causing both venous and arterial dilatation, thus reducing both the amount of blood returning to the heart (venous return/preload) and the pressure against which the left ventricle must work to pump blood around the body (afterload). It therefore reduces the pressure on the failing ventricle and enables the heart to pump more effectively. It also pools fluid in the peripheral circulation and so reduces pulmonary congestion. The usual concentration is 50 mg of GTN in 50 mL of 0.9% saline. This frequently comes pre-mixed. Other concentrations are used less often. If using 50 mg in 50 mL it would be normal to prescribe it as 0–10 mg per hour, aiming to adjust the dose (usually increasing) every 15 minutes, but trying to keep the systolic blood pressure above 100 mmHg.

The starting rate depends very much on the initial blood pressure. It would be detrimental to the patient if their blood pressure was suddenly lowered, especially if they are usually hypertensive, so they need to be monitored carefully, preferably in a coronary care unit or high-dependency unit. The patient in our clinical scenario commences on 2 mg per hour of GTN which is slowly increased, reducing her systolic blood pressure to 120 mmHg. The next drug to consider is intravenous diamorphine (2.5–5 mg) or morphine sulphate (5–10 mg). See Box 6.7.

Box 6.7   Diamorphine (2.5–5 mg) and morphine sulphate (5–10 mg)

These drugs work in two ways:

- first, they are potent venodilators that help to reduce cardiac work (by reducing preload);
- second, they reduce anxiety.

Acute left ventricular failure is a high adrenergic state – the patient's adrenal glands are releasing as much adrenaline (epinephrine) and noradrenaline (norepinephrine) as they can which, although initially helpful in maintaining a good blood pressure, eventually becomes counterproductive. It causes an already struggling heart to work even harder by beating faster, and by causing vasoconstriction it further increases the afterload. This is why patients with acute left ventricular failure characteristically feel cold peripherally (vasoconstriction) and yet feel sweaty (too much endogenous epinephrine/adrenaline). Diamorphine and morphine are effective in reducing the sympathetic drive and relaxing the patient. The patient in our scenario receives 2.5 mg of diamorphine, which visibly relaxes her within five minutes.

The last drug administered is furosemide, usually at a dose of 40–80 mg (see Box 6.8). Our patient's left ventricular failure is due to a reduction in the heart's pumping capability – not to fluid overload. A profound diuresis may be problematic and lead to hypotension. For this reason furosemide is the least important of the drugs discussed so far. However, in a patient with chronic heart failure who is oedematous, or in a patient who has developed heart failure after receiving too much intravenous fluid or blood postoperatively, furosemide is the mainstay of treatment and multiple doses are frequently needed.

Box 6.7   Furosemide

Furosemide is a loop diuretic, but also an effective venodilator. Caution should be exercised when using furosemide in this situation because although it will have an early positive effect (venodilation) it will (within the hour) cause a diuresis that may drop blood pressure significantly.

The patient should start to improve relatively quickly, certainly within 30 minutes. If they do not, then it is imperative to completely re-assess, to ensure the diagnosis is correct, and possibly increase the treatment and seek assistance from a senior doctor.

HOT TIPS

In true *acute* left ventricular failure, intravenous GTN is the primary treatment. Diamorphine and furosemide can be used in small doses to reduce sympathetic drive and to cause venodilation.

In *acute-on-chronic* heart failure or heart failure secondary to too much intravenous fluid, furosemide is the mainstay of treatment. Diamorphine and GTN have lesser roles to play, but can still be useful.

If, when you assess the patient, his or her blood pressure has dropped significantly (systolic blood pressure below 100 mmHg or mean arterial pressure < 70 mmHg), then GTN, diamorphine and furosemide are relatively contraindicated because they will all lower the blood pressure further, leading to cardiovascular collapse. In this situation the patient will require CPAP, assessment by an intensive-care physician and possibly inotropic support, which is beyond the scope of this chapter and certainly beyond the normal ward situation.

HOT TIPS

Investigations such as ABGs and chest x-rays are useful but you shouldn't wait for them before starting treatment.

If intravenous access is delayed or difficult and systolic blood pressure is over 100 mmHg, give two puffs of sublingual GTN. Repeat after 2 minutes if necessary and provided systolic blood pressure is still over 100 mmHg.

Until cardiac enzymes are back from the laboratory, give the patient appropriate acute treatment for acute coronary syndrome (aspirin, clopidogrel, enoxaparin) provided there are no contraindications.

Ongoing continuous monitoring of heart rate, heart rhythm, and SpO_2 are indicated with our patient. It is important to ensure the following are recorded: respiratory rate (over a whole minute), blood pressure, saturations (SpO_2) and heart rate and rhythm, preferably using a cardiac monitor. These would normally be performed half hourly or hourly depending on how stable the patient is. Vital signs should also include a 'patient at risk' score.

A fluid chart should be commenced with hourly fluid input and output recorded, particularly if the patient has been catheterised. Initially it is helpful to calculate the ongoing fluid balance on an hourly basis, but once the patient has improved this can be reduced to four hourly. Any changes and deterioration should be promptly reported to the clinical team caring for the patient and re-assessment undertaken. See Chapter 3 on monitoring of acutely ill ward patients.

Conclusions

The patient described in the case scenario received 15 litres oxygen via a mask and non-rebreathe mask, which increased her oxygen saturation to 96% and reduced her respiratory rate. Intravenous GTN was commenced soon after this, along with 2.5 mg diamorphine and 40 mg of furosemide, and produced visible relaxation, improved peripheral perfusion (warm hands), a lower blood pressure, a lower respiratory rate and pulse, and lower oxygen requirements within 20 minutes. You can breathe a sigh of relief and go to rescue the next patient – the night is not over yet!

HOT TIPS

If the patient continues to deteriorate, or has persistently low oxygen saturations or becomes hypotensive commence CPAP (see Chapter 8) and call for an urgent review by an intensive care physician.

References and further reading

Darcie, H. (2005). Heart failure post-myocardial infarction: a review of the issues. *Heart*, **91**, ii3–ii6.

Munro, J., Edwards, C.R.W. (1995). *Macleod's Clinical Examination*. London, Churchill Livingstone.

Struthers, A.D. (2005). Pathophysiology of heart failure following myocardial infarction. *Heart*, **91**, ii14–ii16.

Varela-Roman, A., Gonzalez-Juanatey, J.R., Basante, P., *et al.* (2002). Clinical characteristics and prognosis of hospitalised inpatients with heart failure and preserved or reduced left ventricular ejection fraction. *Heart*, **88**, 249–54.

7 Chronic obstructive pulmonary disease

Simon Merritt

In the UK around 900,000 people are currently diagnosed with chronic obstructive pulmonary disease (COPD), although allowing for gross under diagnosis it is thought that the true number is closer to 1.5 million (National Institute for Health and Clinical Evidence, 2004); see Box 7.1.

Up to one in eight hospital admissions are due to COPD (NICE, 2004). Unfortunately, especially since it is preventable, it is responsible for 30,000 deaths per year in England and Wales (NICE, 2004).

Box 7.1   Why is COPD underdiagnosed?

There are a number of reasons, not least the feeling among smokers that their symptoms are self-induced and 'par for the course' so why bother a doctor about them. Other reasons include a relatively large reserve in lung capacity, meaning considerable lung destruction must occur prior to the development of significant symptoms, and misdiagnosis as asthma or bronchitis.

By the end of this chapter you will be able to:

- define chronic obstructive pulmonary disease (COPD)
- assess and monitor a patient with COPD
- know how to manage a patient with COPD in the ward environment.

Background and definitions

COPD is defined by the British Thoracic Society and NICE (National Institute for Health and Clinical Excellence) as 'being characterised by airflow obstruction'. The airflow obstruction is usually progressive, not fully reversible, and does not change markedly over several months. The disease is caused predominantly by cigarette smoking' (NICE, 2004). However, this definition fails to point out, firstly, that COPD is preventable and, secondly, that some of the newer inhaled therapies actually improve markers of airway obstruction, such as FEV_1 (forced expiratory volume in 1 second) and degree of hyperinflation.

COPD is diagnosed based on a history of smoking, shortness of breath, a cough, a respiratory examination and spirometry which demonstrates airflow obstruction. An exacerbation of COPD is defined by NICE as a 'sustained worsening of the patient's symptoms from his or her usual stable state that is beyond normal day-to-day variations, and is acute in onset'. Commonly reported symptoms include 'worsening breathlessness, cough, increased sputum production and change in sputum colour' and the 'change in these symptoms often necessitates a change in medication' (NICE, 2004; p. 131). An exacerbation of COPD carries with it a 14% 3-month mortality and a 34% re-admission rate over the same time period (NICE, 2004). Its significance should, therefore, never be underestimated.

Case Scenario

A 65-year-old man was admitted to the medical assessment unit (MAU) with a 6-day history of progressive shortness of breath and a cough productive of thick green sputum. Although his Ventolin™ inhaler had helped with his breathing initially, it seemed to be making no difference now. Normally he was able to walk to his local newsagents without stopping (500 metres), but on the day he came to MAU he could manage no more than 5 metres.

He had been diagnosed with chronic obstructive pulmonary disease by his GP 2 years previously and had been commenced on a salbutamol (Ventolin™) and eformoterol (Oxis™) inhaler. His last spirometry, 8 months ago, revealed a forced expiratory volume (FEV_1) of 1.1 L and a forced vital capacity (FVC) of 2.0 L (see Box 7.2). He suffers from at least three chest infections per year, although none as bad as this one. Unfortunately he continues to smoke 10 cigarettes per day and has done for the last 45 years.

Although he has already received treatment from the admitting medical senior house officer prior to coming to the ward, his shortness of breath has worsened and he has become a little confused. The staff nurse caring for him is concerned and has for him to be reviewed.

If you were the doctor or nurse asked to review this patient what assessment and observations would you perform, and how would you stabilise him?

Pathophysiology and aetiology

The damage in COPD is secondary to a smoking-induced chronic lung inflammation which causes airway narrowing and diffuse damage to the lung parenchyma (the substance of the lung). In the larger airways there is an increase in the size and number of the mucous glands, leading to increased production of thick mucus. Examination of the medium-sized airways reveals thickened and excessively contracted smooth muscle, while the walls of the smaller airways are oedematous and infiltrated with inflammatory cells. The alveoli are variably damaged or destroyed. The extent of these changes differs in every patient.

Box 7.2 Forced expiratory volume (FEV$_1$) and forced vital capacity (FVC)

FEV$_1$ is the amount of air that the patient can exhale in 1 second. It is reduced in COPD because of the narrowed airways.

FVC is the total volume of air that the patient can exhale after a maximal inspiration. It is usually maintained in early COPD, but decreases as the disease progresses due to air trapping and lung destruction.

Age, sex, height and ethnicity all effect FEV$_1$ and FVC. Tables of normal values have been produced and are readily available, as are simple programs designed for use on both desk top computers and PDAs. One such program can be found at: www.patient.co.uk/showdoc/40002357

Exacerbations

COPD exacerbations are commonly due to viral and bacterial infections of the tracheobronchial tree and to air pollution (NICE, 2004). Typically the patient produces more mucous than usual, which is usually thicker and discoloured (green suggests a bacterial infection). Commonly implicated viral organisms are rhinovirus (common cold), influenza, parainfluenza and coronavirus, while bacterial pathogens include *Haemophilus influenza*, *Chlamydia pneumoniae*, *Streptococcus pneumoniae* and *Moraxella catarrhalis*. The cause of the exacerbation may be unidentifiable in up to 30% of cases (NICE, 2004). The pathophysiology of a COPD exacerbation comprises a catabolic state, airway narrowing, an increase in V/Q mismatch (see Box 7.3) and an increase in both the volume and purulence of sputum. It is diagnosed predominantly from the patient's history, although a chest x-ray, arterial blood gas and lung function tests can also be useful.

Box 7.3 Ventilation–perfusion V/Q

V = ventilation of lung.
Q = perfusion (by blood) of the lung.

In normal lungs most of the alveoli are both ventilated and perfused, giving normal V/Q matching which is essential for efficient gas exchange. In COPD there is variable destruction of both alveoli and pulmonary blood vessels, resulting in areas of lung that are either ventilated but not perfused or vice versa, causing V/Q mismatch. This results in inefficient gas exchange and (when advanced) severe hypoxia.

HOT TIPS

The full NICE guidelines for COPD are available on line at:
www.nice.org.uk/guidance/index.jsp?action=downloadando=29303

Assessment

The assessment, as well as the management, of a patient with an exacerbation of COPD should be performed using the **ABCDE** method.

On arrival in medical assessment unit, the staff nurse should attach a cardiac and blood pressure monitor and an oxygen saturation probe and undertake a full set of vital sign recordings (for more on monitoring see Chapter 3).

> **HOT TIPS**
>
> It is helpful, though not imperative, to perform your examination by first inspecting the patient and their surroundings, then palpating, percussing and finally auscultating. The assessment of the patient from the above case history will be detailed here, it important to note however that, in an emergency situation, assessment and treatment are occurring simultaneously rather than one after the other as described below.

A—Airway

You find the patient lying down on his bed (which is clearly making it harder for him to breathe); he is very agitated and refuses to wear his oxygen mask. His lips, tongue and the tips of his fingers have turned a blue/grey colour. However, he is talking in full sentences, albeit non-sensical ones, and you can hear his expiratory wheeze from the end of the bed. Since he is alert and talking you assess his airway as intact, but are a little concerned regarding his confusion and so decide to keep a very close eye on his level of consciousness. Any change in this may impact on his airway.

B—Breathing

His respiratory rate is 25 breaths per minute and his oxygen saturation is 94% on 40% oxygen, via a Venturi mask (when he keeps it on). Inspection of his chest reveals a decrease in chest expansion when he takes a breath in. Palpation of his trachea reveals it to be central. Percussion produces a rather hyper-resonant note, like tapping on a hollow wall. When auscultating his chest you notice that his breath sounds are quieter than you would expect and that he has long polyphonic expiratory wheezes (see Box 7.4).

C—Circulation

Assessment of this patient's circulation begins with the observation that the blue/grey discolouration of his fingertips and lips has diminished, and his hands are now warm to touch and appear well perfused. His palms are erythematous (red). His pulse rate is 96 beats per minute and feels very strong; the character of this pulse is 'bounding'. A bounding pulse and erythematous palms can be an indication of carbon dioxide retention. His blood pressure is elevated at 150/90 mmHg and jugular venous pressure (JVP) is normal at 3 cm. His heart sounds, although quiet, are also normal. Mild peripheral oedema is noted.

Box 7.4 **Added breath sounds (based on Murray and White 1999 and Douglas *et al.*, 2005)**

Crackles (crepitations): Non-musical or popping sounds mainly heard during inspiration caused by:

- re-opening of occluded small airways such as in pulmonary fibrosis and pulmonary oedema., or
- air bubbling through secretions such as in bronchiectasis and consolidation.

They can either be fine or coarse in nature, although differentiating them is not of the utmost importance. *Fine crackles* sound like very fine Velcro™ being undone and suggest the presence of pulmonary oedema or fibrosis. *Coarse crackles* sound like a supermarket plastic bag being crunched and suggest bronchiectasis or consolidation. In the acute situation it can be difficult to determine whether crackles are fine or coarse so the above is useful only if combined with the other examination findings. Asking the patient to cough is essential when crackles are auscultated, because they are not deemed significant if they disappear on coughing.

Wheezes: Musical or whistling sounds produced by air passing through narrowed airways such as in asthma and COPD. They mainly occur on expiration.

Pleural rub: Creaking sounds produced by movement of inflamed pleural surfaces, for example in pleurisy. They are usually associated with pleuritic pain.

HOT TIPS

Assessment must be ongoing. It is important to continually re-assess, especially if the condition of the patient changes or he or she receives any treatment. Remember ABCDE.

D—Disability

It has already been noted that this patient is confused. Therefore it is unsurprising that formal assessment of his alertness and mental disability reveals his Glasgow Coma Score to be 14/15 and 'A' on the AVPU scale (see Box 7.2; and see Chapter 44 on how to perform a GCS).

Box 7.5 **AVPU assessment**

A—Alert
V—Responds to **V**erbal stimuli
P—Responds to **P**ainful stimuli only
U—Unresponsive

Finally, the patient is systematically exposed to ensure that there are no other physical signs. There are none. His temperature is 38.2°C.

Investigations

A departmental chest x-ray had already been done and revealed flattened diaphragms and hyper-expanded lung fields. There was no indication of any other pathology. The arterial blood gas was performed on 40% oxygen (delivered via Venturi mask). The results are shown in Box 7.6.

Box 7.6	Arterial blood gas results at 40% oxygen
PaO$_2$	16.2 kPa
PaCO$_2$	6.9 kPa
pH	7.32
Saturations	98%
Base excess	+2
Bicarbonate	26 mmol/L

They reveal a mild acute respiratory acidosis, with a high PaO$_2$, which may in part be due to over-enthusiastic oxygen therapy. The oxygen concentration should therefore be reduced.

HOT TIPS

Respiratory failure type 1:
PaO$_2$ of less than 8 kPa.
In type 1 respiratory failure the PaCO$_2$ is either normal or low.
If left untreated it has the potential to progress to type 2.

Respiratory failure type 2:
PaO$_2$ of less than 8 kPa.
Elevated PaCO$_2$ (i.e. over 5.5 KPa).
If the PaCO$_2$ is sufficiently elevated then a respiratory acidosis can develop, which has adverse prognostic implications.

Severity

Worrying features, specific to this case include confusion, which may lead to poor compliance with treatment, and the presence of a bounding pulse and red palms, indicating possible carbon dioxide retention. Paradoxically a normal (> 95%) oxygen saturation is almost as concerning as a low one in this situation. Many patients with moderate to severe COPD have chronically low levels of oxygen and their bodies have, to some extent, adapted to this. Therefore, a saturation of 90–93% should be the target, elevating it above this level increases the risk of carbon dioxide retention and respiratory acidosis (NICE, 2004). The mechanism by which this occurs is a combination of a decrease in the central drive to breathe (a tendency to hypoventilate, causing a reduction in respiratory rate) and also a worsening of the ventilation–perfusion mismatch in the lungs. High concentrations of oxygen may result in areas of the lung that are ventilated but not perfused by blood (i.e. increasing V/Q mismatch). See Box 7.3 for an explanation of V/Q mismatch. It is important that medical staff administer oxygen to hypoxic patients with COPD. However it needs to be done in a controlled manner, with frequent monitoring of arterial blood gases and frequent clinical assessments.

Management

A—Airway

It has already been established that this patient's airway is intact. It is helpful in any patient who is having breathing difficulties to sit them upright because this considerably improves the mechanics of breathing.

HOT TIPS

Although high-flow oxygen has the potential to cause harm in COPD by sometimes leading to a high carbon dioxide level, its use is occasionally necessary. In the short term a profound hypoxia is more likely to result in serious harm to the patient than a high carbon dioxide level. Therefore in the emergency situation (i.e. whilst waiting for senior assistance to arrive) sufficient oxygen should be administered to increase the saturation to 90% (but not higher), without thought for the carbon dioxide level.

B—Breathing

We already know that the patient in the scenario is suffering from a mild respiratory acidosis, thought to be secondary to excess oxygen, therefore it would be wise to reduce the concentration until his saturations drop to 90%. In this case, the oxygen was reduced to 28% via a Venturi mask. It is important to repeat the arterial blood gas 20–30 minutes after altering the oxygen concentration to ensure that the PaO_2 remains over 8 kPa and that the pH is improving (becoming less acidotic).

If these variables are not improving then the use of non-invasive ventilation (NIV) should be considered. This is discussed further in Chapter 8. However, with the use of standard therapy (as discussed below), which includes controlled oxygen therapy, 20% of acidotic COPD patients will normalise their pH without the need for NIV (NICE, 2004). See the algorithm for acute respiratory failure in Fig. 7.1.

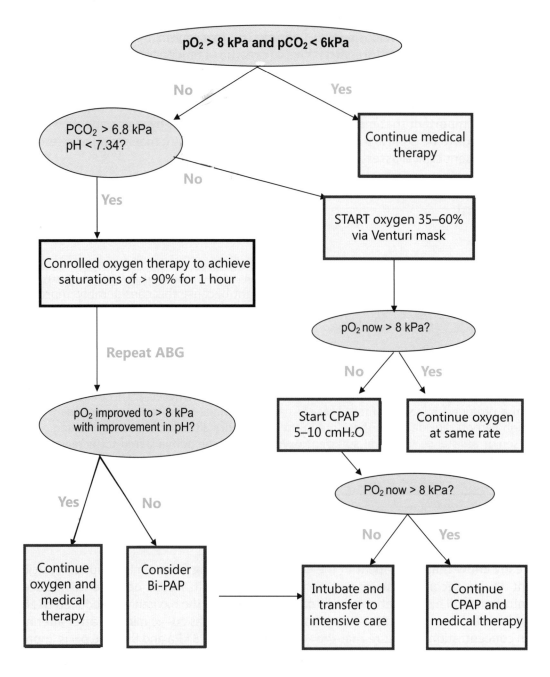

Figure 7.1 Algorithm for acute respiratory failure (adapted from ATS/ERS COPD guidelines, 2004). Bi-PAP, bi-level positive airway pressure; CPAP; continutous positive airway pressure.

ABGs need to be monitored on a regular basis until the patient's condition has stabilised.

Salbutamol and ipratropium nebulisers would be the next treatment to start (see Box 7.7). They are useful in treating bronchoconstriction which is one of the many problems in COPD. Bronchodilators can also help to reduce air trapping, and therefore hyper-expansion; this reduces the sensation of breathlessness and improves the patient's tidal volume and minute ventilation. A recent study by Nair *et al.* (2005) concluded that in COPD there was no difference in outcome (including length of hospital stay or recovery of lung function) when using 5 mg compared to 2.5 mg of nebulised salbutamol.

Salbutamol has relatively short-lasting effects and can be repeated on an almost continuous basis in the acute phase. The effects of ipratropium last for 4–6 hours, therefore it should be administered four to six times daily.

Box 7.7   Bronchodilators

Salbutamol: A beta$_2$-agonist which is usually administered via a handheld inhaler or a nebuliser. In selected cases it is used intravenously. However there is very rarely an indication to do this in COPD. It works via stimulation of beta$_2$-adrenoreceptors in the airway, and results in relaxation of bronchial smooth muscle. Common side effects include tremor, tachycardia and hypokalaemia.

Ipratropium bromide: This antimuscarinic drug can be taken via a handheld inhaler or nebulised. It works by competitively inhibiting muscarinic receptors on the airway smooth muscle, leading to bronchodilation by reducing vagal tone. Possible side effects consist of dry mouth, dilated pupils, urinary retention and constipation, but they are rarely troublesome.

For the patient in our scenario, a nebuliser containing 2.5 mg salbutamol and 500 µg ipratropium bromide is commenced. Once this nebuliser has finished, you re-assess him and find that his respiratory rate has decreased a little and his oxygen saturations have improved. However, he remains quite wheezy so he has another 2.5 mg of salbutamol immediately, and he is prescribed both drugs to be nebulised 4-hourly on the drug chart with extra doses of salbutamol as required. Chest physiotherapy (see Chapter 12) is another useful adjunct to treatment of the COPD exacerbation, especially to aid expectoration and teach more efficient and comfortable ways of breathing.

HOT TIPS

It is essential that this nebuliser is driven on air and not oxygen to avoid the problems with carbon dioxide retention described earlier. Supplemental oxygen can be given simultaneously using nasal prongs – usually at a rate of between 1 and 4 litres.

C—Circulation

Circulation is not usually a major problem in the patient with an exacerbation of COPD except for the tachycardia commonly associated with nebulised salbutamol. However, it is good practice to establish intravenous access and take routine bloods for full blood count, urea and electrolytes, CRP and blood cultures in all acutely unwell patients. In this confused and drowsy patient, in whom compliance may be an issue, it would be wise to give the first dose of antibiotics intravenously.

Antibiotics are not always needed in a COPD exacerbation; their prescription should depend on the presence of at least one of the following: a history of a change in colour of the sputum to green, an increase in its volume or purulence, consolidation on the chest x-ray, a temperature in excess of 37.5°C or a significant elevation in white blood cell count ± CRP. Unless the patient is very unwell, oral dosing of amoxicillin, clarithromycin or doxycycline would normally be reasonable. Steroids are a useful adjunct in the treatment of a COPD exacerbation, and can be administered either orally (e.g. prednisolone) or intravenously (e.g. hydrocortisone). Ideally prednisolone is given orally at a dose of 30 mg daily for 7–14 days (NICE, 2004).

The poor baseline level of lung function means that patients with an exacerbation of COPD can take a considerable time to get better, however the treatment described above will usually serve to stabilise most patients. The unwell COPD patient requires close monitoring and continual re-assessment by the medical team; any further deterioration must be spotted early and treated appropriately.

NIV in a COPD exacerbation

This topic is thoroughly covered in Chapter 8, therefore only a few pertinent points are covered here. NIV is an effective and often life-saving treatment option and should be available in all hospitals admitting acutely unwell patients with COPD. It should be used in the presence of a persistent respiratory acidosis which has proved unresponsive to controlled oxygen therapy and nebulised bronchodilators (NICE, 2004). Ideally prior to instituting NIV a decision should be made as to whether the patient is suitable for admission to the intensive care unit for intubation and ventilation; this decision should be taken by the senior doctor present after consultation with the patient (if possible) and with their family. This decision is usually based on the patient's level of pre-morbid functioning and the presence or absence of comorbidities. If there is any doubt about the patient's wishes, in an ideal world, the patient would be intubated and ventilated for a limited period, with treatment withdrawn at a later date if it becomes futile.

There are usually concerns with admission to intensive care and difficulties weaning in this group of patients. There is some evidence to the contrary; for example, Esteban *et al.* (2002) found that the patients receiving mechanical ventilation due to decompensated COPD had a significantly lower mortality than patients receiving mechanical ventilation because of acute respiratory failure of other aetiologies. The same authors also found a reduced length of mechanical ventilation compared to patients with acute respiratory distress syndrome (ARDS).

Aminophylline

See Box 7.8. Intravenous aminophylline has a very limited role to play in the treatment of COPD exacerbations. It really is a last resort in a very severe exacerbation when all other treatment has failed. The evidence base for its use in acute COPD is limited and a Cochrane review found that, compared to placebo, theophylline produced no significant differences in pulmonary function or symptom scores in exacerbations of COPD (NICE, 2004). In the few occasions when it is used, care must be taken to ensure that the loading dose is omitted if the patient already takes oral aminophylline, and that blood levels are checked on a daily basis. It is worth repeating that controlled oxygen therapy, the appropriate frequency of salbutamol and ipratropium nebulisers and NIV, if indicated, should be used as first-line treatments.

Box 7.3 Aminophylline

Aminophylline belongs to a class of drugs known as theophyllines, which work by inhibiting an enzyme called phosphodiesterase. They cause relaxation of bronchial smooth muscle and therefore bronchodilation. They may also have effects on diaphragmatic contractility, and cardiac output. Sanders *et al.* (1980) suggested that, in addition to bronchodilating, aminophylline also appears to increase the respiratory drive. It seems, however, that this is of relatively little importance. Aminophylline is only a weak bronchodilator. It has many drug interactions and a narrow therapeutic ratio so side effects are common. They include tachycardia, nausea, heart arrhythmias and convulsions.

Conclusions

This patient in the scenario was treated by reducing his oxygen concentration to 28% via a Venturi mask, and with nebulised salbutamol (2.5 mg) and ipratropium (500 µg). Routine bloods, including blood cultures, were taken and an initial dose of antibiotic (amoxycillin and clarithromycin) and steroids was given intravenously. Despite an initial improvement in his clinical condition after 1 hour his blood gases had deteriorated (pH 7.25). It was also noticed that he had become drowsier. After consultation with the outreach team and the medical registrar on call, he is commenced on NIV (see Chapter 8).

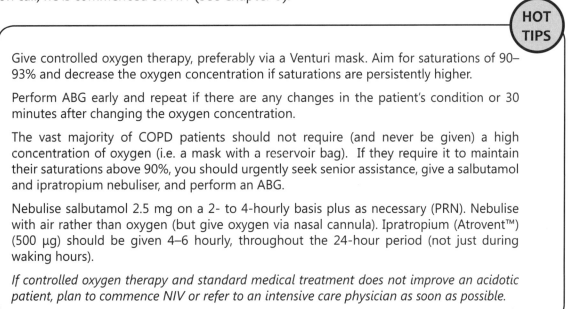

HOT TIPS

Give controlled oxygen therapy, preferably via a Venturi mask. Aim for saturations of 90–93% and decrease the oxygen concentration if saturations are persistently higher.

Perform ABG early and repeat if there are any changes in the patient's condition or 30 minutes after changing the oxygen concentration.

The vast majority of COPD patients should not require (and never be given) a high concentration of oxygen (i.e. a mask with a reservoir bag). If they require it to maintain their saturations above 90%, you should urgently seek senior assistance, give a salbutamol and ipratropium nebuliser, and perform an ABG.

Nebulise salbutamol 2.5 mg on a 2- to 4-hourly basis plus as necessary (PRN). Nebulise with air rather than oxygen (but give oxygen via nasal cannula). Ipratropium (Atrovent™) (500 µg) should be given 4–6 hourly, throughout the 24-hour period (not just during waking hours).

If controlled oxygen therapy and standard medical treatment does not improve an acidotic patient, plan to commence NIV or refer to an intensive care physician as soon as possible.

References and further reading

Douglas, G., Nicol, F. and Robertson, C. (eds) (2005). *Macleod's Clinical Examination*, 11th edn. Churchill Livingstone, Edinburgh.

Esteban, A., Anzueto, A., Frutos, F., *et al.* (2002). Characteristics and outcomes in adult patients receiving mechanical ventilation: A 28 day international study. *Journal of the American Medical Association*, **287**, 345–55.

National Institute for Health and Clinical Excellence (2004). Chronic obstructive pulmonary disease: National clinical guideline on management of chronic pulmonary disease in adults in primary and secondary care. The National Collaboration Centre for chronic conditions. *Thorax*, **59** (suppl.1), 1–232. Available at: thorax.bmj.com/content/vol59/suppl.1/ (last accessed November 2009).

Murray, S.E. and White, B.S. (1999). *Critical Care Assessment Handbook*. Philadelphia, WB Saunders.

Nair, S., Thomas, E., Pearson, S.B. and Henry, M.Y. (2005). A randomized controlled trial to assess the optimal dose and effect of nebulised albuterol in acute exacerbations of COPD. *Chest*, **128** (1), 48–54.

Sanders, J.S., Berman, T.M., Bartlett, M.M. and Kronenberg, R.S. (1980). Increased hypoxic ventilatory drive due to administration of aminophylline in normal men. *Chest*, **78**, 279–82.

Useful websites

British Thoracic Society
www.brit_thoracic.org.uk

Peakflow information
www. patient.co.uk/showdoc/40002357/

8 Non-invasive ventilation in type 2 respiratory failure

Jayne Fraser

This chapter covers the principles of bi-level non-invasive ventilation. It will enable you to recognise patients who may need non-invasive ventilation (NIV) and explain how to monitor and care for a patient receiving NIV.

Non-invasive ventilation (NIV) enables ventilatory support to be given via a mask into the patient's upper airways, rather than an invasive device that entails inserting a tube into the patient's trachea and bypassing the upper airway (British Thoracic Society, 2002). The use of non-invasive ventilation has been recognised as an important tool in the management of type 1 and type 2 respiratory failure and cardiogenic pulmonary oedema; it is also a means for weaning patients from mechanical ventilation in the critical care environment.

NIV has been reported to reduce hospital mortality and the need for intubation and reduce hospital stay (Brochard *et al.*, 1999; Plant *et al.*, 2000). It can occur outside the intensive care unit and can therefore save 'precious' intensive care unit beds, at a relatively low cost. Patients are able to eat and drink, to cooperate with physiotherapy, and to communicate with staff and their family because they do not require sedation when receiving non-invasive ventilation.

The Royal College of Physicians, the British Thoracic Society and the Intensive Care Society (2008) have produced comprehensive guidelines for the care of patients receiving NIV; this chapter uses these as a guide. It considers bi-level non-invasive ventilation in relation to type 2 respiratory failure.

Bi-level non-invasive ventilation

Non-invasive ventilation used in treating patients in type 2 respiratory failure offers bi-level positive airway pressures (Bi-PAP). This gives a pressure at two levels, on inspiration and expiration. Bi-level NIV has a higher pressure on inspiration and lower on expiration. These two pressures are measured in centimetres of water (cmH_2O).

- *Expiratory positive airway pressure (EPAP):* This is the level on expiration. It keeps the alveoli open when the patient breathes out, and has the same function as CPAP (continuous positive airway pressure) and PEEP (positive end expiratory pressure).
- *Inspiratory positive airway pressure (IPAP):* This is the level given on inspiration. The machine senses when the patient breathes in and blows air into the lungs.
- *Pressure support:* This is the difference between IPAP and EPAP (i.e. if IPAP is set at 10 cmH_2O and EPAP is set at 4 cmH_2O, then pressure support will be 6cmH_2O).

The functions of EPAP, IPAP and pressure support are summarised in Table 8.1.

Table 8.1   Functions of expiratory and inspiratory positive airway pressure (EPAP and IPAP) and pressure support

EPAP	IPAP	Pressure support
Keeps the alveoli partly inflated	Supports inspiratory effort	Reduces the effort of breathing and allows patients to relax and rest
Improves alveolar gas exchange	Improves tidal volume	–
Improves oxygenation	Improves carbon dioxide removal	–
Increases lung volume	–	–

The definitions of forced expiratory volume and forced vital capacity are given in Box 8.1.

Box 8.1 FEV_1 and FVC

Forced expiratory volume (FEV_1): The volume of air that can be exhaled in 1 second. It is reduced in COPD because of the narrowed airways.

Forced vital capacity (FVC): The total volume of air that can be exhaled after a maximal inspiration. It is usually maintained in early COPD, but decreases as the disease progresses.

Age, sex, height and ethnicity all affect FEV_1 and FVC. Tables of normal values have been produced and are readily available, as are simple programs designed for use on desk-top computers and mobile computer devices. One such program can be found at: www.patient.co.uk/showdoc/40002357/

Patient selection

Non-invasive ventilation should be considered in patients with an acute exacerbation of COPD with a respiratory acidosis. Suggested physiological parameters (Royal College of Physicians, 2008) are:

- pH < 7.35
- pCO_2 > 6.0.

First-line treatment

Controlled oxygen therapy – at a flow to maintain oxygen saturations of 88–92% (Royal College of Physicians, 2008) – should be started. This is because a low pH and high carbon dioxide can be a consequence of being given too much oxygen in the ambulance or in the hospital environment (Plant *et al.*, 2000b). Maximal medical therapy should be prescribed and administered and should consist of (Royal College of Physicians, 2008):

- nebulised salbutamol
- nebulised ipratropium
- steroids
- antibiotics (if there is an indication of new infection)
- chest x-ray.

Case Scenario

A 65-year-old man was admitted to the Medical Assessment Unit (MAU) with a 6-day history of progressive shortness of breath and a cough productive of thick green sputum. Although his Ventolin inhaler had helped with his breathing initially it seemed to be making no difference now. Normally he was able to walk to his local newsagent without stopping (500 metres) but on the day he came to the MAU he could manage no more than 5 metres. He had been diagnosed with chronic obstructive pulmonary disease (COPD) by his GP around 2 years previously and had been commenced on a Ventolin and eformoterol inhaler. His last spirometry, 8 months ago, revealed a forced expiratory volume (FEV_1) of −1.1 and a forced vital capacity (FVC) of 2.0.

He suffers from at least three chest infections per year, though none has been as bad as this one. Unfortunately he continues to smoke 10 cigarettes per day and has done so for the last 45 years. The patient was treated with a reduction in his oxygen concentration to 28% via a Venturi mask, and administered nebulised salbutamol and ipratropium.

Routine bloods, including blood cultures, were taken and an initial dose of antibiotic (as per local Trust guidelines) and steroids were given intravenously. Despite what appeared to be an initial improvement in his clinical condition, worsening arterial blood gases revealed a pH of 7.25, with a pCO_2 of 9.3 kPa. It was also noticed that he had become more drowsy. After consultation with the critical care outreach team and the medical registrar on call it was decide to commence non-invasive ventilation.

The arterial blood gases should then be repeated and if the patient remains acidotic (pH < 7.35) then escalation of treatment should be considered. This should occur within the first hour of deterioration or arrival at hospital.

Intubation or NIV?

The Royal College of Physicians guidelines (2008) say that the choice of treatment needs to be made sooner rather than later and patients who are suitable for invasive ventilation should be moved to a critical care area after the first hour if there is no improvement in their arterial blood gas analysis. Those with a pH of < 7.25 should be considered for intubation and full ventilation, but if this is not appropriate then NIV may be suitable. Other patients, however, who are not suitable candidates for invasive ventilation, should remain in an appropriate designated location where NIV will be prescribed as their ceiling of treatment. Before commencing, a treatment plan should be made in case NIV is not effective in stabilising the patient; this should be documented in the patient's notes, paying particular attention to the following:

- the severity of the underlying disease
- the reversibility of the acute illness
- the previous level of disability
- the patient's wishes.

Local guidelines should be in place to help ascertain which patients are suitable for non-invasive ventilation, and also consider the contraindications (not all are absolute) (Plant *et al.*, 2000a; Conti *et al.*, 2002; Lightowler *et al.*, 2003). These are shown in Box 8.2.

Box 8.2   Clinical inclusion and exclusion criteria for NIV (Royal College of Physicians, 2008)

Inclusion criteria
  Primary diagnosis of COPD
  Able to protect airway*
  Conscious and cooperative*
  Potential for recovery to acceptable quality of life (acceptable to the patient)
  Patient's wishes

Exclusion criteria
  Facial trauma, burns, recent facial or upper airway surgery
  Upper gastrointestinal surgery
  Fixed obstruction of the upper airway
  Inability to protect airway
  Life-threatening hypoxaemia
  Haemodynamic instability requiring inotropes or pressers
    (unless in a critical care unit)
  Severe comorbidity
  Patient moribund
  Confusion, agitation or severe cognitive impairment
  Vomiting
  Bowel obstruction
  Copious respiratory secretions
  Undrained pneumothorax

*Consider NIV if unconscious and endotracheal intubation deemed inappropriate or NIV to be provided in critical care setting.

Non-invasive ventilation is *not* the treatment of choice for patients whose primary diagnosis is heart failure or pneumonia, but it may be used in COPD patients with these complications if escalation to intubation and ventilation is deemed inappropriate.

Starting treatment

Once a patient has been selected as suitable for non-invasive ventilation, the chest x-ray should be reviewed to rule out a pneumothorax. A chest drain may need to be inserted if a pneumothorax is present. Patient cooperation and compliance is crucial to the success of NIV. Patients will often have severe dyspnoea and difficulty speaking and may be exhausted from the effort of breathing. They may be frightened and apprehensive about trying it. All these problems are potentially reversible and can be overcome by giving the patient calm, clear instructions and information. Spending time at the beginning of treatment saves valuable nursing time later on. Many patients find adapting to the mask the most difficult part of the process. However, in recent years the masks available have improved considerably. The patient should be measured up for a mask using the manufacturer's guidelines – do not be tempted to guess the size because an ill-fitting mask can be uncomfortable and may leak excessively or be too tight.

Ideally two healthcare professionals, one of whom is trained to use non-invasive ventilation, should be present to secure the mask and monitor the bi-level NIV machine. Once the patient is comfortable with the mask held against his or her face, it can be strapped to the head. Do not attach it too tightly (you should be able to move the mask at the chin but not at the nose) and be careful it does not blow into the patient's eyes. The bi-level system on some machines compensates for leakage around the mask itself and also records the amount of leaking.

The pressure of the mask sometimes causes irritation and soreness, especially on the bridge of the nose and the chin, so these areas need to be assessed regularly. A protective dressing can be applied to any areas that begin to look red and sore.

It is of utmost importance that the patient is comfortable wearing the mask, therefore low pressures are set at first so the patient can get used to the feel of blowing air.

Starting pressures are:

- IPAP: 10 cmH$_2$O.
- EPAP: 4 cmH$_2$O.
- Pressure support: 6 cm.

Please refer to your own Trust guidelines for further information on setting the particular machine you are using.

Humidification through the bi-level NIV machine is not needed as long as patients are kept well hydrated, either with oral fluids or with intravenous fluids, or given during breaks off the ventilatory support. A fluid input and output chart is essential. Refer to the physiotherapist for advice and treatment to help the patient with expectorating any sputum. Nursing care of patients receiving non-invasive ventilation is summarised in Box 8.3.

Monitoring

Close and thorough clinical assessment is of paramount importance when caring for a patient receiving non-invasive ventilation. Physiological monitoring is not a substitute for clinical assessment. Observation of the patient on the ventilator should be made regularly and charted according to your individual Trust's guidelines.

Box 8.3   Nursing care of patients receiving non-invasive ventilation

- Reassurance – take your time when commencing.
- Measure the patient for the mask – *do not guess*!
- Remember the mask does not need to be very tight.
- Make sure patients have a means of communication and are located near the nurses' station.
- Observe pressure areas on the patient's face for redness and apply a protective dressing if necessary (be particularly careful if a nasogastric tube is present).
- Move the tube on a regular basis.
- Wash the mask with soap and water when washing the patient's face.
- Remember the patient's hydration and nutritional status.
- Give the patient a break if possible for meals, drugs and nebulisers (nasal cannula to give oxygen can be used for periods off NIV).
- Refer to the chest physiotherapist.

The following clinical features should be assessed:

- chest wall movement
- coordination of respiratory effort with the ventilator
- use of accessory muscles
- general assessment (is the patient sweating, clammy or dyspnoeic?)
- auscultation of the chest
- patient comfort
- neurological status (any signs of confusion or tiredness?).

The patient receiving non-invasive ventilation should be on a cardiac monitor with continuous monitoring of their:

- heart rate and rhythm
- respiratory rate
- blood pressure
- conscious level (use AVPU as in Box 2.1)
- oxygen saturation (measure via pulse oximetry (SpO_2) continuously for at least 24 hours and aim to keep it at 88–92% with supplemental oxygen therapy; Schwartz *et al.*, 2004).

These observations should be documented at least hourly on the patient's observation chart and a track and trigger score should also be recorded (see Chapter 1 on critical care outreach). It is important to consider these vital signs alongside the patient's arterial blood gas measurements. The frequency of subsequent measurements will depend on the patient's progress (see Chapter 40 on taking an arterial blood gas using a radial stab).

Once non-invasive ventilation has been commenced, patients should be clinically assessed and arterial blood gases repeated after 1 hour, or after each pressure change, and again at

> **HOT TIPS**
>
> Blood gas analysis (ABG) should always be interpreted alongside clinical assessment of the patient. Patients often compensate and look worse clinically than the arterial blood gases may indicate. This can lead to a sudden patient collapse if the clinical signs of deterioration are not noted and addressed early.

4 hours and 12 hours. If no improvement is seen and the patient still has a respiratory acidosis after treatment, then check the parameters as detailed in Box 8.4 (remember to use your own hospital's guidelines as different parameters can be adjusted on different machines).

Non-invasive ventilation should continue for as long as possible during the first 24 hours (Royal College of Physicians, 2008).

Box 8.4   Preventing and dealing with treatment failure in non-invasive ventilation (British Thoracic Society, 2002)

Is the treatment of the underlying condition optimal?

- Check the medical treatment prescribed and that it has been given
- Consider physiotherapy for sputum retention

Have any complications developed?

- Consider a pneumothorax, aspiration pneumonia, etc.

$PaCO_2$ remains elevated

Is the patient on too much oxygen?
- Adjust FiO_2 to maintain SpO_2 between 85% and 90%

Is there excessive leakage?
- Check the fit of the mask

Is the circuit set up correctly?
- Check the connections have been made correctly
- Check the circuit for leaks

Is the patient synchronising with the ventilator?
- Observe the patient
- Consider increasing EPAP

Is ventilation inadequate?
- Observe chest expansion
- Increase IPAP

$PaCO_2$ improves but PaO_2 remains low

- Increase FiO_2.
- Consider increasing EPAP

Titrating treatment to blood gas analysis

Arterial blood gas monitoring, as well as the clinical condition of the patient, will guide the practitioner on changing the pressure support, by altering the IPAP and EPAP levels.

> **HOT TIPS**
>
> When adjusting pressures, remember to maintain pressure support. If EPAP is increased then IPAP should also be increased. If pressure support is decreased then the work of breathing will get harder.

Table 8.2 can be used as a guide to optimise non-invasive ventilation and hopefully reduce the duration of the treatment (but these are only a guide, you must adhere to your own hospital's guidelines).

Table 8.2   Titrating the pressures on the non-invasive ventilator

If no improvement in PCO_2

Increase IPAP slowly by 2 cm at a time to a maximum of 20 cm (increases pressure support)

Repeat ABGs to assess effectiveness of pressure changes

If no improvement, is the patient having too much oxygen? Consider reducing FiO_2

If PO_2 remains low and PCO_2 improves

Increase FiO_2

Increase EPAP (only on expert advice) to a maximum of 8 cm

Repeat ABGs to assess effectiveness of pressure changes

Remember if EPAP is increased also increase IPAP to maintain pressure support

If patient shows signs of tachypnoea and fatigue

Increase IPAP to increase pressure support and reduce the work of breathing

Maintain close observation to measure effectiveness of changes

There may be other parameters that can be adjusted on the non-invasive ventilator but these will depend on the make of equipment being used. All personnel using a non-invasive ventilator should be trained and deemed competent in its usage and be aware of hospital guidelines. The figures given in this chapter can be used for guidance, but may vary from hospital to hospital.

Weaning

Ideally the patient should remain on bi-level non-invasive ventilation for as long as possible during the first 24 hours; if the patient's condition allows, however, breaks should be given off the machine for meals, drinks and nebulisers. If after 24 hours the patient's condition has improved and he or she is no longer acidotic the bi-level non-invasive ventilator can be taken off for extended periods of time during the day, at first. Oxygen can be administered via nasal speculum to maintain oxygen saturations at an agreed level with the medical team. It is important to continue to assess the patient, paying particular attention to their respiratory rate, oxygen saturations and conscious level. Some patients may need to continue non-invasive ventilation at night, but often the patient will be able to tell whether they can manage without the machine and wean themselves.

Conclusions

After 24 hours the condition of the patient in the case scenario condition had improved. He was no longer acidotic. The bi-level non-invasive ventilator was taken off for a couple of hours in the morning and again in the afternoon. The following day, the time off the ventilator was extended to 4 hours in the morning and afternoon. During this period of weaning the patient received oxygen via nasal speculum at 1 litre per minute and this maintained his oxygen saturations at 88–92%. On the third day he had non-invasive ventilation at night only. He continued to be assessed, with particular attention given to his respiratory rate, oxygen saturations and conscious level, and he reported that he was finding breathing much easier. He remained stable. An ABG was again performed to assess his progress after a period off non-invasive ventilation and no deterioration was noted in his pH or PCO_2. It was decided to stop non-invasive ventilation with a view to recommence it if he deteriorated further.

Respiratory support in the ward environment is more common in today's health service and has been shown to reduce mortality in patients who are not suitable for invasive ventilation. For further information, please refer to the British Thoracic Society guidance (2002) and the Royal College of Physicians *Concise Guidance to Good Practice* (2008) and your own hospital's local policy. Critical care colleagues will always be available to assist, such as the critical care outreach team or the intensive care team.

References and further reading

British Thoracic Society (2002). Non-invasive ventilation in acute respiratory care. *Thorax*, **57** (3), 192–211.

Brochard, L., Mancebo, J., Wysocki, M., *et al.* (1995). Non-invasive ventilation for acute exacerbation of chronic obstructive pulmonary disease. *The New England Journal of Medicine*, **333**, 817–22.

Conti, G., Antonelli, M., Navalesi, P. *et al.* (2002). Non-invasive vs conventional mechanical ventilation in patients with chronic obstructive pulmonary disease after failure of medical treatment in the ward: a randomised trial. *Intensive Care Medicine*, **28**, 1701–07.

Lightowler, J.V., Wedzicha, J.A., Elliot, M.W. *et al.* (2003). Non-invasive positive pressure ventilation to treat respiratory failure resulting from exacerbations of chronic obstructive pulmonary disease: Cochrane systematic review and meta-analysis. *British Medical Journal*, **326**, 185–87.

Plant, P., Owen, J. and Elliott, M. (2000a). Early use of non-invasive ventilation for acute exacerbations of chronic obstructive pulmonary disease on general respiratory wards: a multicentre randomised controlled trial. *Lancet*, **355**, 1931–35.

Plant, P., Owen, J. and Elliott, M. (2000b). One year period prevalence study of respiratory acidosis in acute exacerbations of COPD: implications for the provision of non-invasive ventilation and oxygen administration. *Thorax*, **55**, 550–54.

Royal College of Physicians, British Thoracic Society, Intensive Care Society (2008). Chronic obstructive pulmonary disease: non-invasive ventilation with bi-phasic positive airways pressure in the management of patients with acute type 2 respiratory failure. *Concise Guidance to Good Practice Series, No 11*. London, Royal College of Physicians.

Schwartz, A.R., Kacmarek, R.M. and Hess, D.R. (2004). Factors affecting oxygen delivery with bi-level positive airways pressure. *Respiratory Care*, **49**, 270–75.

Useful websites

British Thoracic society
www.brit-thoracic.org.uk/ClinicalInformation/NoninvasiveVentilation/
NIPPVNIVinAcuteRespiratoryFailureGuideline/tabid/132/Default.aspx

Royal College of Physicians
www.rcplondon.ac.uk/pubs/brochure.aspx?e=258

9 Pulmonary embolism

Gaurav Agarwal

Pulmonary embolism (PE) is defined as a clot (or clots) of blood that compromise circulation in the pulmonary vasculature (Swearingen and Keen, 2001). Although there are rarer causes – like fat and air embolism, which could strictly speaking still qualify under the umbrella term PE – we will restrict this discussion to the assessment and management of patients with pulmonary thromboembolism (Kumar and Clark, 2002).

Causes of pulmonary embolism

Deep venous thrombosis (DVT) is by far the commonest cause of pulmonary embolism (British Thoracic Society, 2003). Stasis of blood in the pelvic or large limb veins, microvasculature endothelial injury and hypercoagulability of blood results in the formation of a blood clot (thrombus). This then breaks off and travels to the right side of the heart and so makes its way to the pulmonary vasculature. Very rarely (if there is an atrial or ventricular septal defect) the clot can traverse through to the left side of the heart and into the systemic circulation, resulting in compromised circulation. Some thrombi are associated with organ damage (such as cerebrovascular accident, if the embolus reaches the brain).

Other causes of pulmonary embolism

- Right ventricular thrombosis (usually after a myocardial infarction).
- Air (such as traumatic pneumothorax).
- Fat (after major long bone trauma).
- Amniotic fluid (in pregnant women).
- Septic emboli (such as in bacterial endocarditis).

History

Probe specifically about the risk factors listed below and ask for any family history of coagulation disorders. A sudden onset of pleuritic chest pain and dyspnoea, in the absence of another obvious diagnosis, gives a strong suspicion of pulmonary embolism.

Risk factors (British Thoracic Society, 2003)

- Clinical deep venous thrombosis (DVT).
- Previous proven DVT or PE.
- Pregnancy, post-partum, oral contraceptive pill, hormone replacement therapy.
- Recent immobilisation or major surgery.
- Recent lower limb trauma or surgery.
- Recent long haul air travel.
- Malignancy.

Symptoms (one of those marked * is present in almost all cases of pulmonary embolism)

- Shortness of breath (dyspnoea).*
- Chest pain (pleuritic).*
- Coughing up blood (haemoptysis).
- Syncope, dizziness, collapse.
- Palpitations.

Vital signs (signs marked * are suggestive of large pulmonary embolism)

- Tachypnoea.
- Tachycardia.
- Hypotension.*
- Elevated jugular venous pressure (JVP).
- Cyanosis (look carefully for).*
- Hypoxemia.*

Chest examination

- Pleural rub.
- Evidence of small pleural effusion.

Cardiac/neurological/abdominal examination (usually normal, but look for these specifically)

- Signs of recent surgery.
- Tender, red or swollen calf.

Investigations

Chest radiograph

This is often normal. Sometimes a small pleural effusion may be detected. Very rarely there is a wedge-shaped infarct (opacification, with the apex of the wedge being more central and base more peripheral).

Electrocardiogram

This could be normal or it could show sinus tachycardia. There may be evidence of a right-heart strain pattern (right bundle-branch block and T-wave inversion in V1 to V4). In large PEs, there may be an S-wave in lead I and a Q wave and T-wave inversion in lead III. This is referred to as an S1Q3T3 pattern.

> Echocardiography can reliably diagnose clinically massive pulmonary embolism.

Arterial blood gas analysis

Low PaO_2 (due to poor oxygenation) and low $PaCO_2$ (due to 'blowing off' off of carbon dioxide) as a result of tachypnoea is common. In large pulmonary embolisms, lactate may be raised due to poor peripheral tissue perfusion leading to anaerobic metabolism.

> Allen's test should be performed before an ABG is carried out to avoid digital ischaemia in case of an anomalous absent radial or ulnar artery. See Box 9.1.

D-dimers

Other than troponins, no other blood test has been the target of such extensive debate in medicine! If used intelligently, D-dimers are brilliant for excluding the diagnosis of pulmonary embolism, provided the clinical probability is low. There is little value in doing a D-dimer if the clinical probability is moderate or high; you should instead proceed to definitive imaging straight away (British Thoracic Society, 2003).

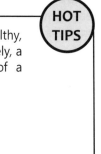

> An alveolar (A)–arteriolar (a) gradient (A—a) of less than 2 kPa in a young, healthy, non-smoking adult woman virtually excludes a pulmonary embolism. Conversely, a gradient of more than 2 kPa adds weight to the clinical probability of a diagnosis of pulmonary embolism.
>
> A—a gradient = FiO_2 (%) – (PaO_2 + $PaCO_2$ × 1.25) kPa
>
> *For example:*
>
> A—a gradient = 21 – (13 + 3 × 1.25) = 4.25 kPa

Emergency imaging

When a patient is haemodynamically unstable, it is difficult to perform definitive imaging studies. Delays can be fatal, which is why echocardiography is useful for looking for right heart strain. It offers the advantage of corroborative evidence before thrombolysis is attempted.

Box 9.1   **Allen's test (based on Murray and White, 1999)**

1. Ask the patient to clench his or her hand tightly for several seconds.

2. Compress the radial or ulnar artery and ask the patient to open the hand.

3. Colour should return quickly to the palm if the non-compressed artery is patent.

4. If colour does not return quickly, do not take arterial blood gases from this arm as circulation to the limb might be compromised.

The alveolar–arterial gradient will be raised by more than 2 kPa.

Definitive investigation with CTPA (computerised tomogram pulmonary angiography)

This is a contrast-enhanced study of the pulmonary vasculature that outlines filling defects as a result of emboli. If CTPA is unavailable or inaccessible then a ventilation–perfusion (V/Q) scan can be done at the nuclear medicine department of your hospital. Look for perfusion defects that are not matched with ventilation defects (if any). This is not as sensitive a test as CTPA and it often takes longer to perform and is more difficult to interpret, especially if the chest radiograph was abnormal. An indeterminate probability scan should always be followed by a CTPA if the clinical suspicion is high (British Thoracic Society, 2003).

Treatment

Once the diagnosis is suspected, it is mandatory – in the absence of a contraindication – to start treatment-dose heparin. Low-molecular-weight heparin (LMWH) as a single subcutaneous daily injection (1.5 mg/kg) is suggested. Once the diagnosis is confirmed, oral warfarin should be started in combination with the heparin injections. Once a stable INR (international normalised ratio) is reached, heparin injections are discontinued; warfarin is continued for a period of at least 3 months, often 6 months, and may be life-long in recurrent disease. Careful attention must be paid to monitoring the INR and adjusting the daily dose of warfarin. The GP surgery and anticoagulation clinic service are invaluable in this regard.

Occasionally, inferior vena cava filters are required. These are used either if there is a failure of or a contraindication to anticoagulation. If there has been a massive pulmonary embolism resulting in haemodynamic compromise, then urgent thrombolysis using recombinant tissue plasminogen activators is suggested (British Thoracic Society, 2003). Rarely, in such situations, pulmonary embolectomy may be required if there is either a failure of or contraindication to thrombolysis.

HOT TIPS

Low-molecular-weight heparin is not a clot-buster, but it prevents enlargement of existing clots and inhibits development of new clots.

Prevention

- Prophylactic once-daily subcutaneous LMWH injection.
- Removal of the agent that increases risk of pulmonary embolism (if feasible).
- Use of full-length compression stockings.
- Early mobilisation.
- Thrombophilia screen in patients with a family history of thromboembolic disorder.

Case Scenario

A 40-year-old woman is admitted to a medical ward with a right leg 'cellulitis' for intravenous antibiotics. She has been previously healthy and has never smoked in her life. You are the medical foundation year 1 doctor on call for wards, and the ward sister calls you at 2 A.M. because the patient has suddenly started complaining of shortness of breath and right-sided pleuritic chest pain. Her blood pressure has dropped to 90/60 mmHg and her respiratory rate increased to 26 breaths per minute. Her SpO_2 is 92% on room air and heart rate 120 beats per minute. She is apyrexial.

How would you rapidly assess this patient?

Think of the steps you would follow before reviewing the guidance below!

The patient would be assessed using the **ABCDE** approach.

A—Airway

The patient's airway is patent.

B—Breathing

THe respiratory rate is high. If the patient is cyanosed, initiate high-flow oxygen therapy immediately and perform an arterial blood gas analysis.

C—Circulation

Urgent fluid resuscitation is needed as well as a portable chest x-ray and an echo. Recombinant tissue plasminogen activator should be obtained from the 'locked drugs cabinet' as soon as possible. A 12-lead ECG is required.

D—Disability

If mentation is altered, the patient must be very hypoxic.

E—Exposure and Environment

Ensure that the patient is on a cardiac monitor and is in an environment where thrombolysis (if required) is safe. Meanwhile, review the notes to rule out any absolute contraindications to thrombolysis and contact a senior colleague. Consider transferring the patient to a high dependency unit if available.

References and further reading

British Thoracic Society (2003). Guidelines for the management of suspected acute pulmonary embolism. *Thorax*, **58**, 47–84.

Kumar, P. and Clark, M. (2002). *Clinical Medicine*, 5th edn. London, WB Saunders.

Murray, S.E. and White, B.S. (1999). *Critical Care Assessment Handbook*. Philadelphia, WB Saunders.

Swearingen, P.L. and Keen, J. (2001). *Manual of Critical Care Nursing: Nursing Interventions and Collaborative Management*, 4th edn. Mosby, USA.

Useful websites

British Thoracic Society
www.brit-thoracic.org.uk

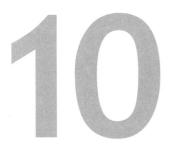

Pneumonia

Gaurav Agarwal

This is an acute inflammatory reaction of the lower respiratory tract, often resulting in patchy consolidation on the chest radiograph, and carrying a 1 in 10 mortality rate among patients requiring hospital admission. The commonest symptoms are fever with chills and rigors and the production of discoloured sputum (Kumar and Clark, 2002).

Classification and causes

Community-acquired pneumonia (CAP) (British Thoracic Society, 2001)

This is the commonest (default) type of pneumonia. The causative organism is *Streptococcus pneumoniae* in 70% of cases; others are *Haemophilus influenzae* and *Staphylococcus aureus* (mortality is high with methicillin-resistant *Staphylococcus aureus*, MRSA). The so-called atypical pneumonias (presenting with diarrhoea, abnormal liver function tests or no consolidation on the chest radiograph) are caused by *Mycoplasma*, *Chlamydia* and *Legionella*. Viruses like influenza, varicella and cytomegalovirus (and, rarely, fungi) also cause pneumonia.

Hospital-acquired pneumonia

This type of pneumonia develops in patients who have been in hospital for more than 48 hours. The organisms responsible, therefore, are those that are more commonly encountered within a hospital rather than in the community. *Staphylococcus aureus* (including MRSA), *Klebsiella*, *Pseudomonas* (which causes green phlegm, green wound discharge, etc.), *Escherichia coli*, *Proteus* and anaerobes are some common causative organisms in this setting.

Aspiration pneumonia

This is common in patients who have lost protection of their airway, for example in intoxicated, stroke patients and neuromuscular disorders such as multiple sclerosis or myasthenia gravis. The anaerobes from the gut or oropharynx cause this type of pneumonia.

Pneumonia in the immunocompromised patient

In diabetic patients, patients who are post-chemotherapy, HIV patients and in those with malignancies, pneumonia could often be the reason for death if it were not managed aggressively enough early on. Any organism can cause this type of pneumonia but, in addition, keep an eye out for fungi, especially if no clinical improvement is noticed after 2 days of standard therapy.

History

The onset is usually over a few days, but can be less than 1 day in immunocompromised patients. The British Thoracic Society (2004) suggests assessing the severity of the pneumonia using the CURB-65 tool (see Box 10.1). This will give an indication as to whether hospital management is indicated.

Box 10.1   **Severity assessment CURB-65 tool (British Thoracic Society, 2004)**

C—Confusion (score 1 if new onset)
U—Urea (score 1 if > 7 mmol/litre)
R—Respiratory rate (score 1 if more than 30 breaths per minute)
B—Blood pressure (score 1 if systolic blood pressure < 90 mmHg or diastolic < 60 mmHg)
65—65 years old (score 1 if age is more than 65)

If the score is <2, then the pneumonia is not severe and may be suitable for out of hospital management, and if the score is >2, then pneumonia should be managed in hospital and will probably need intravenous antibiotics at least for the first day or two. A score of 3 or 4 suggests that urgent hospital referral is needed.

Symptoms

- Shortness of breath (dyspnoea).
- Pleuritic chest pain.
- Fever with chills and rigors.
- Coughing up streaks of blood with yellow, green or brown phlegm.
- Non-specific systemic symptoms such as anorexia, malaise and nausea.
- Confusion (an important cause for confusion in the elderly population).

Vital signs

- Tachypnoea.
- Fever.
- Tachycardia.
- Hypotension.
- Cyanosis (look carefully for).
- Hypoxemia.

Chest examination

- Inspection (decreased chest expansion on the side of the disease).
- Palpation (tenderness on the affected side).
- Percussion (dullness on affected side).

- Auscultation (bronchial breathing – with a gap in between inspiration and expiration – and increased vocal resonance on the affected region of the lung).
- Pleural rub (sometimes heard).
- Small pleural effusion (evidence of).

Cardiac, neurological and abdominal examination

- Usually normal.

Investigations

Chest radiograph

There is patchy consolidation, pleural effusion and rarely cavitation. A normal-looking chest radiograph does not exclude the diagnosis of pneumonia – it could be atypical or *Pneumocystis carinii* pneumonia (PCP), so go with history and clinical suspicion rather than just the chest radiograph.

Blood tests

Carry out a full blood count (neutrophilic leucocytosis is the commonest), urea, creatinine, electrolytes (hyponatremia suggests an atypical infection), liver function tests, C-reactive protein, arterial blood gas analysis and blood cultures. Suspected atypical pneumonia patients should have appropriate serology sent off as well.

Sputum

Send for microscopy and culture or sensitivity. Often a saline nebuliser may help induce sputum.

Arterial blood gas analysis

Often hypoxemia is evident. Severe hypoxia merits the use of non-invasive ventilation.

Pleural fluid

This can be invaluable if a diagnostic tap is sent off before antibiotics are started. Check lactate dehydrogenase (LDH), glucose and pH and send some for cultures as well.

Bronchoalveolar lavage

This is useful in an immunocompromised or critical care patient.

Blood cultures

Although not routinely needed, they should be taken in patients that require hospital admission.

Treatment

Treatment should comprise the following (British Thoracic Society, 2001; 2004):

- **Oxygen therapy:** to treat hypoxia.
- **Fluid rehydration:** either oral or intravenous, as needed, plus antipyretics and analgesia.

- **Antiemetics:** and other symptomatic therapy as needed.
- **Antibiotics:** oral or intravenous depending on the CURB-65 score (see below).
- **Medical prophylaxis:** against deep venous thrombosis, unless contraindicated (e.g. dalteparin 5000 units once daily by subcutaneous injection).

Choice of antibiotics

The choice is often driven by local protocols, so familiarise yourself with your local microbiology guidelines. Often a penicillin should be used as first-line therapy in community-acquired pneumonia, a macrolide in atypical pneumonia, and a combination of a penicillin and beta-lactamase inhibitor in severe pneumonia along with a macrolide.

Care must be taken to make sure that the moment blood cultures have been taken, the intravenous antibiotics are given, either by yourself or a colleague – just prescribing on the drug chart does not mean it will be given straightaway!

Complications

- Pleural effusion (may need to insert a chest drain).
- Empyema (if a chest drain fails to resolve this, a surgical procedure may be required).
- Lung abscess (aggressive, longer-duration antibiotic therapy is usually curative).
- Type I respiratory failure: this can then lead on to type II respiratory failure (non-invasive ventilation should be started early in patients with severe disease, particularly those who are at risk of type II respiratory failure).

Prevention (British Thoracic Society, 2001)

- Pneumonia jabs and flu vaccines for all at-risk individuals.
- Encourage and help people to quit smoking.

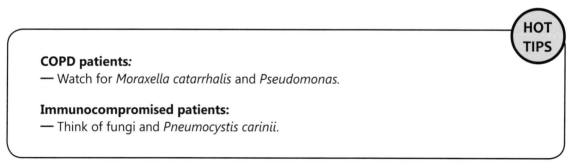

HOT TIPS

COPD patients:
— Watch for *Moraxella catarrhalis* and *Pseudomonas*.

Immunocompromised patients:
— Think of fungi and *Pneumocystis carinii*.

> ### Case Scenario
>
> A 50-year-old man is admitted to a medical ward with cough and fever and diagnosed with upper respiratory tract infection. You are the medical foundation year 1 doctor on call for wards and the ward sister calls you at 8 P.M. because the patient has started coughing up blood-streaked sputum and is very worried.
>
> His blood pressure has dropped to 88/60 mmHg and his respiratory rate has increased to 32 breaths per minute. His SpO$_2$ is 95% on room air and heart rate is 120 beats per minute. He is apyrexial.
>
> *How would you rapidly assess this patient?*
>
> *Think of the steps you would follow before reviewing the guidance below!*

Scenario review

The patient would be assessed using the **ABCDE** approach.

A—Airway
The patient's airway is patent.

B—Breathing
High respiratory rate. If the patient is cyanosed, initiate high-flow oxygen therapy immediately and perform an arterial blood gas analysis.

C—Circulation
Urgent fluid resuscitation is needed for low blood pressure. A portable chest x-ray is also needed.

D—Disability
If mentation is altered, the patient is likely to be very hypoxic.

E—Exposure and Environment
Apply 'fan therapy' and 'tepid sponging' if the patient's temperature is very high. Follow this with definitive treatment of pneumonia if the CURB-65 score is indicative of a severe pneumonia (and inform your senior immediately).

References and further reading

British Thoracic Society (2001). Guidelines for the management of community-acquired pneumonia in adults. *Thorax*, 56 (Suppl.4), 1–64.

British Thoracic Society (2004). Guidelines for the management of community-acquired pneumonia in adults – An update. Available at: http//www.brit-thoracic.org.uk/Portals/0/Clinical%20Information/Pneumonia/Guidelines/MACAPrevisedApr04.pdf (last accessed November 2009).

Kumar, P. and Clark, M. (2002). *Clinical Medicine*, 5th edn. London, WB Saunders.

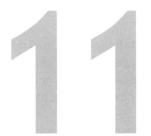

Neurological diseases affecting breathing

Alistair Challiner

Two conditions that may be encountered on acute medical wards are Guillain–Barré syndrome and myasthenia gravis. Both conditions cause muscle weakness, but the important factors to be concerned with are respiratory muscle weakness that causes hypoventilation and loss of control of swallowing reflexes, giving risk to aspiration and pneumonia.

These are life threatening, therefore both conditions may need admission to intensive care unit and intubation if symptoms deteriorate, and it is essential to know what these signs are and how to monitor them.

At the end of this chapter you should be able to:

- review Guillain–Barré and myasthenia gravis from the respiratory perspective
- identify critical illness neuropathy as a complication in post-intensive care patients.

Case Scenario

A 26-year-old woman was admitted to hospital with headache, nausea and weakness and numbness in her legs, causing her to collapse several times. In hospital, as no obvious signs were found and the CT scan was clear, the medical staff assumed this was related to anxiety and that she was exaggerating her symptoms. The numbness and weakness in her legs became worse, ascending higher, and she became breathless.

She was referred to the intensive care unit and a neurologist referral made. The neurologist diagnosed Guillain–Barré syndrome, supported by loss of reflexes in the legs, weakness and numbness by clinical examination and lumbar puncture CSF analysis showed an increased protein level. Her ABG was normal but vital capacity measurement was 1.5 litres. She was able to swallow.

She was admitted to the high-dependency unit and treated with immunoglobulin infusions for 5 days. She improved, particularly with respect to respiratory function, and hence did not need ventilation. She made a full recovery following rehabilitation over several months to regain her ability to walk.

Guillain–Barré syndrome

This is caused by an inflammatory neuropathy affecting the nerves – not the muscle. The myelin sheath that covers the nerves is reduced, causing decreased conduction; this is due to an autoimmune response. Triggers include infections like those with *Campylobacter* or herpes viruses, 1–3 weeks previously. Other causes include malignancy. There is no obvious cause in 40% of cases.

The disease starts in the legs and ascends up the body. Motor and sensory nerves can be involved as can autonomic nerves, causing arrhythmias and hypotension. In severe cases a flaccid paralysis occurs including that of the respiratory muscles. The symptoms can last for several months, and 85% of cases make a full recovery.

Diagnosis

Diagnosis is by history and clinical examination. The key features are a symmetrical ascending motor paralysis, with loss of reflexes. The cerebrospinal fluid (CSF) shows increased protein levels, but normal cell counts.

Management

Management is supportive and includes preventing deep vein thrombosis (DVT) and infections. Immunomodulating therapy with immunoglobulin can improve symptoms, as can plasma-phoresis (a modified haemofiltration technique to remove antibody load). Vigilance in monitoring respiratory function is vital, in case the patient requires respiratory support with a ventilator in the intensive care unit. Ventilation may be required for weeks or months, necessitating a tracheostomy.

Myasthenia gravis

Antibodies against acetylcholine receptors cause myasthenia gravis, whereby the motor nerve stimulates a voluntary muscle. This causes weakness that increases the more the muscle is used (seen as increased fatigue and weakness over the course of the day).

Diagnosis

Symptoms include drooping of the eyelids, nasal speech and difficulty swallowing. There is no sensory component to this disease. It can be caused by a tumour of the thymus gland or related to other autoimmune diseases such as thyroid and rheumatoid arthritis.

Management

Treatment is with drugs that increase the level of acetylcholine such as pyridostigmine, as well as immunosuppression with steroids, for example. Deterioration can be caused by a worsening of the condition (myasthenic crisis) or by effective over-dosage of the pyridostigmine (cholinergic crisis). Worsening of the condition may be brought on by changes in medication or infection. The patient may require ventilation if severe.

Pyridostigmine causes an increase in acetylcholine levels by reducing its breakdown, thus increasing its concentration at the receptors and enhancing muscle function. Very high levels of acetylcholine in cholinergic crisis produce a neuromuscular block similar to that brought about by anaesthetic muscle relaxants, causing sweating, fever, salivation, small pupils and muscle weakness with twitching of the muscles. These symptoms, except muscle weakness, are due to blockade at autonomic (parasympathetic) receptors, which also use acetylcholine.

Patients with myasthenia gravis who are undergoing surgery may have elective admission to the intensive care unit postoperatively because of the risk of respiratory inadequacy.

Respiratory muscle weakness

Simple clinical observation, peak flow, saturations and blood gases should not be relied on in isolation as they are not sufficiently specific. For this reason, it may be too late to determine when ventilation is necessary.

The most effective way of monitoring patients with muscle weakness is to measure their forced vital capacity (FVC). This is the volume of air that can be breathed out after taking a maximal deep breath. It is normally in the region of 5–6 litres, but when it gets to 15 mL/kg (around 1 litre) ventilation may be required. This should be measured regularly according to severity such as every 1–2 hours. Clinical signs such as being unable to speak, tachypnoea, drooling, shallow breaths and exhaustion are another indication for ventilation.

A patient who is deteriorating should be transferred to the high dependency unit or intensive care unit for closer observation and readily available ventilation.

The forced vital capacity is measured with a respiratory function device such as a vitalograph, but such equipment is not normally available in the acute medical environment. It is more common to use a Wright flowmeter attached to an anaesthetic face mask, usually obtained from the operating theatre or intensive care unit.

Disordered swallowing or bulbar signs

Signs of this include an abnormal voice (particularly nasal sounding) and difficulty swallowing water or regurgitating water nasally. The risk is aspiration pneumonia. Anaesthetic assessment is required and the patient should be nil by mouth, due to the risk of aspiration.

Critical illness neuropathy/myopathy

This condition can result from prolonged admission on the intensive care unit and may be present in patients discharged from intensive care to the ward (see post-intensive care unit patient Chapter 29). The symptoms are predominantly generalised muscle weakness.

The causes are unclear but are related to immunosuppression, sepsis, and the use of drugs such as muscle relaxants and steroids. The patient may have weakness of all limbs, and will therefore need supportive nursing care, prophylaxis for deep vein thrombosis, and intensive physiotherapy. Mostly these patients make a full recovery.

Conclusions

This chapter provides an overview of the neurological conditions that affect breathing, which are sometimes seen in acute care wards. Key points to remember are that the patient's airway must be monitored and protected and that their respiratory function and strength must also be closely monitored. Deterioration in either of these areas requires urgent critical care input.

References and further reading

Bersten, A.D., Soni, N., and Oh, T.E. (eds) (2004) *Oh's Intensive Care Manual*, 5th edn. Philadelphia, Butterworth-Heinemann,

Useful websites

Guillain–Barré support group
www.gbs.org.uk

Myasthenia Gravis Association
www.mgauk.org

Support Group for Myasthenia patients
www.patient.co.uk/support/Myasthenia-Gravis-Association.htm

12 Physiotherapy in the acutely ill

Sarah Elliott

Physiotherapy is a healthcare profession that is found in all areas of health and is primarily concerned with human function, movement and maximising potential. Respiratory care is just one branch of physiotherapy, and because of our extensive knowledge of anatomy, physiology and pathology – alongside excellent assessment, handling and communication skills – we are ideally suited to the treatment of acutely ill patients within intensive care, high-dependency and ward settings.

Not only do physiotherapists deal with the treatment of acute respiratory problems, but they also identify potential problems, undertake preventative measures, and act as educators in disease management and smoking cessation. Physiotherapy assessment always involves assessment of the whole patient because it is ineffective to intervene with a process that is as personal as breathing without attending to the person as a whole.

This chapter aims to provide a brief overview of respiratory physiotherapy including team structure, referrals, the on-call service, assessment and a selection of treatments.

Physiotherapy department and teams

Within an acute hospital, physiotherapy will be divided into specialist teams such as respiratory care. Each team consists of a highly specialised team leader, many of whom have extended skills beyond the normal boundaries of physiotherapy, for example in arterial stabs, chest x-ray requests and interpretation, tracheostomy care and prescribing. Other members of the team may include both senior and junior physiotherapists, some who work on a rotational basis in order to gain experience in all fields of physiotherapy care, and physiotherapy assistants who support the qualified staff. Please refer to local procedures for referrals to physiotherapy, but generally, referrals for physiotherapy will be accepted from medical staff, qualified nursing staff and other qualified allied health professionals (such as occupational therapists, speech and language therapists, dieticians and pharmacists). Referral may be:

- via a referral form
- verbally (while the therapists are visiting the wards)
- via the pager system
- via the telephone.

It is important that as many details as possible as well as the reason for referral are included to allow physiotherapists to prioritise their workload. If you are unsure, consult the ward physiotherapist to discuss, or (if they are in place) refer to the physiotherapy referral guidelines. An example of referral guidelines is shown in Box 12.1.

Box 12.1   **Respiratory physiotherapy team referral guidelines**

DO **REFER**

Surgical
— All major abdominal surgery, pre-operatively if possible
— ENT surgery such as radical neck dissection and laryngectomy
— Vascular surgery such as femoral–popliteal bypass
— Through foot and toe amputations

Respiratory
— Ventilated patients
— Atelectasis
— Worsening SpO_2 or arterial blood gases
— Unable to clear secretions effectively
— Exacerbation of chronic obstructive pulmonary disease
— Rib fractures
— Chest infection
— Breathlessness

Mobility
— Patients whose normal level of mobility is impaired due to current medical or surgical conditions (and which is unlikely to resolve without rehabilitation)
— Patients who have stairs at home and who need to be assessed prior to discharge home

DO *NOT* **REFER**
— Minor or laparoscopic surgery
— Amputations (please refer to Amputees Physiotherapy Team)
— Pulmonary oedema
— Pulmonary emboli
— Raised respiratory rate due to acidosis
— Patients whose mobility is limited by medical conditions (e.g. pain, vomiting, diarrhoea)
— Long-term immobility (e.g. contractures, wheelchair bound)

N.B. IF YOU ARE UNSURE, CONSULT YOUR WARD PHYSIOTHERAPIST

On-call or out of hours service

The majority of physiotherapy departments offer an out of hours (overnight and weekends) emergency respiratory service for patients who would deteriorate without respiratory physiotherapy when full active management is being planned. There are two categories of patients:

- *Ongoing treatment*: these patients have already been assessed by their physiotherapist and designated as at risk of deterioration in their condition if not treated out of normal working hours. For these patients, a planned visit or telephone check will be carried out.
- *Call out*: these are patients referred by senior medical staff due to an acute episode. As most physiotherapists are on call at home, referral should be made as early as possible to allow a swift response, with a comprehensive handover of the patient's current clinical condition. The physiotherapist may request interventions such as pain relief and nebulisers while on route. These requests should be responded to promptly to facilitate more effective treatment.

Following discussion with the referring doctor, the on-call physiotherapist has the professional autonomy to delay attendance to a call out if the patient does not fulfil the criteria as an 'emergency'. A full explanation will be given and the patient will be assessed the following working day. For full details, refer to local policy and procedure or consult a lead respiratory physiotherapist.

Physiotherapy intervention

Assessment

Accurate assessment is the linchpin of physiotherapy and a respiratory assessment should include:

The database
This will include history of the present case, past medical history, drug history, smoking history, social and family history. This information will be gathered from medical notes, nursing staff, the patient and their relatives.

Investigations
These might include chest x-rays, CT scans and lung function tests, and will be reviewed by the physiotherapist. If indicated, some senior physiotherapists are able to request these investigations autonomously but this will vary between hospitals.

Observations
Usually from the patient's charts. If relevant, physiotherapists will measure them directly. They include: heart rate, blood pressure, oxygen saturations, respiratory rate, fluid balance, urine output, temperature, central venous pressure and arterial blood gases. Physiotherapists with extended skills are able to carry out arterial stabs.

Apparatus (especially oxygen)

Questions to be asked include: Does the patient require oxygen? Is it prescribed? Is it humidified? Is it the correct delivery method? Physiotherapists also review intravenous infusions, wound drains and chest drains.

Patient observation

This should occur before the patient is aware of the physiotherapist's presence and includes observation of the breathing rate and pattern, posture, colour, chest shape and hands.

Subjective assessment

Following introductions, the patient is given the opportunity to define his or her problems, symptoms and the influence of these factors on their lifestyle; respect for a patient's opinions is a potent motivating factor and can help build rapport. Specific questions may address levels of pain and the presence of a cough: Is this cough normal? Are you producing any sputum? What colour is it? Is that normal or has it changed? Do you get breathless? How far can you walk? Further questioning may cover the patient's social history including their home situation, employment, hobbies and activities of daily living (ADLs).

Objective assessment

This may include auscultation, percussion note, chest expansion and breathing pattern. The effectiveness and sound of the patient's cough is noted, documenting the colour, consistency and quantity of sputum. A musculoskeletal assessment may be carried out if appropriate, and may include joint range of movement (ROM), muscle tone and strength, assessment of normal movement, gait and the ability to carry out daily tasks such as transfers and toileting.

Following a thorough assessment, the physiotherapist can, through clinical reasoning, identify the patient's problems.

Aims of respiratory physiotherapy

The main aims of respiratory physiotherapy are:

- to increase lung volume
- to improve gas exchange
- to decrease the work of breathing
- to clear secretions.

Other physiotherapy-related problems may be identified, such as:

- decreased mobility and function
- decreased range of movement
- decreased strength
- altered tone.

Other problems may be identified that require further medical intervention such as:

- fluid overload or depletion
- poor oxygen therapy
- drugs review
- pain management
- neurological assessment.

Referrals to other professions may also be instigated, including:

- occupational therapy
- speech and language therapy
- dietetics
- outreach team
- community physiotherapy team
- social services.

Once the problems have been identified, through analytical problem solving, a treatment plan using evidence-based theories can be established and agreed with the patient, including time frames and goals.

Treatment

Treatments for the identified problems may include:

1. Physiotherapy techniques to increase lung volume

Positioning

This is used to facilitate maximal inspiration (Draper and Ritson, 2004) with functional residual capacity (FRC) increasing in the following positions: supine, slumped sitting, half-lying, side-lying inclined towards prone, sitting upright, standing (Jenkins *et al.*, cited by Hough, 1991).

Controlled mobilisation/exercise

Dull and Dull (cited by Hough, 1991) advocate that exercise is the optimum treatment for increasing lung volume and should always be considered in the first instance. However, it should be graded to ensure diaphragmatic breathing is achieved and this is not always feasible in the acutely ill adult.

Breathing exercises

The aim is to achieve maximal inspiration, to recruit collateral ventilation. Patients are requested to carry out a few at a time (three to five) which means they must be repeated hourly to ensure maximum effort is achieved (Hough, 1991).

Incentive spirometry

This device gives visual feedback on the performance of deep-breathing exercises.

Intermittent positive pressure breathing (IPPB)

This is also known as 'the bird'. It assists breathing through the use of a pressure-cycled ventilator. The device, once triggered by the patient's own inhalation, delivers positive pressure on inspiration and then allows passive expiration. The pressure, flow rate and trigger sensitivity can be altered according to the individual patient's needs.

2. Physiotherapy techniques to increase gas exchange

Positioning

This is best applied to patients with unilateral lung pathology. In side-lying with the affected lung uppermost, the lower and better-ventilated lung is then also better perfused, thus improving V/Q (ventilation–perfusion) matching (Winslow *et al.*, cited by Hough, 1991). Acute respiratory distress (ARD) patients, who are extremely hypoxic, may be nursed prone as this aids the recruitment of lung tissue (Draper and Ritson, 2004); this is usually only performed within the intensive-care setting.

Exercise

Ventilation and perfusion become more even throughout the lung (Hough, 1991).

3. Physiotherapy techniques to decrease the work of breathing

Positioning

The aim is to support the patient's position to encourage relaxation of the upper chest and shoulders, which in turn eases the load on their inspiratory muscles. Positions include: high-side lying, sitting upright in chair with arms supported on pillows, relaxed standing and forward-lean sitting. O'Neill and McCarthy (cited by Hough, 1991) explain that in this position the diaphragm is domed and therefore works with greater efficiency.

Breathing control

This is controlled tidal breathing with the upper chest and shoulders relaxed. It is best taught as a coping strategy as part of pulmonary rehabilitation when the patient is well.

Relaxation

Relaxation and stress-reduction strategies are useful tools for reducing muscle tension and anxiety. Simple things like positioning, the use of the voice and reassurance, as well as specific relaxation techniques, all help.

4. Physiotherapy techniques to clear secretions

Hydration

Effective hydration, either by oral or intravenous routes, will decrease sputum viscosity (Blanshard, cited by Hough, 1991) and allow effective mucociliary action.

Humidification

Any patient whose own respiratory system has been bypassed, or who has thick secretions or who is using oxygen via a face mask (generally over 5 litres, but check hospital policy) should receive humidification.

Exercise/mobilisation

As exercise increases lung volume, collateral ventilation is recruited which aids movement of secretions in the distal airways. Clarke (cited by Hough, 1991) identified that active exercises are particularly beneficial and can be incorporated into the general rehabilitation of the patient. Additionally, Mier *et al.* (cited by Hough, 1991) identified that mucus transport increases with exercise.

Breathing exercises

These were identified as beneficial by Anderson *et al.* (cited by Hough, 1991). They may also be described as thoracic expansion exercises with the aim of gaining maximal breath in followed by relaxed expiration (Draper and Ritson, 2004). To boost collateral ventilation, patients may be requested to carry out an inspiratory 'hold' (to hold their breath for 3 seconds at full inspiration) or a 'sniff' (sniffing air through the nose at full inspiration). They can be used in conjunction with manual techniques and positioning.

Active cycle of breathing

This is a cycle of breathing exercises including thoracic expansion exercises (as above), breathing control (relaxed tidal breathing) and forced expiratory technique (FET) (Pryor and Prasad, 2002). FET is described by Draper and Ritson (2004) as a gentle but forced breath out through an open mouth following a breath in; care should be taken not to invoke bronchospasm (Menkes and Britt, cited by Hough, 1991).

Positioning (postural drainage)

Gravity-assisted positions may be adopted to aid drainage of secretions from affected areas (Hough, 1991). However, in acute settings head down positions are best avoided due to the number of contraindications which include: hypertension, dyspnoea, recent surgery and cardiac failure (Draper and Ritson, 2004).

Manual techniques (percussion)

Slow rhythmic clapping on the patient's chest can moderately aid mucociliary transport (Van der Schans *et al.*, cited by Hough, 1991). This can sometimes lead to dependency by the patient on the physiotherapist (Hough, 1991), therefore, it is mainly used on patients with lower levels of consciousness.

Suction (endotracheal tube, tracheostomy, nasopharyngeal, oropharyngeal, minitracheostomy)

Suction is a procedure that uses negative pressure to remove excessive or retained secretions from the main airway of patients who are not otherwise able to effectively clear those secretions. It may need to be preceded by other treatment techniques to ensure secretions are accessible in the upper airway (Hough, 1991). See Chapter 40 on suctioning tracheostomies.

Cough assist

This is a device that delivers a positive pressure breath, followed in quick succession by a switch to negative pressure. It is used mainly with neuromuscular or fatigued patients with an ineffective cough (Draper and Ritson, 2004).

Other treatments

Other treatments available to clear secretions include use of positive expiratory pressure (PEP) masks, the 'flutter' and the technique of autogenic drainage. However, these are more likely to be used with chronic sputum producers such as patients with bronchiectasis and cystic fibrosis, and they are infrequently used in acute settings.

Once the treatment has been carried out it will be evaluated for its effectiveness, and modified if necessary. The patient will then be left with a plan that may include independent activities and will be reviewed at a given time, when the process begins again. Once the problem has been resolved the patient will be discharged from physiotherapy.

The following case study aims to summarise a physiotherapy intervention through a cyclic procedure of assessment, identification of the problems, treatment intervention, re-assessment and future plans. All the findings would be documented in the medical notes and discussions carried out with relevant personnel.

Case Scenario

At 8 P.M. the on-call physiotherapist is asked to review a 54-year-old woman following a laparotomy a few hours earlier, who has decreasing saturations of oxygen. Assessment showed the following:

Database: She is a known smoker of 30 cigarettes per day for over 20 years. She suffers from mild asthma and uses her Ventolin™ inhaler as required. Occasionally she clears sputum plugs. She is normally independently mobile with no shortness of breath on exertion.

Investigations: Chest x-ray shows total right lung opacity with raised hemidiaphragm. Arterial blood gases (on 60% oxygen) yield: pH 7.43; $PaCO_2$ 4.8; PaO_2 7.6; bicarbonate 25.4; base excess 1.8.

Observations: Her temperature 38.7°C, heart rate 125 beats per minute, blood pressure 135/85 mmHg, respiratory rate 35 breaths per minute, SpO_2 87%.

Apparatus: She is on patient-controlled morphine, 60% humidified oxygen via a face mask, has intravenous fluids running, and has a catheter and wound drain.

Patient observation: She is slumped in the bed, with rapid apical breathing and looks pale.

Subjective assessment: She is afraid to take a deep breath or cough, and rates pain at 9/10.

Objective assessment: Expansion is decreased on her right side. On auscultation, normal breath sounds are heard on the left side, and bronchial breathing right side.

Consider the following regarding the patient in this case scenario.

Problems
- Pain.
- Hypoxaemia (decreased gas exchange).
- Decreased lung volume on right side (due to sputum plug as at risk due to smoking and asthma history).
- Increased work of breathing.
- Anxiety.

Treatments

- Request medical review for pain management.
- Explain the physiotherapist's role and explain interventions to lessen her anxiety.
- Position her so she is left-side lying to aid V/Q matching and drainage of secretions and to increase lung volume. Also ensure she is well supported with pillows to decrease the work of breathing.
- Apply saline nebuliser (oxygen driven) to loosen secretions.
- Teach her to carry out thoracic expansion exercises, noting her lung expansion; when secretions are audible in the upper airways, encourage her to support her abdominal wound in order to achieve effective cough.
- If adequate expansion is not possible through breathing exercises or if the patient becomes fatigued, consider progressing to intermittent positive pressure breathing (IPPB).

Re-assessment

- **Observations**: SpO_2 improved to 96%. Respiratory rate 20 breaths per minute. Heart rate 101 beats per minute.

- **Patient observation**: Good position in bed with the shoulder girdle relaxed. Respiratory rate even and settled.

- **Subjective assessment**: Patient feels much better after clearing secretions. No longer frightened to cough. Pain 5/10 and improving.

- **Objective assessment:** Patient cleared two large plugs of thick yellow secretions. On auscultation, normal breath sounds on the left side, slight bronchial breathing remains in right lower zone. Expansion: right equals left.

Analysis of treatment

The patient has improved gas exchange and lung volume post-physiotherapy, which is clearly evidenced using objective markers. She is now independently performing breathing exercises and clearing sputum. With thorough explanations and reassurance, work of breathing and anxiety have lessened.

Plan

Overnight, regular saline nebulisers are to be prescribed. The patient is encouraged to continue with breathing exercises. She is to be positioned in left-side lying or upright position. Ward physiotherapists are to review the following morning, to re-assess and treat any identified problems. Progression of treatment may include review of breathing exercises and modify or progress if identified, weaning of oxygen therapy, active exercises or controlled mobilisation and referral to members of the multidisciplinary team if required.

References and further reading

Draper, A. and Ritson, P. (2004). Respiratory physiotherapy treatment. In: B. Harden (ed.) *Emergency Physiotherapy*. Edinburgh, Churchill Livingstone.

Hough, A. (1991). *Physiotherapy in Respiratory Care*. London, Chapman and Hall.

Pryor, J.A and Prasad, S.A. (eds) (2002). *Physiotherapy for Respiratory and Cardiac Problems*, 3rd edn. Edinburgh: Churchill Livingstone.

ABCDE

Circulation

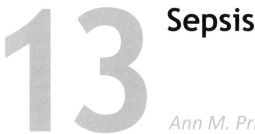

Sepsis

Ann M. Price and Sally A. Smith

S epsis continues to have a high mortality rate despite advances in treatment (Dellinger *et al.*, 2004). A consensus conference was held to examine the current evidence in the treatment of sepsis in a bid to reduce mortality and improve patient outcomes (see the Surviving Sepsis website). There is now a clear set of guidelines that should be followed in the treatment of sepsis. This chapter focuses on the initial treatment of severe sepsis within the ward setting.

At the end of this chapter you should be able to:

- define sepsis, severe sepsis and septic shock
- identify the signs and symptoms of sepsis
- understand the pathophysiology underpinning sepsis
- describe the initial management of a patient with sepsis.

Definitions

Sepsis is often a progressively worsening condition if left untreated. Three common terms are used to describe it, namely sepsis, severe sepsis and septic shock. The following list is based on criteria of Flynn and McLeskey (2005) and Dellinger *et al.* (2008):

Sepsis and severe sepsis

Sepsis is the systemic response to infection including two or more of the following aspects (Survive Sepsis, 2007):

- Temperature above 38.3°C or below 36°C.
- Tachycardia > 90 beats per minute.
- Tachypnoea (> 20 breaths per minute).
- White blood cells < 4 or > 12 g/L.
- Altered mental state.
- Glucose > 6.6 mmol/L (unless diabetic).

Severe sepsis presents with the signs of sepsis with additional organ dysfunction such as hypotension, oliguria, lactic acidosis and confusion.

Septic shock

Septic shock presents with the signs of severe sepsis where hypotension is unresponsive to fluid challenges, perfusion abnormalities continue and inotropic support to maintain blood pressure is needed. Many factors should be eliminated when trying to identify the cause of sepsis. Possible causes include vascular lines (e.g. central venous catheter), intra-abdominal pathology, pneumonia, urinary tract infection, wound infection and trauma. The Survive Sepsis Team (www.survivesepsis.org) have produced an easy-to-use version of the severe sepsis screening tool to identify sepsis and its possible causes (see Fig. 13.1).

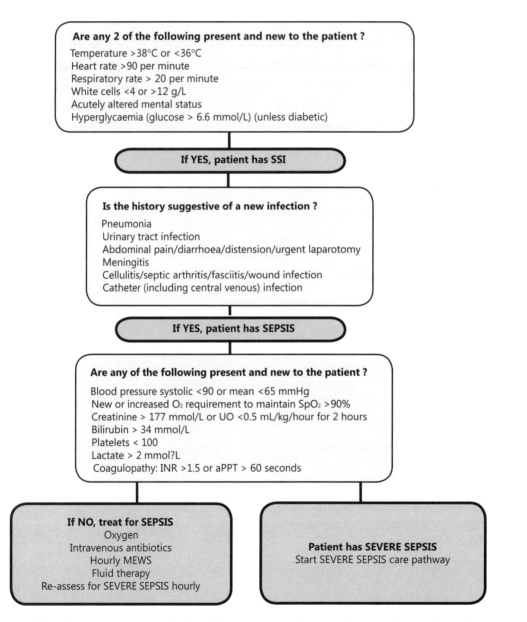

Are any 2 of the following present and new to the patient ?

Temperature >38°C or <36°C
Heart rate >90 per minute
Respiratory rate > 20 per minute
White cells <4 or >12 g/L
Acutely altered mental status
Hyperglycaemia (glucose > 6.6 mmol/L) (unless diabetic)

If YES, patient has SSI

Is the history suggestive of a new infection ?

Pneumonia
Urinary tract infection
Abdominal pain/diarrhoea/distension/urgent laparotomy
Meningitis
Cellulitis/septic arthritis/fasciitis/wound infection
Catheter (including central venous) infection

If YES, patient has SEPSIS

Are any of the following present and new to the patient ?

Blood pressure systolic <90 or mean <65 mmHg
New or increased O_2 requirement to maintain SpO_2 >90%
Creatinine > 177 mmol/L or UO <0.5 mL/kg/hour for 2 hours
Bilirubin > 34 mmol/L
Platelets < 100
Lactate > 2 mmol?L
Coagulopathy: INR >1.5 or aPPT > 60 seconds

If NO, treat for SEPSIS
Oxygen
Intravenous antibiotics
Hourly MEWS
Fluid therapy
Re-assess for SEVERE SEPSIS hourly

Patient has SEVERE SEPSIS
Start SEVERE SEPSIS care pathway

Figure 13.1 Severe sepsis screening tool (from www.survivesepsis.org with permission).

Case Scenario

A 75-year-old woman is admitted after surgery for a perforated bowel due to diverticular disease. You notice that she is pyrexial, tachycardic and hypotensive. Her urine output has reduced to less than 20 mL per hour and she has not responded to a fluid challenge.

Pathophysiology

Sepsis is a very complex phenomenon which is believed to be initiated by the release of cytokines and inflammatory mediators as a response to infection (Flynn and McLeskey, 2005). This causes several reactions within the body that lead to the dysfunctions seen in sepsis.

1. Vasodilation of blood vessels leads to hypotension – this limits blood flow to vital organs causing dysfunction and eventual failure.

2. Capillaries become more permeable, leading to fluid leaking from vascular space into interstitial and intracellular spaces, causing oedema, worsening hypotension and restricting organ perfusion further. This may also affect the function of the lungs leading to acute respiratory distress syndrome (ARDS).

3. Initially the myocardium tries to compensate with a 'hyperdynamic' response to the sepsis, but myocardial function is depressed and may progress to cardiac failure.

4. The clotting cascade is affected in a variety of ways causing abnormal platelet aggregation and overactive coagulation. This leads to the formation of micro-clots within the circulation that impede blood flow to the vital organs. This can progress to disseminated intravascular coagulation (DIC) which can cause major bleeding problems.

5. The body is unable to utilise energy sources as normal, resulting in metabolic acidosis (often seen as lactic acidosis). This means that the cells are starved of energy and metabolise abnormally leading to cell damage; the body tries to compensate by finding alternative sources of energy, which may lead to high blood sugars and insulin resistance.

It is vital that the early signs of sepsis are recognised and treated to prevent the sepsis cascade and deterioration to septic shock which is very difficult to reverse.

Monitoring and management

The Surviving Sepsis Campaign (Survive Sepsis 2007; Dellinger *et al.*, 2008) has highlighted clear steps in the management of severe sepsis which will be outlined here. Following the European Intensive Care Society meeting in Barcelona in 2002, the surviving sepsis guidelines were endorsed as part of an international effort to reduce mortality in severe sepsis and septic shock by 25% by 2009 (Dellinger *et al.*, 2004; Survive Sepsis, 2007). It comprises the creation of evidence-based guidelines sponsored and endorsed initially by 11 international organizations (Dellinger and Vincent, 2005) and further refined in 2008 (Dellinger *et al.*, 2008).

The Institute for Healthcare Improvement (IHI) distilled the guidelines into two care bundles – the *resuscitation* bundle (a set of tasks to be achieved within 6 hours of the onset of presenting with sepsis) and the *management* bundle (to be completed within 24 hours). It has been suggested that the resuscitation bundle can be further refined into two components – those aspects of care not requiring a central line and the use of central venous access to guide early goal-directed therapy (EGDT) (Survive Sepsis, 2007).

The specific set of actions within the first hour following onset has been termed 'Sepsis 6' (Daniels *et al.*, 2008; see Box 13.1) and includes fluid management, oxygen therapy, fluid balance, antibiotics, blood cultures and lactate. The resuscitation care bundle, which outlines the interventions and clinical targets for the first 6 hours after diagnosis of severe sepsis (Daniels *et al.*, 2008), is described in more detail below. The management care bundle that describes the specific process and care to be delivered for the next 24 hours, usually in the intensive care unit (Survive Sepsis, 2007) is beyond the scope of this text. For further information please refer to the Survive Sepsis websites.

Observations

Patients who are at risk of severe sepsis should be continuously monitored, with vital sign recordings taken 1–2 hourly, including blood pressure, mean blood pressure, pulse, central venous pressure (where present), urine output and 4-hourly temperature. This will ensure prompt recognition of the deteriorating patient.

Initial resuscitation

Initial resuscitation during the first 6 hours is to achieve a mean arterial blood pressure (MAP) of > 65 mmHg using initially fluid resuscitation of 20 mL/kg of either 0.9% saline or Hartmann's, up to a maximum of 60 mL/kg. If the patient remains hypotensive, a central venous line should be inserted aiming for a central venous pressure 8–12 mmHg. A central venous ($ScvO_2$) or mixed venous oxygenation (SvO_2) can be taken, aiming for > 70%. Haemoglobin levels should be checked and blood transfusion considered if levels are less than 7 g/dL. If $ScvO_2$ is < 70% despite CVP within limits then norepinephrine or dobutamine should be commenced. Any patient who displays signs of severe sepsis should be referred to the critical care team urgently and as soon as possible (Daniels *et al.*, 2008; see also www.survivesepsis.org).

Diagnosis

Blood cultures should be taken from peripheral site and from any invasive lines that have been in situ more than 48 hours, ideally *before* commencing antibiotics. Other specimens and investigations should be undertaken as indicated (e.g. urine, cerebrospinal fluid or CT scan, ultrasound). All these aim to accurately identify the cause of the sepsis. An arterial lactate and arterial blood gas sample must be obtained straight away. Some blood gas machines will

Box 13.1   **Sepsis 6 (Survive Sepsis, 2007; Daniels *et al.*, 2008; from www.survivesepsis.org with permission)**

TO BE DELIVERED WITHIN THE FIRST HOUR FOLLOWING THE ONSET OF SEPSIS

Oxygen: Give 15 litres via non-rebreathe mask; arterial blood gases; take care with COPD patients.

Blood cultures: Take before starting antibiotics using peripheral vein with aseptic technique; also from any indwelling device. Consider other cultures. Consider CT, ultrasound and drainage if localised source of infection is suspected.

Antibiotics: Initially broad spectrum as per local policy. Give within 1 hour of time zero (3 hours for the emergency department); each hour of delay increases mortality by 7.6%. Consider any existing antibiotic therapy and seek microbiological advice.

Fluids: Ideally two large-bore cannulae. Hartmann's solution initially at 20 mL/kg (may require further boluses up to 60 mL/kg). If using colloids, decrease volumes to one-third. Consider a central venous catheter now.

Lactate and haemoglobin: Check quickly on arterial blood gas analysis. Transfuse if Hb < 7.0 g/dL until above this level. Check lactate within first hour and repeatedly thereafter as a guide to improving perfusion to current therapy. Lactate > 2 indicates sepsis, whereas > 4 indicates severe sepsis (and level 2 care and support should be sought). Lactate may be elevated in patients with hepatic failure due to impaired clearance. Some hospitals are using procalcitonin as an alternative.

Urinary catheter and hourly urine output measurements: (catheter not necessary if patient is fully mobile and self voiding). Insert urinary catheter and commence hourly measurements with urometer. An existing catheter does not need to be replaced. Output target is 0.5 mL/hour/kg. Monitor response to fluid challenges to see if output is improved transiently or sustained.

provide a lactate, but otherwise it is essential to send a sample promptly to the laboratory for analysis. These investigations are sensitive indicators of perfusion and oxygenation.

Intravenous antibiotics

Antibiotics should be commenced within 1 hour of recognition of severe sepsis in the hospital setting (3 hours if in emergency department).

Controlling the source of infection

Several options should be considered to control the source of the infection: drainage of abscesses, removal of invasive devices, debridement of tissue, and definitive control usually through surgical intervention.

Other therapies

Other therapies that are used within the critical care environment include steroids, recombinant human activated protein C, blood products (only transfuse if haemoglobin is less than 7 g/dL, mechanical ventilation, sedation, tight glucose control and renal replacement therapy. These are specialist interventions which are beyond the scope of this chapter. Consider consulting the critical care team about any patient who is in septic shock or does not improve following the administration of these resuscitation care bundle elements.

HOT TIPS

Report the following quickly if they are not achieved or are deteriorating:

— Mean BP > 65 mmHg
— Systolic BP > 90 mmHg
— Pulse < 100 beats per minute
— Temperature > 36°C to < 38°C
— Urine output > 0.5 mL/kg/hour

Remember that some causes of sepsis are preventable and non-essential invasive lines should be removed as soon as possible. Phlebitis scores should be recorded daily and lines removed or changed when indicated.

Conclusions

Sepsis, severe sepsis, and septic shock are still major causes of mortality in the western world. Some episodes can be prevented by simple observation and prompt action. Deterioration can be minimised by swift implementation of the sepsis regimen as outlined here, even within the ward setting.

References and further reading

Daniels, R. (2008). Personal communications.

Daniels, R., McNamara, G., Nutbeam, T. and Laver, K. (2008). *Survive Sepsis Manual*. Sutton Coldfield, Heart of England Foundation Trust.

Dellinger, R.P., Carlet, J.M., Masur, H., *et al.* (2004). Surviving Sepsis Campaign: Guidelines for the management of severe sepsis and septic shock. *Critical Care Medicine*, **32** (3), 858–73.

Dellinger, R.P., Levy, M.M., Carlet, J.M., *et al.* (2008). Surviving Sepsis Campaign: International guidelines for management of severe sepsis and septic shock. *Critical Care Medicine*, **36**, 296–327; published correction appears in *Critical Care Medicine* **36**, 1394–96.

Flynn, M.B. and McLeskey, S. (2005). Shock, systemic inflammatory response syndrome, and multiple organ dysfunction syndrome. In: P.G. Morton, D.K. Fontaine, C.M. Hudak, B.M. Gallo (eds) *Critical Care Nursing: A Holistic Approach*, 8th edn. Philadelphia, Lippincott Williams and Wilkins.

Survive Sepsis (2007). The official training programme for the surviving sepsis campaign, 1st edn. Sutton Coldfield, Heart of England Foundation Trust. Available at: www.survivesepsis.org (last accessed November 2009).

Useful websites

Surviving Sepsis
www.survivesepsis.org
www.survivingsepsis.org

Institute for Health Improvement
www.ihi.org

14 Hypovolaemic shock

Tim Collins

Clinical shock can be evident in any patient admitted to hospital. The underlying physiology, causes and treatment of this life-threatening condition are often complex and challenging for the healthcare professional. Hypovolaemic shock is a common cause of inadequate tissue perfusion, and results in widespread cellular hypoxia and altered homeostasis. Prompt assessment, recognition and management will improve outcome because hypovolaemic shock is a significant cause of death both within hospital and in the pre-hospital environment. This chapter aims to explore the underlying pathophysiology of hypovolaemia, as well as strategies that can be used to assess and manage this life-threatening condition. It will:

- explore the physiology and resultant abnormal homeostasis of hypovolaemic shock
- discuss the clinical presentation of a patient suffering from hypovolaemic shock and relate this to underlying physiology
- identify the potential causes of hypovolaemic shock
- look at the assessment and management of a critically ill patient presenting with hypovolaemia.

Pathophysiology

The circulating fluid volume of an adult is 70 mL/kg (Baskett and Wilson, 1992) hence total blood volume is in the region of 4 to 5 litres. Hypovolaemic shock results when circulating fluid volume is reduced, causing a reduction in cardiac output and a low perfusion state (Collins, 2000). This low perfusion state causes widespread cellular hypoxia and lactic acidosis, which will ultimately cause multiorgan failure and death if not promptly resolved. Hypovolaemia has many causes but is frequently associated with haemorrhage. Haemorrhage can be classified as being either internal or external. Internal haemorrhage may occur following a postoperative bleed, rupture of an abdominal aortic aneurysm, abdominal or thoracic trauma or a traumatic bone fracture. Driscoll *et al.* (1999) states that estimated blood loss of up to 800 mL has been associated with traumatic fracture of the humerus, 5000 mL with fracture of the pelvis, 2000 mL with fracture of the femur and 1000 mL with traumatic fracture of the tibia. Internal haemorrhage can often be more difficult and complex to diagnose than external haemorrhage, in which excessive blood loss is visible and often creates the 'white patient–red floor syndrome External haemorrhages are often related to traumatic injuries or gastrointestinal bleeds. Multiple trauma patients will nearly always present with hypovolaemia leading to shock that often results in death; unfortunately, trauma is the leading cause of death in young adults (Lawrence *et al.*, 2000).

Hypovolaemic shock is not solely caused by haemorrhage and can also be caused by dehydration and fluid loss from extracellular compartments. Conditions that may cause hypovolaemia following fluid loss include: severe diarrhoea and vomiting, excessive nasogastric tube loss, fever, bowel obstruction, burns, pancreatitis, diabetic ketoacidosis, third space fluid shift movements, and inappropriate diuretic therapy. Lost fluid in these situations will mainly consist of plasma rather than whole blood, as in the trauma or haemorrhaging patient (Kreimeier, 2000). See Box 14.1.

Box 14.1   Causes of hypovolaemic shock

External haemorrhage (e.g. arterial bleed)
Internal haemorrhage (e.g. ruptured spleen, ruptured internal blood vessel)
Trauma
Fractures
Severe vomiting and diarrhoea
Bowel obstruction
Pancreatitis
Peritonitis
Burns
Third space fluid shift movements
Inappropriate diuretic therapy

Consequences of hypovolaemia

The reduction in circulatory volume leads to a lower cardiac preload and venous return, which – if severe – will result in hypotension and poor systemic perfusion (Kreimeier, 2000). As part of the body's compensatory mechanisms to abnormal homeostasis, it will initially instigate compensatory strategies to counteract the fluid loss. This is known as the *compensatory* stage of hypovolaemia; if the fluid loss continues and action to resolve the condition does not occur, the compensatory mechanisms of the body will fail, resulting in severe hypotension: this is known as the *de-compensatory* or *progressive* stage of clinical shock (Collins and Plowright, 2007).

During the compensatory stage, which occurs with vascular loss of 15–30% of total blood volume, the body will firstly release catecholamines such as adrenaline (epinephrine) and noradrenaline (norepinephrine) into the systemic blood circulation (Bersten and Soni, 2003). This will bring about peripheral vasoconstriction in an attempt to promote perfusion to the vital aerobic organs like the brain, heart and lungs. Reduced peripheral circulation follows and the patient will present with cool peripheries, reduced amplitude of distal pulses, delayed capillary refill time (over 2 seconds) and reduced urine output while the body diverts perfusion away from the non-essential organs (Collins and Plowright, 2007). The increased catecholamine release and reduced cardiac output causes tachycardia, which is an attempt to counteract the effects of a reduced preload and cardiac output. If the hypovolaemia continues, then the body's compensatory mechanisms begin to fail and the patient enters the progressive or decompensated phase of shock. This is where the blood loss has exceeded 30% of body blood volume and the patient's compensatory mechanisms no longer function adequately. There is dramatic deterioration in the patient's condition and severe hypotension. If the patient does not have immediate treatment, multi-organ failure and death are imminent. The classes of hypovolaemic shock are given in Box 14.2.

Box 14.2 **Four classes of hypovolaemic shock and the observations associated with blood loss (based on Collins, 2000 and Gonce Morton *et al.*, 2003)**

CLASS 1: Up to 15% blood loss

Circulatory volume equates to 70 mL/kg in adults and 80 mL/kg in neonates

Usually few clinical signs as the body's compensatory mechanisms are activated to cope with the blood loss

Patients who are young and fit can tolerate significant blood loss before vital signs become abnormal

CLASS 2: 15–30% blood loss

Tachycardia (weak and thready pulse)

Hyperventilation

Vasoconstriction (delayed capillary refill of > 2 seconds)

Cool or diaphorectic skin

Oliguria (below 0.5 mL/kg/hour)

Concentrated urine

Confusion and agitation

Poor peripheral pulses

$SvO_2 < 60\%$

Haemodynamics: low cardiac output and high systemic vascular resistance (SVR)

Reduced central venous pressure (CVP)

Elevated lactate

N.B. Changes in all observations except for blood pressure

CLASS 3: 30–40% blood loss

Dramatic deterioration in all vital signs

Severe tachycardia and hypotension develops as above

Reduced oxygen saturations

Oliguria leading to anuria

Mental stupor

$SvO_2 < 55\%$

Metabolic acidosis

CLASS 4: Above 40% blood loss

Immediate threat to life

Cardiorespiratory arrest impending

Drastic surgery and treatment required

Assessment and management of patients in hypovolaemic shock

As with any critically ill patient, the standard **ABCDE** approach should be utilised in assessing a patient suspected of hypovolaemic shock. The patient should be attached to continuous monitoring of their heart rate, oxygen saturations, and non-invasive blood pressure. Vital signs include respiratory rate, urine output, and any other fluid losses, such as blood loss or vomit; drains should also be recorded. Fluid input must be recorded, and balance calculations made every 4 hours. The frequency of vital sign recordings must be assessed on an individual basis, but they should be at least hourly in the acute phase, and must include a 'track and trigger' score. A patient requiring aggressive fluid resuscitation must not be left until he or she is more stable.

Treatment for hypovolaemia involves optimising ventilation and oxygenation by administering oxygen therapy, and correcting the cause of hypovolaemia and fluid resuscitation. Urgent surgery in the operating theatre may be needed if bleeding is suspected. It is imperative that early referral is made to senior surgical and anaesthetic personnel, including referral to the critical care outreach team. It is essential that early aggressive treatment and assistance is obtained for patients suffering from hypovolaemic shock because cell damage and death can occur rapidly in this life-threatening condition. See Box 14.3 for the signs and symptoms of hypovolaemia.

Box 14.3   Signs and symptoms of hypovolaemia

Rapid, weak and thready pulse
Tachypnoea
Delayed capillary refill (over 2 seconds) (see Box 9.1)
Cold, pale, diaphorectic peripheral digits (vasoconstriction)
Weaker peripheral pulses
Oliguria (reduced below 0.5 mL/kg/hour and concentrated)
Confusion and agitation
Reduced Glasgow Coma Score (see Chapter 45) or AVPU (see Box 2.1)
Visual signs of blood loss
Excessive blood loss from wound drains
Hard, distended and painful abdomen
History of recent surgery or trauma (fractures)
Blood results:
    — falling haemoglobin
    — arterial blood gases show metabolic acidosis
    — elevated lactate level (normal < 1.5)
Low central venous pressure
SvO_2 of < 60%
Cardiac output measurements show:
    — low cardiac output
    — high systemic vascular resistance
Reduced oxygen saturations (poor signal may be associated with vasoconstriction)
Hypotension (late sign)
Decreased pulse blood pressure

Management plan

The management of patients with hypovolaemia focuses on restoring circulatory volume and correcting the cause of the fluid loss. All shocked patients should be given high-flow oxygen via a non-re-breathe face mask, with the aim of improving arterial oxygen-carrying capacity and oxygen delivery (DO_2) to the tissues (Bersten and Soni, 2003). If respiratory or airway compromise is present then early intubation should be considered, particularly if a patient is becoming confused and agitated due to hypoxia which is impeding fluid resuscitation and haemodynamic monitoring.

Fluid resuscitation

It is widely recognised that optimising preload and increasing circulatory fluid volume is paramount for patients and several litres of fluid may be needed to achieve this. In uncomplicated hypovolaemia, such as dehydration from extracellular fluid losses, the instigation of intravenous fluid therapy may quickly correct the hypovolaemia. However, in cases of haemorrhage, the correction of shock can be far more complex and challenging. It also needs to be remembered that an increase in blood pressure may not mean that the bleeding has stopped.

It is widely accepted that the fluid used to correct any deficit should be the same type of fluid lost (Roth *et al.*, 2005). In uncomplicated hypovolaemia, such as extracellular fluid losses including vomiting and diarrhoea, an appropriate crystalloid fluid with electrolytes (e.g. Hartmann's or 0.9% normal saline) may replace missing fluid and essential electrolytes. In the case of bleeding patients, blood transfusion will be required; this often involves the administration of packed red blood cells, which will increase the haemoglobin and subsequent oxygen-carrying capacity (Bersten and Soni, 2003). A multicentre, randomised-controlled trial conducted by Hebert *et al.* (1999) found that it appears safe for intensive care patients to have a maintenance haemoglobin of 7–9 g/dL compared to a more traditional level of 12 g/dL. However, this is contraindicated in patients with acute coronary syndromes and lactic acidosis (Hebert *et al.*, 1999). Given the fact that patients in hypovolaemic shock often present with a lactic acidosis due to anaerobic perfusion, a haemoglobin of 10 g/dL is normally aimed for.

Transfusing blood usually takes the form of packed red blood cells to provide oxygen-carrying capacity; it does not include essential clotting factors and fluid. When blood is lost and replaced with packed cells and intravenous fluids, a dilutional coagulopathy will develop as clotting factors bleed out, therefore it is essential to consider administering fresh frozen plasma (FFP) and platelets in a haemorrhaging patient, otherwise the coagulation deficiencies will prolong and worsen any haemorrhage. See Fig. 14.1 for a summary of hypovolaemic shock.

In addition to providing red blood cells and clotting factors for a bleeding patient, it is essential to use intravenous fluid to enhance the circulating fluid volume (Bersten and Soni, 2003). Over the last few decades there has been considerable debate about the type of fluid that should be used for fluid resuscitation (often referred to as the 'colloid versus crystalloid debate'). A Cochrane systematic review by Alderson *et al.* (2003) reviewed over forty randomised controlled trials in an attempt to address the debate about the superiority of colloids over crystalloids in fluid resuscitation in the critically ill. This meta-analysis found no difference in reduction in mortality when either crystalloids or colloids were used for hypovolaemia. The debate still rages on as some practitioners believe that colloids (gelatins, starches, albumin) are more effective in hypovolaemia because they have a higher molecular weight (over 30 kDa) than crystalloids (normal saline) and stay in the intravascular compartment for longer, enhancing available circulatory volume by increasing intravascular oncotic pressure (Woodrow, 2005). The alternative argument is that crystalloids are cheaper and have fewer adverse side effects than colloids and, as there is no conclusive research that colloids improve survival, crystalloids will suffice (Whinney *et al.*, 2000). Despite the ongoing debate, it cannot be stressed enough that aggressive intravenous fluid resuscitation with either a colloid or a crystalloid is essential for any patient suffering from hypovolaemia.

Initially when blood volume is lost the body compensates by moving extracellular fluid into the vascular compartment. This fluid is similar to crystalloid solutions, hence replacement of losses with crystalloids replaces vascular and extravascular fluids in a 1 to 3 ratio. Hence 1 litre of blood loss needs about 3 litres of crystalloid to replace it.

Colloids have molecules that do not diffuse through the capillary walls, which means the fluid stays in the vascular space, replacing blood loss on a 1 to 1 basis. However, over time the colloid molecules (e.g. gelatine) lose their effect and pass out of the vessels. Naturally occurring colloids, such as albumin, can pass out of blood vessels in normal conditions, and greater vessel permeability increases this considerably, as in severe shock states.

Fluid challenge

A fluid challenge is required for any patient suspected to be suffering from hypovolaemia and displaying the signs and symptoms listed previously. A fluid challenge may be with either a crystalloid or a colloid but it needs to be administered quickly and have a significant volume to help counteract the signs of volume depletion. If the signs and symptoms of hypovolaemia are seen, a fluid challenge of 500 mL (suggest 0.9% normal saline or local protocol) is given over 10 minutes (see Fig. 14.2 for when to give a fluid challenge).

If the patient has myocardial impairment as the cause for hypotension then the fluid challenge should be reduced to 250 mL (Smith, 2003; Collins and Plowright, 2007). It is important to remember that the most common cause for hypotension is hypovolaemia and a fluid challenge is vital for restoring organ perfusion (Smith, 2003). Following the fluid challenge, the patient should be re-assessed for heart rate, capillary refill, blood pressure and urinary output; if there is no or little improvement then a further fluid challenge is required (this may need to be repeated a number of times). Regular assessment of signs of fluid overload should be undertaken (for instance, auscultation of the lungs for crepitations) to limit further intravenous fluid boluses.

Ideally, fluid challenges should be aided by measuring the central venous pressure (CVP). This is performed as described above but with reference to the CVP value and observing the change in CVP after the fluid challenge. If the CVP does not rise or transiently increases to the original value after 10 minutes then the fluid challenge should be repeated. If the CVP is very high (over 15 mmHg) then expert opinion is required. When the CVP stays raised after 10 minutes, the patient can be assumed to be adequately filled. CVP value does not work like a 'fuel gauge' but measures the compliance of the vascular system, which is increased in hypovolaemic patients.

Remember if the cause of the fluid depletion is due to haemorrhage then administer blood and clotting products and ensure early referral to the surgical team (Fig. 14.2).

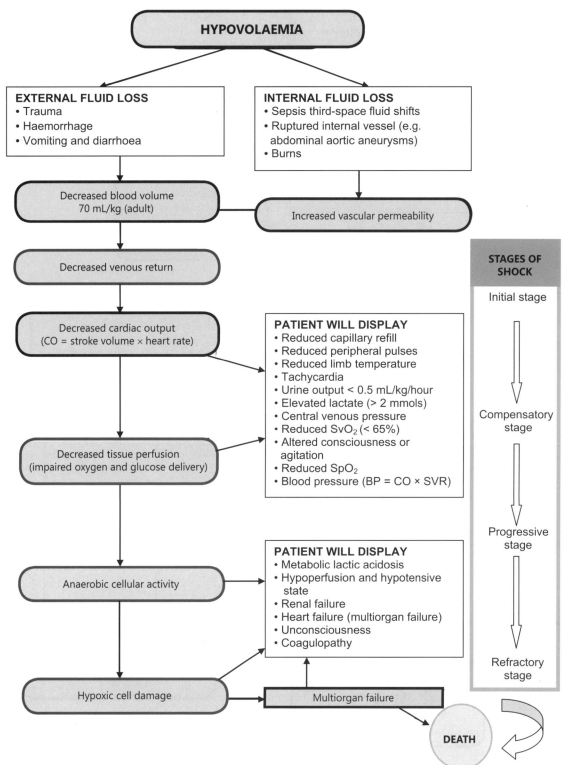

Figure 14.1 Summary of hypovolaemic shock.

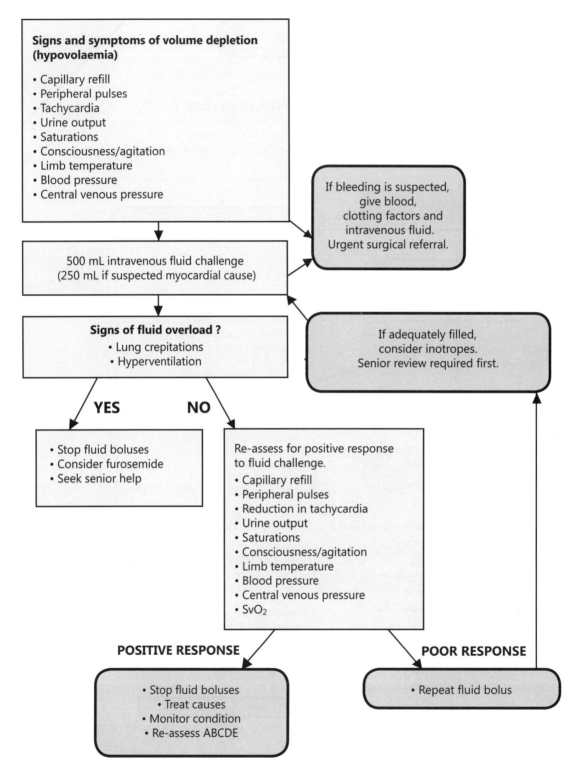

Figure14.2 When to give a fluid challenge.

Conclusions

Patients suffering from hypovolaemia should be assessed using the ABCDE approach. Early treatment is essential and involves maximising oxygen delivery, fluid resuscitation and haemostasis, and may or may not involve urgent surgery in the operating theatre. All patients with hypotension should be considered to be hypovolaemic until proven otherwise and an intravenous fluid challenge should be administered.

References and further reading

Alderson, P., Schierhout, G., Roberts, I. and Bunn, F. (2003). Colloids versus crystalloids for fluid resuscitation in critically ill patients. *The Cochrane Database of Systematic Reviews. 3.*

Baskett, P. and Wilson, I. (1992). The diagnosis of treatment of haemorrhagic shock. *World Federation of Societies of Anaesthesiologists*, **1**(4), 1–2.

Bersten, A. and Soni, N. (2003). *Oh's Intensive Care Manual*, 5th edn. London, Butterworth Heinemann.

Collins, T. (2000). Understanding shock. *Nursing Standard*, **14**(49), 35–41.

Collins, T. and Plowright, C. (2007). Identifying and managing life-threatening situation. In: F. McArthur-Rouse and S. Prosser (eds). *Assessing and Managing the Acutely Ill Adult Surgical Patient*. London, Blackwell.

Driscoll, P., Skinner, D. and Earlam, R. (1999). *ABC of Major Trauma*, 3rd edn. London, Blackwell.

Gonce Morton, P., Fontaine, D., Hudak, C. and Gallo, B. (2003). *Critical Care Nursing: A Holistic Approach*. 8th edn. Philadelphia, Lippincott.

Hebert P., Wells, G. and Blajchman, M. (1999). A multicentre, randomised-controlled trial of transfusion requirements in Critical Care., *New England Journal of Medicine*, **340**, 409–17.

Kreimeier, U. (2000). Pathophysiology of fluid imbalance. *Critical Care*, **4** (Suppl.2), s3–7.

Lawrence, P., Bell, R. and Dayton, M. (2000). *Essentials of General Surgery*, 3rd edn. Philadelphia, Williams and Wilkins.

Roth, M., Garcia, F. and Chaudhry, A. (2005). First aid: bleeding and hypovolaemic shock. *Student British Medical Journal*, **13**, 139–41.

Smeltzer, S. and Bare, B. (2000). *Brunner and Suddarth's Textbook of Medical–Surgical Nursing*, 9th edn. Philadelphia, Lippincott.

Smith, G. (2003). *ALERTTM: A Multiprofessional Course in Care of the Acutely Ill Patient*. Portsmouth, University of Portsmouth Learning Media Development.

Whinney, R., Cohn, S. and Zacur, S. (2000). Fluid resuscitation for trauma patients in the 21st century. *Current Opinion Critical Care*, **6**, 395–400.

Woodrow, P. (2005). *Intensive Care Nursing*, 2nd edn. London, Routledge.

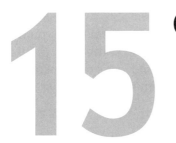

Cardiogenic shock

Russell Canavan

Cardiogenic shock has a high mortality of 40% in the first year (Cowie *et al.*, 2000) but those who survive generally have a good quality of life. Important new advances have radically improved prognosis and reinforced the need for timely intervention. Most cases of cardiogenic shock are caused by acute myocardial infarction and have a mortality of 57%, but can be reduced to 38% with early reperfusion (Hochman *et al.*, 1999) such as thrombolysis or coronary angioplasty. The majority of survivors have, according to New York Heart Association (2002; see Table 15.1), grade 1 heart failure (minimal) and are therefore able to enjoy a good quality of life.

By the end of this chapter you should be able to:

- understand the pathophysiology and causes of cardiogenic shock
- know how to assess a patient with cardiogenic shock
- understand and explain the management in the ward.

Definition and causes

Cardiogenic shock is defined as a low cardiac output state leading to inadequate tissue perfusion in the presence of adequate left ventricular filling. The most common cause is acute myocardial infarction. Other causes include pericardial, myocardial, and endocardial (valvular) disease, pericardial tamponade, or dissecting aneurysm.

Although it does not fulfil the above definition for cardiogenic shock, pulmonary embolism is often considered in the same category. This is also true for right ventricular infarction, in which the problem is primarily poor left ventricular filling, but clinically appears as the pattern of cardiogenic shock.

Pathophysiology

In all cases of cardiogenic shock there is a failure to eject blood from the heart, leading to hypotension and, therefore, inadequate cardiac output (Porth, 2002). The preload of the heart increases as blood accumulates that has returned to the heart but is not able to be pumped forward. This is due to impaired ejection of blood from the heart during systole. This pump failure means there is impaired perfusion of peripheral tissues and major organs. The sympathetic nervous system is activated because of the reduction in blood pressure and leads to an increase in heart rate and vasoconstriction (cool peripheries) in an effort to improve stroke volume (Murray and White, 1999).

Table 15.1 New York Heart Association Classification (from the Committee of the New York Heart Association, 1994, with permission)

Class	Patient symptoms
Class I (mild)	No limitation of physical activity Ordinary physical activity does not cause undue fatigue, palpitation, or dyspnoea (shortness of breath)
Class II (mild)	Slight limitation of physical activity Comfortable at rest, but ordinary physical activity results in fatigue, palpitation, or dyspnoea
Class III (moderate)	Marked limitation of physical activity Comfortable at rest, but less than ordinary activity causes fatigue, palpitation or dyspnoea
Class intravenous (severe)	Unable to carry out any physical activity without discomfort Symptoms of cardiac insufficiency at rest If any physical activity is undertaken, discomfort is increased

Assessment

This clinical pattern is common to a number of other disorders, and must be differentiated from other forms of shocks, such as hypovolaemic, anaphylactic and septic (see Chapters 13 and 14). Initial assessment is best carried out using the **ABCDE** approach. A patient with cardiac problems is likely to require supplementary oxygen. They may have a degree of pulmonary oedema (see Chapter 6). Assess the patient's oxygen saturations and respiratory function and attach them to a monitor that records oxygen saturations and heart rhythm. Vital signs should be recorded according to how unwell the patient is and how abnormal the vital signs are. Acutely unwell patients may require hourly observations, some more frequently. Once the patient's airway and breathing have been assessed and managed, their circulation needs to be assessed and any difficulties treated.

Patients in cardiogenic shock are cold peripherally and they are sweaty. They have a low blood pressure, often a tachycardia, dyspnoea (secondary to pulmonary oedema), and may have chest pain or dysrhythmias or be anxious and fatigued (Murray and White, 1999). Of particular note is the raised jugular venous pressure (JVP) which differentiates cardiogenic shock from other forms of shock. If a central venous catheter (CVC) line is in situ then a high central venous pressure value such as 15 mmHg or more is another characteristic feature.

Clinical assessment may miss the features of pulmonary embolus and right heart failure (see Chapter 9). This is important because in these conditions the left ventricle is not adequately filled.

A chest x-ray is useful for detecting pulmonary oedema and an enlarged heart; arterial blood gases will assess acid–base balance and hypoxia; a 12-lead ECG helps to identify abnormalities (Murray and White, 1999). The echocardiogram is key to assessing the patient although it may not be available at the onset. However, echocardiograms can identify treatable conditions such as mitral regurgitation (secondary to chordal rupture) or a ventricular septal defect (VSD).

In the ward setting, it is imperative that the patient is placed on a cardiac monitor. The patient's heart rate, blood pressure, respiratory rate and oxygenation need to be recorded at regular intervals. It may be difficult to obtain an accurate oxygen saturation trace, due to peripheral shut down; but an ear probe may help. High-flow oxygen should also be administered using a non-rebreathe mask.

Case Scenario

A 50-year-old man with type 2 diabetes mellitus is admitted with chest pain. He is sweaty and unwell.

A—Airway
He is maintaining his airway.

B—Breathing
His respiratory rate was raised at 28 breaths per minute and oxygen saturation was 85% FiO_2 0.21 increasing to 96% FiO_2 0.85 (where FiO_2 is the fraction of inspired oxygen). Auscultation revealed bi-basal crepitations to mid-zones.

C—Circulation
Pulses were barely palpable peripherally and his blood pressure was 85/40 mmHg. Capillary refill time was 5 seconds.

D—Disability
He is alert and orientated.

E—Exposure and Environment
He is overweight and sweaty but there are no specific findings. He has a high 'track and trigger' score requiring referral to the medical team and intervention.

Treatment

Treatment involves administering high-flow oxygen via a non-rebreathe mask to improve hypoxia and breathlessness; reducing preload and JVP through use of diuretics or nitrates; treating hypotension with inotropes (see Box 15.1); and giving analgesia to reduce pain and anxiety. Diuretics need to be used with caution as they can drop blood pressure further and, if the underlying cause is not addressed, can lead to dehydration. Once the immediate concerns (airway, breathing and circulation management) have been addressed and the patient has been stabilised, then early assessment by a cardiologist with early reperfusion has been shown to significantly improve survival (Hochman *et al.*, 1999). Also, early correction of surgical lesions (VSD or chordal rupture) will give a favourable outcome.

As a temporary measure inotropes can help to improve cardiac output, but they do not improve the long-term outcome if the underlying condition is not treated (see Box 15.1). There is little evidence to differentiate between inotropes, but dobutamine causes a less chronotropic response (increase in heart rate) and is often favoured. Milrinone has the added advantage of being a vasodilator and can reduce preload and afterload. Nitrates can improve coronary perfusion but they need to be used with caution because they can drop the blood pressure further.

Box 15.1   Terms and definitions (based on McKinley and Robinson, 2001)

Inotropes
  Affect heart contractility.
  Positive inotropes increase contractility (e.g. dobutamine, epinephrine).
  Negative inotropes decrease contractility (e.g. lidocaine).

Chronotropes
  Affect heart rate.
  Positive chronotropes increase heart rate (e.g. atropine, isoprenaline).
  Negative chronotropes decrease heart rate (e.g. verapamil, digoxin, adenosine, beta-blockers).

Preload
  The amount of fluid returning to the ventricle.
  Drugs that reduce preload include diuretics, nitrates and morphine.
  Fluids increase preload.

Afterload
  The amount of resistance that the ventricle is pumping against.
  Drugs to *decrease* afterload (vasodilation) include amrinone and hydralazine.
  Drugs to *increase* afterload (vasoconstriction) include norepinephrine.

In diffuse coronary artery disease, the intra-aortic balloon pump (IABP) can improve peripheral perfusion and also improve diastolic filling of the coronary arteries. It is an invasive device that acts in a similar way to inotopic support, but also increases coronary artery perfusion. The IABP is a specialised treatment that often needs referral and transfer to a cardiac centre; therefore its usefulness in the acute situation is limited.

Left-ventricular assist devices are surgically implanted devices used in specialist centres. They increase the left ventricular output mechanically and are often used as a bridge to transplant. They buy the patient time when they are on a waiting list for heart transplant. Again, early referral to assess for suitability is needed and they are not always useful in the acute situation.

References and further reading

Committee of the New York Heart Association (1994). *Nomenclature and Criteria for Diseases of the Heart and Great Vessels*, 9th edn. Boston: Little Brown and Co.

Cowie, M.R., Wood, D.A., Coats, A.J.S., *et al.* (2000). Survival of patients with a new diagnosis of heart failure: A population based study. *Heart*, **83**, 505–10.

Heart Failure Society of America and New York Heart Association (2002). *The Stages of Heart Failure Classification*. Available at: www.abouthf.org.questions_stages.htm (last accessed November 2009).

Hochman, J.S., Sleeper, L.A., Webb, J.G., *et al.* (1999). Early revascularization in acute myocardial infarction complicated by cardiogenic shock. Shock investigators: Should we emergently revascularize occluded coronaries for cardiogenic shock. *New England Journal of Medicine*, **341** (9), 625–34.

McKinley, M.G. and Robinson, C.F. (2001). Shock. In: M.L. Sole, M.L. Lamborn and J.C. Hartshorn (2001). *Introduction to Critical Care Nursing*, 3rd edn. Philadelphia, WB Saunders.

Murray, S.E. and White, B.S. (1999). *Critical Care Assessment Handbook*. Philadelphia, WB Saunders.

Porth, C.M. (2003). *Essentials of Pathophysiology: Concepts of Altered Health States*. Philadelphia, Lippincott, Williams and Wilkins.

Useful websites

Heart Failure Society of America
www.abouthf.org

British Heart Foundation
www.bhf.org.uk

16 Management of critically ill patients with malignancy

Angus Turner

Patients with malignancy who become critically ill require special consideration if they are to be managed correctly. That said, the principles of assessment, resuscitation and referral are the same as when dealing with other groups of patients and are described in full elsewhere. The aim of this chapter is not to be an exhaustive text on all critical illnesses related to malignancy. Instead, it will try to cover the common scenarios and highlight the areas that often cause anxiety and confusion.

Critically ill patients with malignancy cover a vast range of issues – from specialist oncological, through to general medical, surgical and ethical. It is not unusual to become involved on the ward with these patients when emotions are running high, when adequate information is not available, when key senior personnel are not contactable, and when proper communication has not occurred and decisions need to be made.

To make matters more challenging, treatment and prognosis are continuously changing and improving for many malignancies. Specialists in treating malignancy are at risk of becoming frustrated when communicating with other disciplines that are, understandably, not up to date. In the worst case scenario, this lack of knowledge can be perceived as prejudice.

Assessing and understanding the situation

Malignancy

The term *malignancy* includes all malignant solid tumours (cancers and sarcomas) and haematological malignancies (leukaemias and lymphomas). You cannot manage a critically ill patient with malignancy, or communicate properly, unless you understand the language that will be used to describe them.

Palliative

Palliative means different things to different people. The term needs special attention because it is commonly used in two very different contexts: palliative *care* and palliative *therapy*.

Palliative care

This refers to an approach in which the primary aim is to relieve symptoms and improve quality of life. This might include some palliative 'therapy' (see below). When the palliative care team becomes involved, there has been an acceptance that the patient is not going to survive his or her illness. This is invariably in the context of a limited life expectancy, which may be as short as a few hours or as long as a few months. It is generally accepted that a critical illness in these patients should be treated as a terminal event and should be managed with symptom control rather than resuscitation.

Palliative therapy

This means that a patient is receiving active 'anti-cancer' treatment (e.g. chemotherapy, radiotherapy, surgery) with the aim of improving their quality of life by the relief of symptoms. It has been accepted that the treatment will not be curative. The life expectancy, in this instance, varies tremendously from a few weeks to many years. A good example is the palliative treatment of bone metastasis from breast cancer – a situation that may be stable for many months. The prognosis for patients receiving palliative therapy can be the same as patients without a malignancy. In other words, the presence of an 'incurable cancer' should not necessarily be a bar to full active treatment, including organ support on the intensive care unit.

Know the patient, know the disease

Patients with malignancy who become critically ill are more difficult to manage. In addition to the usual problems of their critical illness and comorbidities, their malignancy adds a number of very important variables that impact significantly on management. As well as the usual thorough history and examination, it is vital to seek out as much information as possible from all sources.

Diagnosis and stage

Different malignancies behave in different ways. Although this seems obvious, it is important to get it right. The difference between squamous cell and small cell cancer of the lung has important implications for its assessment, treatment and prognosis. Similarly stage IA Hodgkin's disease is a very different beast from stage IVB.

Treatment received and response

The amount of treatment received by a patient can be an important indicator to prognosis. A patient with acute myeloid leukaemia with neutropenic sepsis after the first cycle of chemotherapy, prior to a bone marrow transplant, has a good prognosis. The prognosis is grave with the same critical illness following rescue chemotherapy, after the transplant has failed.

Prognosis and level of communication

A knowledge of the expected prognosis is an essential tool to help tailor appropriate therapy (e.g. admission to the intensive care unit). Although the prognosis might be known to the specialists treating the patient's malignancy, this information must be readily available to all professionals managing the critical illness. It is surprising how often the prognosis is not appreciated by the patient or their friends and family. Insight into this is important to avoid awkwardness during discussions.

Functional status and general health and comorbidities

It is important not to lose sight of a 'holistic' approach to treating critically ill patients with malignancy. A patient with congestive cardiac failure and a poor exercise capacity presenting with tumour lysis syndrome and renal failure after chemotherapy for lymphoma is a good example. This patient probably has a worse prognosis from the concomitant illnesses than from the malignancy and its complications. A proper history, including a full systems review and exercise tolerance and functional capacity, must not be overlooked.

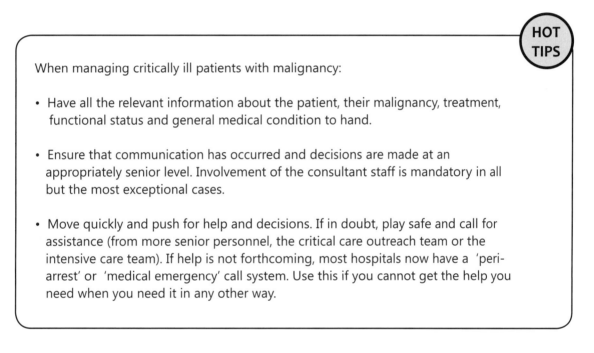

HOT TIPS

When managing critically ill patients with malignancy:

- Have all the relevant information about the patient, their malignancy, treatment, functional status and general medical condition to hand.

- Ensure that communication has occurred and decisions are made at an appropriately senior level. Involvement of the consultant staff is mandatory in all but the most exceptional cases.

- Move quickly and push for help and decisions. If in doubt, play safe and call for assistance (from more senior personnel, the critical care outreach team or the intensive care team). If help is not forthcoming, most hospitals now have a 'peri-arrest' or 'medical emergency' call system. Use this if you cannot get the help you need when you need it in any other way.

Common critical illnesses in patients with malignant disease

Specific critical illness scenarios affecting patients with malignant disease need specialist knowledge to diagnose and treat. Most oncology and haematology units will have protocols in place to deal with these situations. However, the initial assessment and resuscitation needs to be performed using the same principles that apply to other patient groups.

Neutropenic sepsis

This is a medical emergency, usually seen in patients being treated for haematological malignancies. It is defined as an absolute neutrophil count of less than 1×10^9/L with a pyrexia of over 38°C, or clinical signs of septicaemia or site of infection. Specialist advice must be sought immediately, along with ongoing management of the septicaemia. Neutropenic sepsis is the commonest problem resulting in critical illness in patients with malignancy.

Cardiovascular failure

Sepsis is the most important cause of cardiovascular collapse in this context and should always be considered, if not treated speculatively. However, there are other specific causes of cardiovascular collapse that should be considered:

- dehydration, especially in the presence of diarrhoea, which can occur with some chemotherapy regimens (e.g. 5-fluocytosine)
- pericardial tamponade
- myocardial failure, which can be a result of disease infiltration or chemotherapy (e.g. anthrocyclines).

Respiratory failure

There are many routes by which a patient with malignancy can develop respiratory failure. These include:

- pulmonary infection
- pulmonary oedema
- pleural effusions and/or massive ascites
- airway obstruction
- neurological causes such as:
  — malignancies of the brain leading to compromise of the respiratory centre or post-ictal respiratory depression
  — cervical cord compression
  — secondary to opioid analgesia.

Patients with malignant disease have a worse prognosis than other groups if they are treated with invasive artificial ventilation. Therefore, it is very important to ensure that all potentially reversible factors have been dealt with. Examples include draining pleural effusions, treating infection, using steroids or epinephrine nebulisers to ease airway obstruction, and targeted fluid balance. Non-invasive positive pressure ventilation (NIV) is becoming more sophisticated and more widely available and confers a better prognosis. In many situations NIV should be the first-line therapy if respiratory support is needed (for more about this, see Chapter 8) (Larché et al., 2003).

Renal failure

Tumour lysis syndrome

This syndrome occurs due to massive tumour breakdown following chemotherapy, or even steroid therapy for bulky sensitive malignancies, especially leukaemias and lymphomas;

occasionally it can occur prior to therapy. The cell breakdown causes the patient to become acidotic, hyperkalaemic, hyperuricaemic, hyperphosphataemic and hypocalcaemic, and renal failure frequently occurs. Prompt resuscitation and specialist treatment, coupled with appropriate referral for renal dialysis, means that the prognosis is often good (Davidson *et al.*, 2004).

Of course patients with malignant disease will also present with unrelated medical and surgical problems (e.g. patients with cancer will still suffer myocardial infarctions or appendicitis) and their malignancy will need consideration, either to limit therapy appropriately in advanced, incurable disease, or to be excluded as an insignificant consideration because their disease has a potentially good prognosis.

The role of the intensive care unit in treating critically ill patients with malignant disease

The decision whether or not to refer a patient with malignant disease to the intensive care unit (ICU) can be easy or can be fraught with dilemmas. In cases where the patient is so unwell that any delay might compromise his or her chances of survival, assessment and referral should be able to be made by any member of the team. Examples are critical airway obstruction or severe neutropenic sepsis. When the situation allows, it is important that a proper full history is taken, information gathered and senior input obtained prior to referral to the intensive care unit. Although this is occasionally regarded as unnecessary, such an approach avoids exposing the patient to inappropriate, dangerous or invasive interventions.

A trial of ward-based therapy is also possible after a proper assessment, again avoiding unnecessary intervention; this could be with the support of the intensive care unit and/or outreach teams. Fig. 16.1 shows an algorithm of referral guidelines that could be considered when caring for critically ill patients with malignancy who may need referral to the intensive care unit.

While every case must be judged on its own merits, some guidelines are useful. The ones illustrated here are used at our own hospital and been found to have performed well when audited. They are based on the following:

- Mortality from multiorgan failure is as high as 90%, even in patients without malignant disease (Knaus *et al.*, 1985).

- Multi-organ failure results in a prolonged stay on intensive care unit of several weeks, and a period of recuperation that lasts several months.

- One- or two-organ failure confers a good prognosis, even in patients with advanced malignant disease, and may be appropriate in the setting of good palliative therapy.

It is not always possible to reliably assess acutely critically ill patients. If there is difficulty in making a confident assessment, then admitting the patient for a trial of support in the intensive care unit is reasonable. A regular review should be made every 48 hours. This is an opportunity to withdraw or continue organ support in the face of objective clinical deterioration or improvement (Thiéry *et al.*, 2005). See Box 16.1 for sample guidelines relating to the intensive care unit.

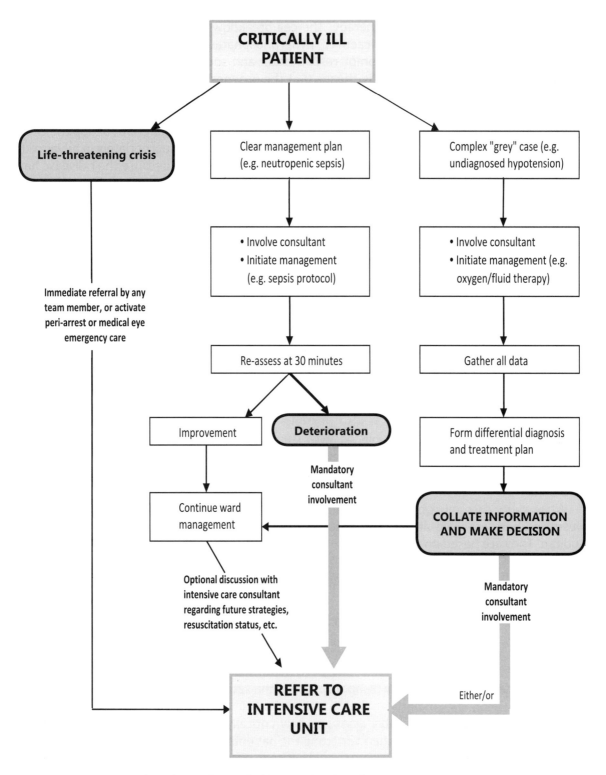

Figure 16.1 Algorithm for referral of critically ill patients with malignancy to the intensive care unit.

> **Box 16.1** **Sample guidelines for considering admission to intensive care**
>
> Consider ward management if the patient is clearly too well or too sick.
> 1–2 established organ failure.
> Should admit *unless* underlying prognosis is < 3 months.
> 3+ established organ failure.
> Should *not* admit unless realistic cure or prolonged survival (over 6 months) from underlying malignancy.
> If in doubt, admit for trial of intensive care therapy.
> Regular review of progress or deterioration.
> Clear plan with regard to limitation of therapy in the face of increasing organ failures.
>
> *N.B. Bone marrow failure, as manifest by low white cell count, anaemia and low platelet count, is usually due to the effect of chemotherapy. In this context, it should not be counted as 'organ failure' as it is predictably reversible without specific therapy (although granulocyte colony-stimulating factor can be used to enhance recovery)*

Consider the following scenarios 1 and 2 (overpage).

> **Case Scenario 1**
>
> You are attending a 65-year-old man with a diagnosis of advanced squamous cell carcinoma of the tongue, with local spread to cervical lymph nodes. He had radical surgery 18 months ago but the tumour has recurred and he has been treated with a full dose of radiotherapy to the affected lymph nodes. His last dose of radiotherapy was 1 week ago.
>
> Over the past 24 hours he has developed stridor. The peripheral oxygen saturations are 65% on high-flow oxygen. His blood pressure is 130/80 mmHg, his heart rate is 110 beats per minute and respiratory rate is 40 breaths per minute.
>
> He has a good urine output and normal renal function. There is no other significant past medical history and he played 18 holes of golf twice a week prior to his diagnosis.

Discussion of scenario 1

This man has respiratory failure secondary to airway obstruction by recurrent cancer. Despite the fact that treatment of single organ failure has a good prognosis on intensive care, it will not be possible to treat this cancer because a full dose of palliative radiotherapy has already been given and there is no further surgical option. The prognosis, even in the absence of airway obstruction, is certainly less than 3 months; therefore the current situation should be treated as a terminal event.

Management plan

If not already aware, the consultant oncologist must be informed of the patient's deteriorating condition. Admission to intensive care is inappropriate and the onus must be on palliative care, symptom control, and achieving as comfortable and dignified a death as possible. An urgent referral to the palliative care team should be made. Initial symptom control can be started with titrated doses of intravenous diamorphine, at 1 mg increments every 5 to 10 minutes to relieve distress. Intravenous steroids (dexamethasone 8 mg) and nebulised epinephrine (0.5 mg) will temporarily reduce the element of airway obstruction caused by oedema, and help to gain control of the situation. Appropriate discussions with the patient and family need to take place. Consider a 'do not resuscitate' order.

Case Scenario 2

A 35-year-old woman is on the haematology ward with neutropenia following the first dose of chemotherapy for acute myeloblastic leukaemia. She is pyrexial at 38.5°C and has had 24 hours of broad-spectrum antibiotics for a chest infection, confirmed clinically and on x-ray. She now has a blood pressure of 75/30 mmHg, a heart rate of 120 beats per minute, a respiratory rate of 35 breaths per minute and a poor urine output.

Arterial blood gases show a PaO_2 of 10 kPa on FiO_2 0.6 and a $PaCO_2$ of 4.0 kPa. The base excess is −8.2, with a serum lactate of 6.0 mmol/L. Her platelet count is 20×10^9/L and her haemoglobin concentration 8.5 g/dL.

Discussion of scenario 2

The prognosis for acute myeloblastic leukaemia is potentially very good, however this woman is at very high risk of progressing rapidly into established multiple organ failure due to septic shock. There is a window of opportunity to reverse the process with prompt, targeted treatment on the intensive care unit. Ideally this should involve the consultant haematologist, but referral to intensive care must not be delayed by this – minutes count. On the other hand, failure to escalate her treatment in a timely manner will probably result in deterioration to multiple organ failure, which would result in her requiring invasive positive pressure ventilation and other organ support measures, such as haemofiltration/dialysis. The prognosis, should this situation occur, is extremely poor and such measures should only be undertaken after significant discussion between senior medical and nursing staff, relatives, and (if possible) the patient.

Management plan

This patient should be urgently reviewed and initial treatment with high-flow oxygen, fluid resuscitation through a large-bore cannula and an urgent antibiotic review should be immediately commenced. Simultaneously, an urgent referral to intensive care must occur and senior haematology assistance requested. Admission to intensive care or high dependency unit is mandatory. Fluid resuscitation (guided by invasive haemodynamic monitoring e.g. arterial line, central venous line ± cardiac output monitor), cardiovascular support with inotropes and vasopressors, non-invasive ventilatory support with non-invasive ventilation (NIV) and urgent review of her antibiotic regimen by a consultant microbiologist should take place. With these measures, a rapid improvement in her septic shock can be achieved. Haematology input will be required with regards to supporting the low platelet count, anaemia and optimising bone marrow recovery (e.g. with granulocyte colony stimulating factor).

Conclusions

Patients suffering from malignant disease and presenting with acute critical illnesses create a unique set of challenges that require knowledge, insight and experience. It is not possible for any one discipline to possess all the skills needed to provide the highest quality of care; therefore, a multidisciplinary team approach is central to a successful outcome. Inherent in this process is the application of thorough basic clinical skills, good communication between specialties, and the prompt involvement of senior medical personnel. Novel therapies have resulted in an improved outlook for many malignancies. With objective and prompt intensive care input, highly satisfactory outcomes can be achieved in a variety of difficult clinical scenarios.

References and further reading

Davidson, M.B., Thakkar, S., Hix, J.K., Bhandarkar, N.D., Wong, A. and Schreiber, M.J. (2004). Pathophysiology, clinical consequences and treatment of tumor lysis syndrome. *American Journal of Medicine*, **116**, 546–54.

Knaus, W.A., Draper, E.A., Wagner, D.P. and Zimmerman, J.E. (1985). Prognosis in acute organ-system failure. *Annals of Surgery*, 202 (6), 685–93.

Larché, J., Azoulay, E., Fieux, F., *et al.* (2003). Improved survival of critically ill cancer patients with septic shock. *Intensive Care Medicine*, 29 (10), 1688–95.

Thiéry, G., Azoulay, E., Darmon, M., *et al.* (2005). Outcome of cancer patients considered for intensive care unit admission: a hospital-wide prospective study. *Journal of Clinical Oncology*, 23 (19), 4406–13.

Useful websites

National Cancer Research Institute
www.ncri.org.uk

Cancer Research, UK
www.cancerresearch.org

British Association of Surgical Oncology
www.baso.org

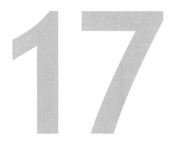

Tachyarrhythmias in the acutely ill

Kuno Budack

Arrhythmias are very common in the acute setting. They can be the cause or a symptom of a disease. Tachyarrhythmias in the acutely ill are a common problem.

By the end of this chapter you should be able to:

- recognise an arrhythmia
- be aware of the appropriate treatment and investigations necessary to give your patient the best chance.

Cardiac output

Cardiac output is the sum of stroke volume (volume ejected with each heart beat) multiplied by heart rate in one minute and is measured in litres per minute (Box 17.1).

Box 17.1 Cardiac output

Cardiac output (CO) is calculated by:

Stroke volume × Heart rate
or
CO = SV × HR

A patient will try to maintain an adequate cardiac output through several responses; one of them is to increase heart rate (see Fig. 17.1). The heart is sensitive to adrenergic influences making arrhythmias familiar sequelae in the unwell patient. Tachyarrhythmias are divided into *narrow* complex (supraventricular) and *broad* complex (ventricular or supraventricular with aberrant conduction). On identification of an abnormal heart rate or rhythm, urgent help is needed. It may be safer to put out an emergency call, as per your Trust's policy, but ideally the responder needs to be someone with advanced life support (ASL) training. The initial management should follow the latest Resuscitation Council UK (2006) guidelines.

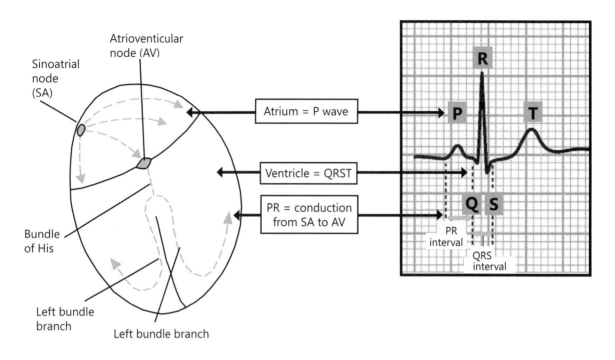

Figure 17.1 Normal conduction of the heart.

Narrow-complex tachycardia

Narrow-complex refers to the width of a QRS complex on a standard 12-lead ECG at 25 mm per second. Anything less than 0.12 seconds (three little squares) is deemed to be *narrow* (Resuscitation Council, 2005). By far the commonest tachyarrhythmia in the unwell patient is a sinus tachycardia (Fig. 17.2).

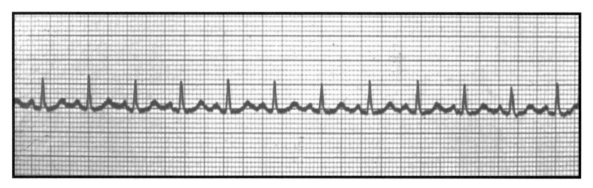

Figure 17.2 ECG of sinus tachycardia.

Abnormal tachycardias include:

- atrial fibrillation/flutter (AF)
- superventricular tachycardia (SVT)
- Wolfe–Parkinson–White (WPW) syndrome.

Possible causes of tachycardia in the acutely ill patient are listed in Box 17.1.

Box 17.2 Possible causes of tachycardia

1. Anything that makes you unwell such as:

    Surgery
    Infection
    Poorly controlled pain
    Trauma
2. Hyperthyroidism

    Always check thyroid stimulating hormone
    If suspected treatment maybe different

3. Electrolyte imbalances

    Always check electrolytes, particularly potassium
    Magnesium is less important but consider replacement when indicated

4. Structurally abnormal heart

    Previous myocardial infarction
    Heart failure
    Valvular heart disease

5. Drugs

Atrial fibrillation

Atrial fibrillation is the most common narrow-complex tachycardia and is irregularly irregular in nature. An irregular, narrow-complex tachycardia is atrial fibrillation until proven otherwise. Predisposing factors are shown in Box 17.2.

Atrial *fibrillation* is an irregular narrow-complex tachycardia (Fig. 17.3). In atrial fibrillation, no P-waves are visible.

Atrial *flutter* is often irregular, but can have a block to conduction that makes it look like a regular narrow-complex tachycardia. Atrial flutter shows a typical *saw-tooth* pattern. See Fig. 17.4.

Box 17.3 Predisposing factors for atrial fibrillation

Age—prevalence increases with age
Gender—men have a higher prevalence than women
Abnormal heart structure
Medical conditions—hypertension, hyperthyroidism, acute illness, drugs
Lifestyle—intake of alcohol, coffee, drugs

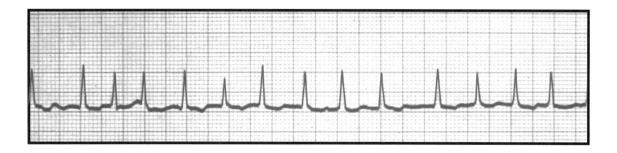

Figure 17.3 ECG of atrial fibrillation.

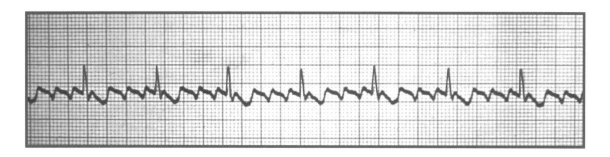

Figure 17.4 ECG of atrial flutter.

The annual risk of stroke attributable to atrial fibrillation increased from 1.5% in Framingham Study participants aged 50 to 59 years to 23.5% for those aged 80 to 89 years (Wang *et al.*, 2003; see Table 17.1). The total mortality rate is approximately doubled in patients with atrial fibrillation compared with those in normal sinus rhythm, and is linked with the severity of underlying heart disease. The major issues in management of unwell patients with atrial fibrillation are to treat the cause. The others are related to the arrhythmia itself and the prevention of thromboembolism.

Table 17.1	Annual stroke risk according to CHADS-2 score			
C—Congestive cardiac failure	1 point	0 points	1.9%
H—Hypertension	1 point	1 point	2.8%
A—Age (> 75)	1 point	2 points	4.0%
D—Diabetes	1 point	3 points	5.9%
S—Stroke (previous)	2 points	4 points	8.5%
	—	5 points	12.5%
	—	6 points	18.2%

Supraventricular tachycardia

Supraventricular tachycardia is a regular narrow-complex tachycardia (Fig. 17.5).

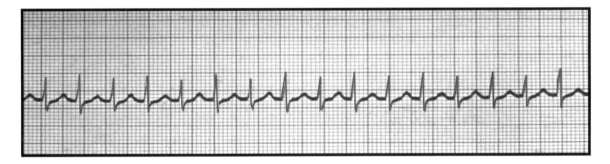

Figure 17.5   ECG of supraventricular tachycardia.

Wolfe-Parkinson-White syndrome (accessory pathway)

Accessory pathways can, in theory, cause any arrhythmia. However, the WPW syndrome is easily recognisable on a resting ECG with controlled rate by a short PQ interval with the typical delta wave (Fig. 17.6).

Diagnosis

The diagnosis of a narrow-complex tachycardia is based solely on the ECG. This can sometimes be difficult, so call someone with experience early on. An easy guide is that every irregular narrow-complex tachycardia is atrial fibrillation, and every regular narrow-complex tachycardia is supraventricular tachycardia (SVT) until proven otherwise.

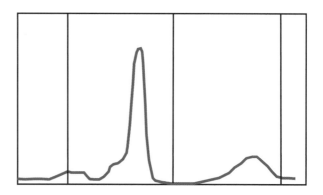

Figure 17.6   ECG of Wolfe–Parkinson–White
syndrome.

Assessment

The ABCDE approach should be used: give oxygen, insert a cannula, monitor the ECG, blood pressure and SPaO$_2$ and record a 12-lead ECG.

Treatment

Always treat the cause. For example, good analgesia reduces the sympathetic overdrive and can already terminate a tachycardia. With severe sepsis it is virtually impossible to terminate a tachyarrhythmia until the underlying sepsis is improving.

- If the patient is haemodynamically *unstable,* consider synchronised cardioversion; sedation may be indicated and specialist help should be sought (e.g. from an anaesthetist).
- If the patient is haemodynamically *stable* (with blood pressure > 90 mmHg, conscious, no chest pain or heart failure) try vagal manoeuvres.

If the patient is haemodynamically stable and does *not* have asthma, then give adenosine. This results in cardioversion of 90% of regular narrow-complex tachycardias (SVTs). If given in atrial fibrillation it will only transiently slow down the rate, which will enable you to make an accurate diagnosis.

- If the tachycardia is still not controlled, consider either atenolol or amiodorone treatment (amiodorone infusion needs central venous access).
- If tachycardia is still not controlled, then consider elective DC cardioversion (synchronised).

The Resuscitation Council (2005) have an adult tachycardia algorithm with pulse, which should be used to guide management.

Broad complex tachycardia

Broad complex refers to the width of a QRST complex on a standard 12-lead ECG at 25 mm per second. Anything more than 0.12 seconds (three little squares) is deemed *broad.* A heart rate of more than 100 beats per minute is considered tachycardic. This includes ventricular tachycardia (VT) and supraventricular with aberrant conduction. Fortunately these are much rarer than narrowomplex tachycardia. A true VT is a peri-arrest arrhythmia with a high morbidity and

Box 17.4	**Possible causes of broad complex tachycardia**

Ischaemic heart disease

Electrolyte disturbances

Structurally abnormal heart (heart failure, valvular disease, other cardiomyopathies, cardiac surgery)

Drugs

Bradyarrhythmias (a complete heart block can trigger VT as an escape rhythm)

mortality. You should treat every broad-complex tachycardia as VT in the acute onset situation until proven otherwise. See Box 17.4 for possible causes of broad-complex tachycardia. The incidence of VT is not well quantified because of the clinical overlap of VT with ventricular fibrillation (VF). Examination of sudden death data provides a rough estimate of VT incidence. Most sudden cardiac deaths are caused by VT or VF, at an estimated rate of approximately 300,000 deaths per year in the United States (American Heart Association, 2007). This translates to an incidence of 0.1–0.2% per year. This is only a rough estimate of VT incidence because many patients have non-fatal VT and because some sudden deaths are associated with VF or bradycardia, rather than VT. Incidence of VT correlates with the prevalence of coronary artery disease.

Diagnosis

Again the diagnosis of a broad-complex tachycardia is based solely on the ECG. It can sometimes be difficult, so call someone with experience early on. As a guide, regular broad-complex tachycardias are usually VT, whereas irregular broad complex tachycardias could be atrial fibrillation with bundle branch block (BBB) or a polymorphic VT (such as torsades de pointes) (Resuscitation Council, 2005).

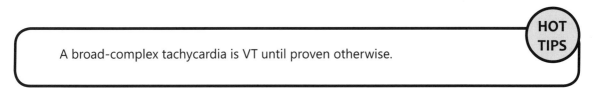

A broad-complex tachycardia is VT until proven otherwise.

HOT TIPS

The likelihood of a broad-complex tachycardia being VT (Fig. 17.6) and not atrial fibrillation with bundle branch block (Fig. 17.7) is increased when:

- the QRS complexes are very broad
- there is a gross cardiac axis shift
- there is concordance in the chest leads (the R waves are all upwards)
- there are capture beats (an 'own' complex captured amongst the VT beats)
- there is a fusion beat (a bizarre QRS complex made up of an 'own' and a VT beat).

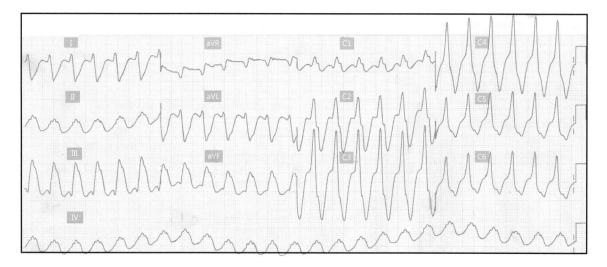

Figure 17.7 ECG of ventricular tachycardia.

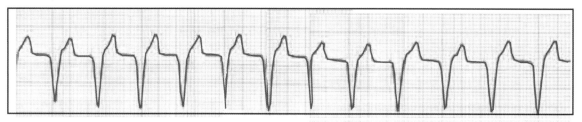

Figure 17.8 Atrial fibrillation with bundle branch block.

Assessment

The ABCDE approach should be used: give oxygen, insert a cannula, monitor the ECG, blood pressure and SPaO$_2$ and record a 12-lead ECG.

Treatment

- If the patient is haemodynamically *unstable,* consider urgent synchronised cardioversion; sedation may be indicated and specialist help should be sought (e.g. anaesthetist).
- If the patient is haemodynamically *stable,* give amiodarone (note: intravenous amiodarone should be given into a central, large vein) and call for expert help.
- If tachycardia is still not controlled, consider elective DC cardioversion (synchronised).

The Resuscitation Council have an adult tachycardia algorithm with pulse (Resuscitation Council, 2005) which should be used to guide management.

> **HOT TIPS**
>
> Every patient with a tachycardia should have:
>
> • it documented on an ECG
> • their electrolytes checked
> • their condition treated primarily.

Every patient with a tachycardia who is haemodynamically unstable (hypotension, heart failure, chest pain, reduced consciousness) should be cardioverted as a matter of urgency, independent of the type of tachycardia. Get help from an ALS provider, and more senior help as required.

Conclusions

Tachyarrhythmias are termed *peri-arrest* as they can deteriorate to cardiac arrest. Quickly determine whether a patient is stable or unstable. If they are unstable, synchronised DC cardioversion is the treatment of choice – irrespective of the type of tachyarrhythmia. It is important to call the cardiac arrest or medical emergency team so that you can get expert help quickly. If the patient is haemodynamically stable, then medical treatment is appropriate. The arrhythmia is nevertheless deemed a *peri-arrest arrhythmia* and expert help should be sought early on.

References and further reading

American Heart Association (2007). *Sudden cardiac death*. Available at: www.americanheart.org/presenter.jhtml?identifier=14 (last accessed November 2009).

Resuscitation Council (2005). *Peri-arrest arrhythmias*. Available at: www.resus.org.uk/pages/periarst.pdf (last accessed November 2009).

Resuscitation Council UK (2006). *Advanced Life Support*, 5th edn. London, Resuscitation Council UK.

Wang, T.J., Massaro, J.M., Levy, D., *et al.* (2003). A risk score for predicting stroke or death for individuals with new-onset atrial fibrillation in the community: The Framingham Heart Study. *Journal of the American Medical Association*, **290**, 1049–56.

Useful websites

American Heart Association
www.americanheart.org

Resuscitation Council UK
www.resus.org.uk

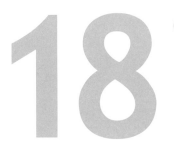

Chest pain

Kuno Budack and Ann M. Price

Chest pain is a very common complaint and may be the cause of a patient being unwell or a direct result of another condition. It is often one of the more difficult situations to deal with in an acute setting. The differential diagnoses are varied and it is impossible to investigate for all possibilities.

The aim of this chapter is:

- to provide you with knowledge about the assessment needed
- to make you aware of the possible causes and the initial treatment for the patient who complains of chest pain.

Diagnosis

A swift but thorough history and physical examination is vital. This usually will give a good impression as to the likely cause of the chest pain. In fact, the right questions, a good examination and a few tests will be able to establish the most likely diagnosis quickly. However a doctor should be called for early in a patient with chest pain.

> **HOT TIPS**
>
> Remember, the diagnosis in most cases will be made by:
>
> — a good history
> — a physical examination
> — a few tests.

The main concern with an acutely ill patient presenting with chest pain is that it may have a cardiac origin – therefore acute myocardial infarction will need to be considered initially. Box 18.1 identifies other possible causes of chest pain that need to be excluded.

Box 18.1	Possible causes of chest pain (based on Murray and White, 1999)

Cardiovascular

Angina pectoris
Acute myocardial infarct
Valvular disease
Pericarditis
Aortic dissecting aneurysm

Pulmonary

Pneumonia
Pulmonary embolism
Pneumothorax

Gastrointestinal

Reflux oesophagitis
Peptic ulcers
Pancreatitis
Cholecystitis

Musculoskeletal

Costochondritis
Trauma/fracture
Rheumatoid arthritis
Cervical/thoracic disc compression

Miscellaneous

Anxiety
Herpes zoster (shingles)
Tumours

Pathophysiology

Chest pain can have a variety of causes as outlined above. It is important to identify the type, severity, position and any radiation, its duration and any other associated symptoms. The patient should be asked to describe the pain and whether anything makes the pain better or worse. For a more detailed explanation of assessment and management of a variety of causes, please refer to Albarran and Tagney (2007).

Box 18.2	Anatomy and physiology review

Refresh your understanding of the anatomical structures and functions of the heart, coronary blood supply, responses to stress and the development of atheroscleroma.

In the acutely ill patient any chest pain should be treated as potentially of cardiac origin. When a patient is acutely ill the body is under increased emotional and physical stress; this may mean that the heart has increased workload and so needs a greater oxygen supply. If the coronary arteries are compromised because of atherosclerotic plaques, the added workload on the heart can lead to myocardial ischaemia and chest pain (angina); in severe cases a myocardial infarction may be precipitated.

Case Scenario

You are called to see a 65-year-old man on a medical ward who has developed chest pain. On arrival you note that he is anxious, sweaty and has central chest pain. He is able to talk to you.

His respiratory rate is 26 breaths per minute and his blood pressure is 160/80 mmHg. He has a tachycardia of 120 beats per minutes. His saturations are 96%.

Assessment and management

Assessment and management of the patient in our case scenario should follow the **ABCDE** method. See Box 18.3 for a treatment summary.

Box 18.3   Treatment summary for cardiac chest pain

Morphine—To relieve pain and anxiety

Oxygen—Use 100% (unless contraindicated)

Aspirin—To impede the clotting process (unless contraindicated, as in gastric ulcer)

Nitrates—To relieve pain (hypotensive patients might suffer further blood pressure drop so consider its use carefully)

Other—Consider antiarrhythmic drugs, ACE inhibitors, beta-blockers and statins as appropriate

A—Airway

In this patient, the airway was patent as he is able to speak.

B—Breathing

His respiratory rate is slightly fast. Any patient with chest pain should be commenced on high-flow oxygen via a non-rebreathe mask so that oxygen delivery to the heart is maximised. Respiratory rate should be recorded half-hourly and saturations should be measured. Remember that the patient is sweaty and may be peripherally shut down, so peripheral saturations may not be accurate. If there is any suspicion that the chest pain has a respiratory cause, then a chest x-ray may be indicated.

C—Circulation

The patient's blood pressure (BP) is slightly raised and he is tachycardic. Ideally, continuous ECG monitoring will be commenced and observations of blood pressure and heart rate should be recorded half-hourly. Temperature readings should be taken. A history should also be taken; the kind of questions to ask are listed in Box 18.4. A physical assessment including palpation, percussion and auscultation should be undertaken. The patient's pulse should be felt and assessed for strength (bounding or weak), capillary refill can be assessed and jugular venous pressure can be estimated. The heart should be auscultated for evidence of any murmurs and the lungs for signs of pulmonary oedema (see Chapter 6 on left ventricular failure). It may be useful to measure blood pressure on both arms to exclude aortic dissection. A 12-lead ECG should be done as a priority and reviewed by a knowledgeable professional. A venous cannula should be inserted and blood tested for glucose and urea and electrolytes and a full blood count.

If myocardial ischaemia is strongly suspected then 300 mg aspirin (as long as there are no contraindications) can be given while thrombolytic therapy is established. Assistance is required from a senior person or the outreach team to review the need for a specialist bed, such as on coronary care unit. If thrombolysis is needed to treat a myocardial infarction then a coronary care bed is essential and will be a priority.

Box 18.4 Questions to ask patients with acute chest pain

Where exactly do you feel the pain?
Lateral pains are unlikely to be due to an acute cardiac event or aortic dissection.

What does the pain feel like?
'Tight' suggests cardiac pain.
'Sharp' suggests inflammation (pleurisy, infection).
'Tearing' suggests dissection.

Does the pain spread anywhere?
Associated arm or jaw pain suggests the heart.
Radiation to the back suggests dissection.

What makes the pain worse?
Anything triggered from the outside (inspiration, pressure) points away from the heart
  and aorta (but does not exclude them).
Pain related to exertion suggests angina.
Pain after a meal could be gastrointestinal (reflux, cholecystitis, pancreatitis).

What helps the pain?
Glyceryl trinitrate (helps angina and reflux).
Sitting up (eases pericarditis).

Do you get anything else with the pains?
Sweating and giddiness are alarm signs.

For patients developing hypotension, cardiogenic shock should be considered (refer to Chapter 15). Arrhythmias can complicate cardiac chest pain and should be treated appropriately (see Chapter 17).

D—Disability

Analgesia to relieve the pain should be given (this is probably why his blood pressure is high). Morphine is often used, but glycerine trinitrate (GTN) tablets or sublingual spray may be indicated if the patient has a history of angina. Both morphine and GTN work by dilating coronary arteries and improving oxygen to the heart muscle. Morphine has the added benefit of reducing anxiety. Conscious level should be assessed because deterioration or increased confusion can indicate a worsening condition, and possibly an imminent cardiac arrest. Suggest keeping the patient nil by mouth if a non-cardiac cause is suspected.

E—Exposure, Environment and Everything Else

The priority for these patients is to reduce their distress. However, it is important to examine the patient fully for any possible injuries, peripheral oedema (which may indicate heart failure) or signs of peripheral vascular disease (which can indicate concurrent cardiovascular disease).

Investigations

ECG

- Look for ischemia, ST depression, infarction, ST elevation, and bundle branch blocks.
- Helps with diagnosis of pericarditis (widespread saddle-shaped ST segment elevation in most leads).
- Helps with diagnosis of pulmonary embolism ($S_I Q_{III} T_{III}$) or right heart strain (right axis shift, right bundle branch block, anterior T-wave inversion).

Chest x-ray

- Check for pneumothorax (loss of lung markings).
- Helps with diagnosis of pneumonia (see Chapter 10).
- Might point towards aortic dissection (mediastinal widening).

Blood tests

Refer to hospital reference ranges (see Box 18.5).
- Full blood count (to look for anaemia and signs of gastric bleeding).
- Urea and electrolytes (to look for imbalances, particularly of potassium).
- Troponin (a sensitive test of myocardial injury if raised above normal value of < 0.03 ng/mL).
- Amylase (to exclude pancreatitis).
- Glucose (to look for undiagnosed diabetes).
- Arterial blood gases (to exclude respiratory problems) (see Chapter 41).

Box 18.5	**Normal blood result ranges (from Bloodbook, 2007)**
Haemoglobin	Males 13–18 g/dL; Females 12–16 g/dL
Potassium	3.5–5.0 mEq/L
Amylase	53–123 units/L
Glucose	70–110 g/dL (or 3.9–7.0 mmol/L)
Magnesium	1.5–2.0 mEq/L

Echocardiogram

- Useful when a new murmur has been detected.
- Can help with diagnosis of aortic aneurysm in the ascending aorta or the aortic root.

Conclusions

Chest pain is a common problem in the acutely ill adult and has potentially life-threatening complications if the cause is not identified swiftly and treated appropriately. The National Institute for Health and Clinical Excellence (NICE) is currently developing guidelines on 'chest pain' and 'acute coronary syndrome' which are due for publication in 2010.

References and further reading

Albarran, J. and Tagney, J. (2007). *Chest Pain: Advanced Assessment and Management Skills*. Oxford, Blackwell.

Blood Book (2007). Blood test reference range chart. Available at: www.bloodbook.com/ranges.html#BLOOD/ (last accessed November 2009).

Hudak, C.M. and Gallo, B.M. (1994). *Critical Care Nursing: A Holistic Approach*, 6th edn. Philadelphia, Lippincott.

Murray, S.E. and White, B.S. (1999). *Critical Care Assessment Handbook*. Philadelphia, WB Saunders.

Useful websites

British Heart Foundation
www.bhf.org.uk

National Institute for Health and Clinical Excellence (NICE)
www.nice.org.uk

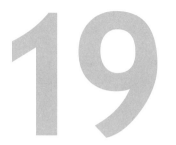

Acute abdomen

Russell Canavan and Ann M. Price

Approximately half of all acute surgical admissions present with abdominal pain (Cole *et al.*, 2006). Thus the acute abdomen is relatively common and presents a special challenge as it comprises of a number of clinical conditions. Often it requires a definitive intervention (for example, surgery) which may be high risk in the acutely ill patient. A methodical approach to resuscitation and timing of a procedure is essential to optimise the patient's chances of survival. The acute abdomen **is the subject of other books, so this chapter gives a typical case example and points to some pitfalls in managing a patient with an acute abdomen.**

At the end of this chapter you should:

- be aware of the main causes of an acute abdomen
- be able to assess and plan initiate treatment.

Background and definitions

The acute abdomen is not a diagnosis in itself but is part of a nebulous group of medical, surgical and gynaecological conditions that require hospitalisation. Often the cardinal feature of the admission is abdominal pain.

Mechanism of condition and therapy

This woman in the case scenario overpage was clearly unwell with an *acute abdomen*. The **ABCDE** approach showed she reached three of the criteria for systemic inflammatory response syndrome (SIRS) (see more about sepsis in Chapter 13) which are likely to be secondary to an abdominal cause. Therefore, she needs urgent assessment and appropriate treatment to prevent any further deterioration. You will need to consider the causes of an acute abdomen and consider which of these are relevant in this woman (see Box 19.1). Although this is a long list, most of the conditions are fairly straightforward to diagnose and their treatment is well

A 46-year-old obese woman attended the emergency department. She arrived vomiting with sudden onset central abdominal pain that radiated through to her back. On arrival she was assessed according to the ABCDE approach.

A—Airway
She was alert and talking (complaining of pain).

B—Breathing
She had a respiratory rate of 24 breaths per minute with saturations of 100% on air. She had a clear chest on auscultation.

C—Circulation
She was dehydrated and flushed. Her pulse was bounding with a rate of 110 beats per minute and she had a blood pressure of 90/40 mmHg.

D—Disability
She was alert and orientated. Her capillary blood glucose came back as 9.8 mmol/L.

E — Environment and Exposure
Exposing the patient revealed no abnormality.

Abdominal examination was performed:
— Inspection: her abdomen was tense but essentially normal.
— Percussion: gave no suggestion of any enlarged organs or ascites
— Palpation: proved difficult as she was voluntarily guarding. However, she was noted to be diffusely tender and her abdomen was soft when distracted. She had no palpable organs.
— Auscultation: active bowel sounds could be heard.

established. The pathophysiology of the acute abdomen is varied depending on the cause and you should refer to other texts for further details (such as McConnell, 2007).

As surgical teams are often asked to manage these patients, it is important not to miss medical conditions that can mimic a surgical abdomen. These include diabetic ketoacidosis, acute myocardial events, biochemical abnormalities and sickle cell disease.

Assessment and management

A thorough assessment is required. Box 19.2 describes the assessment required in acute abdomen. Pregnancy must be excluded in all women of childbearing age. Box 19.3 (overpage) describes bowel sounds and their possible causes.

Box 19.1   Causes of acute abdominal pain (based on Cole *et al.*, 2006)

Liver	Hepatitis
	Liver abscess
	Budd–Chiari syndrome
	Hepatic ischaemia
Gynaecological	Ectopic pregnancy
	Ovarian cyst
	Salpingitis
	Pelvic inflammatory disease
	Fibroids
Pancreatobiliary	Cholangitis
	Cholecystitis
	Pancreatitis
	Biliary leak/perforation
Peritoneum	Primary peritonitis
	Secondary peritonitis
Urogenital	Acute retention
	Obstructive uropathy
	Testicular torsion
Gastrointestinal	Gastritis
	Bowel obstruction
	Gastroenteritis
	Peptic ulcer disease
	Hernia
	Volvulus
	Diverticulitis
	Ischaemic bowel
	Appendicitis
	Intersusception
	Perforation
Medical	Diabetes mellitus
	Addison's disease
	Herpes zoster
Spleen	Rupture
	Infarction
Haematological	Sickle cell disease
	Malaria

...history and history of present complaint
This s... highlight previous episodes of abdominal pain and their outcome. Current history (e.g. rate of onset, precipitating factors) may aid diagnosis. Predisposing factors should become evident (e.g. alcohol, foreign travel, family history).

Physical observation
This includes the **ABCDE** approach and incorporates inspection, percussion, palpation and auscultation of the abdomen using the 4- or 9-quadrant method. Remember to ask about the type and frequency of stools and vomiting, and examine skin turgor.

Haemodynamics
Include blood pressure, heart rate, respiratory rate, urine output, temperature and capillary refill time.

Blood tests
Full blood count (for low haemoglobin and high white cell count), urea and electrolytes (for renal impairment and electrolyte imbalances), clotting, liver function tests, amylase, blood glucose, blood cultures, arterial blood gases, and others as indicated (e.g. pregnancy test).

Others as indicated
Urinalysis, ECG, endoscopy, CT scan, MRI, x-ray, ultrasound.

Irrespective of the cause of the pain, the patient's immediate needs are fluid resuscitation, analgesia, and antibiotics. Two large-bore cannulae should be inserted and fluid should be given according to the response of the heart rate, blood pressure and urine output. Continuous monitoring would be the gold standard, with hourly observation of vital signs and fluid input and output; ideally a urinary catheter will be needed. A central venous line should be considered if the patient's condition does not improve swiftly. If available, a high-dependency bed may be required so that close observation is possible.

A tense or distended abdomen means that the diaphragm cannot function properly, causing 'splinting'; this can lead to respiratory problems, therefore oxygen therapy and respiratory assessment is important.

The choice of analgesic varies with the cause of the abdominal pain; opiates (such as morphine) are thought to cause spasm of the sphincter of Oddi and may increase pain in biliary problems. However, in the acute phase controlling pain with analgesia and assessing response using a pain score will guide treatment. Patient-controlled analgesia (this includes epidurals) can be useful for abdominal pain and referral to the acute pain team or anaesthetist; if pain is poorly controlled, it should be considered.

Early aggressive (usually intravenous) antibiotics are crucial and should be instigated with consideration of the likely cause of the pain, local hospital antibiotic policy and, when needed,

Box 19.3	**Bowel sounds**

Absent sounds: possibly caused by gastrointestinal paralysis (eg ileus or peritonitis).

Overactive or tinkling sounds: possibly caused by gastrointestinal obstruction.

N.B. The usefulness of bowel sounds in the acute situation is controversial.

input from the consultant microbiologist. Once appropriate microbiological investigations have been carried out, such as stool and urine specimens, wound swabs, and blood cultures, if antibiotics are not being effective then specialist advice should be sought.

> **HOT TIPS**
>
> Review an anatomy and physiology book to locate key organs in the abdomen including the spleen, liver, stomach, small and large intestines, ovaries, uterus, kidneys, bladder and aorta.
>
> Also review the 4 or 9 quadrants of the abdomen used in physical assessment.

It is not uncommon for these patients to aspirate if they are vomiting. A large-bore nasogastric tube can be life-saving in this situation (size 14 Fr is suggested). Nasogastric tubes also help to ensure accurate fluid balance because the amount of vomitus can be underestimated (see Chapter 43 on placing a nasogastric tube). If the patient is actively vomiting they should be made nil by mouth; instigate anti-emetics and review the effect. If a patient is to remain nil by mouth or has a poor oral intake it will be important to consider their nutritional requirements (see Chapter 44 for more on meeting nutritional requirements).

> **HOT TIPS**
>
> Early referral to senior clinicians is of paramount importance with patients who remain hypotensive despite fluid resuscitation. See Chapter 2 for more about assessing and monitoring the acutely unwell patient.

The woman in our clinical scenario was critically unwell and needed hourly monitoring, of her vital signs, including her urine output. She remained hypotensive and needed central venous pressure monitoring. In the acute abdomen there is often a definitive procedure that can be done to alleviate the problem, so when the patient is stable enough they should be sent for this. In the case of the woman in our case scenario, the bloods revealed she had an acute pancreatitis with deranged liver enzymes. Using the Glasgow criteria she was classified as severe pancreatitis (see Box 19.4). Abdominal ultrasound demonstrated a dilated common bile duct and the presence of gallstones. Within 48 hours of admission, she underwent an endoscopic retrograde cholangiopancreatogram (ERCP), during which a sphincterotomy was performed and the gallstones were removed. Following her recovery, she was booked for a laparoscopic cholecystectomy.

Box 19.4 **Pancreatitis scores according to Ranson and Glasgow criteria (based on Felstead, 2007)**

Ranson criteria (three or more factors indicates severe disease)

Age > 55 years
> 10% decrease in haemoglobin
White cell count > 16,000 mm^3
Urea > 16 mmol/L
Calcium < 2 mmol/L
Glucose > 10 mmol/L
Fluid loss > 6 litres

Glasgow criteria (three or more factors indicates severe disease)

Age > 55 years
White cell count > 15,000 mm^3
Urea > 16 mmol/L
Calcium < 2 mmol/L
Glucose > 10 mmol/L
Albumin < 32 g/L

Conclusions

The acute abdomen is a common cause for admission to hospital. Most of these patients will have a correctable condition which needs swift diagnosis and treatment to ensure good outcome. Early aggressive resuscitation using the **ABCDE** approach in the unwell patient with careful monitoring can significantly improve outcome. There are a few pitfalls but they can be easily avoided.

References and further reading

Cole, E., Lynch, A. and Cugononi, H. (2006). Assessment of the patient with acute abdominal pain. *Nursing Standard*, 20 (39), 67–75.

Felstead, I. (2007). Upper gastrointestinal surgery. In: F.J. McArthur-Rouse and S. Prosser (eds) *Assessing and Managing the Acutely Ill Surgical Patient*. Edinburgh, Blackwell Publishing.

McConnell, T.H. (2007). *The Nature of Disease: Pathology for Health Professionals*. London, Lippincott Williams and Wilkins.

Murray, S.E. and White, B.S. (1999). *Critical Care Assessment Handbook*. Philadelphia, WB Saunders.

Useful websites

Association of Surgeons of Great Britain and Ireland
www.asgbi.org.uk

British Society of Gastroenterology
www.bsg.org.uk

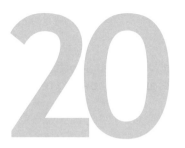

Oesophageal varices

Russell Canavan

Patients with oesophageal varices are at risk of large upper gastrointestinal bleed (a GI bleed). When they bleed, they present in an alarming way and have a very high mortality. A methodical approach to their management can relieve the anxiety of both the patient and the staff managing the patient. Recent advances in the treatment of varices have had a significant impact on the outcome of the disease and should be incorporated in the treatment of the disease.

At the end of this chapter you will be confident:

- in the diagnosis of variceal haemorrhage
- about the management of variceal haemorrhage.

Background and definitions

The portal circulation is normally a low-pressure system that carries 1500 mL per minute of blood from the spleen, stomach, small and large bowel to the liver. If there is a restriction to the blood flow before, within, or after the liver, then the pressure in the system will rise. Portosystemic shunting occurs, and leads to the development of varices. In some patients their underlying liver disease may not be apparent until their first bleed.

It is suggested that you review the anatomy and physiology of the upper gastrointestinal tract.

HOT TIPS

Carry out an anatomy and physiology review. Revise the position of the liver, spleen, gall bladder and portal circulation, the oesophageal veins, and pre-, intra- and post-hepatic obstruction. Identify the structure and function of each.

A 43-year-old man was referred for assessment of 'coffee ground' vomiting. Shortly after arrival, he vomits approximately 1 litre of fresh red blood and is assessed according to the ABCDE approach.

A—Airway
He is agitated but talking to you.

B—Breathing
His respiratory rate is 30 breaths per minute.

C—Circulation
His pulse is 120 beats per minute and is regular. He has a blood pressure of only 80/50 mmHg. His peripheries are cold and his capillary refill time is 5 seconds.

D—Disability
He is alert but confused.

E—Exposure and Environment
There is nothing to note when the patient is exposed.

Abdominal examination was conducted:

Inspection: This gentleman is pale and has multiple spider naevi (defined as small blanching vascular skin lesions that fill centrally; they can be a normal finding but in association with other features imply chronic liver disease). He has abdominal distension and pedal oedema. Some distended veins are noted on his abdomen. You note that he has several tattoos.

Palpation: He has no palpable organomegaly.

Auscultation: He has normal bowel sounds.

Percussion: He has evidence of shifting dullness on palpation.

For more on bowel sounds and their possible causes, see Box 19.3 in the previous chapter.

Pathophysiology, aetiology, mechanism and therapy of the condition

In our case scenario, the clinical examination showed clear signs of portal hypertension. The most likely explanation for the presentation is that this man has portal hypertension resulting in an acute variceal bleed. See Box 20.1 for causes of portal hypertension. In most cases the pathology is hepatic cirrhosis and this carries its own problems. In the developed world the most common cause of this has been alcoholic liver disease, but the demographics are changing. As a result of our modern lifestyle, a large number of patients are now being seen for non-alcoholic fatty liver disease (NAFLD), which can also lead to cirrhosis.

> **Box 20.1 Assessment in acute abdomen (based on Murray and White, 1999 and Cole *et al.*, 2006)**
>
> **Pre-hepatic:** portal vein disease.
> **Hepatic:** liver disease.
> **Post-hepatic:** hepatic vein disease.

Cirrhosis

Cirrhosis can be defined as the histological development of regenerative nodules surrounded by fibrous bands in response to chronic liver injury, which leads to portal hypertension and end-stage liver disease (Schuppan and Adfhal, 2008). In the most common scenario, the patient will have liver cirrhosis as well as a problem with bleeding varices or portal hypertension. The cirrhotic patient may have deranged synthetic and metabolic functions of their liver, possibly including hepatorenal complications (Gines, 2004).

Liver function tests

Liver function tests include those for aspartate aminotransaminase (AST), alkaline phosphatase (ALP) and bilirubin (conjugated and total). These are usually elevated in liver disease (Murray and White, 1999). There is retention of free body water in patients with liver cirrhosis, which leads to a dilution of serum sodium, causing a relative hyponatraemia. This can lead to cerebral oedema and its sequelae.

Hepatic encephalopathy

Hepatic encephalopathy is a syndrome observed in patients with cirrhosis. It is defined as a spectrum of neuropsychiatric abnormalities in people with liver dysfunction, after exclusion of other known brain disease. It is characterised by personality changes, intellectual impairment and a depressed level of consciousness. Grading of the symptoms of hepatic encephalopathy is performed according to the so-called West Haven classification system, as shown in Box 20.2.

Liver proteins and metabolism

The liver has a large role in synthesis of various proteins. The most useful for the clinician in the acute situation is the albumin, and clotting factors. These can be measured and are prognostic when evaluated in combination with other markers. Albumin is usually low and prothrombin

Box 20.2   The stages of hepatic encephalopathy (based on Wolf, 2007)

Stage 0:   Minimal hepatic encephalopathy (previously known as subclinical hepatic encephalopathy)
Lack of detectable changes in personality or behaviour
Minimal changes in memory, concentration, intellectual function, and coordination
Asterixis is absent

Stage 1:   Trivial lack of awareness
Shortened attention span
Impaired addition or subtraction
Hypersomnia, insomnia, or inversion of sleep pattern
Euphoria, depression or irritability
Mild confusion
Slowing of ability to perform mental tasks
Asterixis can be detected

Stage 2:   Lethargy or apathy
Disorientation
Inappropriate behaviour
Slurred speech
Obvious asterixis
Drowsiness and lethargy
Gross deficits in ability to perform mental tasks
Obvious personality changes and inappropriate behaviour
Intermittent disorientation, usually regarding time

Stage 3:   Somnolent but can be aroused
Unable to perform mental tasks
Disorientation about time and place, marked confusion and amnesia
Occasional fits of rage
Present but incomprehensible speech

Stage 4:   Coma with or without response to painful stimuli

time may be prolonged. The Childs–Pugh–Turcotte classification (see Table 20.1) is used to predict severity of liver disease in these patients. Various metabolic functions are carried out in the liver and a basic understanding of these is useful when looking after patients with liver problems. An example of this is the importance of the liver in glucolysis. This can lead to hypoglycaemia in the context of liver failure – an important clinical finding in liver patients who are agitated, drowsy or confused. The liver is also key in the metabolism of many drugs, which should be checked in the appendix of the *British National Formulary* prior to administration. If the metabolic function of the liver deteriorates, the waste products of metabolism can build up and cause hepatic encephalopathy. This problem can be exacerbated by opiates and sedatives that are also metabolised by the liver.

Reversible causes of portal hypertension should be identified and treated as a matter of urgency when the patient is stable enough.

Table 20.1 Childs–Pugh–Turcotte classification (Schuppan and Adfhal, 2008). Add up the scores for each criterion to predict a patient's life expectancy prior to acute deterioration

Parameter	Score 1	Score 2	Score 3
Ascites	None	Moderate	Severe
Encephalopathy	None	Mild	Severe
Prothrombin time (above normal)	< 4 secs	4–6 sec	> 6 sec
Serum bilirubin	< 35 μmol/L	35–50 μmol/L	> 50 μmol/L
Serum albumin	> 35 g/L	30–35 g/L	< 30 g/L

Scoring system

Childs–Pugh A: Score 5–6 (life expectancy 15–20 years)
Childs–Pugh B: Score 7–9 (life expectancy 4–14 years)
Childs–Pugh C: Score 10–15 (life expectancy 1–3 years)

Assessment, monitoring and management based on current evidence

History

It is particularly important to get the diagnosis of chronic liver disease. There are many clues that can help give the likely diagnosis.

- **Alcohol:** Not only whether they drink but how much and for how long. Confirm the amount with a third party if possible.
- **Age:** Neonates, children, teenagers, adults, middle-aged people and elderly people all have differing causes of liver diseases.
- **Ethnicity:** Certain ethnic groups have specific liver conditions associated with them (e.g. Ashkenazi Jews and Gaucher's disease).
- **Past medical history:** e.g. lupus and liver disease.
- **Associated symptoms:** e.g. skin rashes and arthralgia.
- **Viral risk factors:** e.g. living abroad, blood transfusions, injecting drug use history, unprotected sex, healthcare worker and tattoos.
- **Drugs:** prescribed, non-prescribed, social, and herbal.

Look

Make an assessment on the colour and pallor of the patient. They may be losing blood. This may also elicit an assessment of their hydration status (for example, do they have a dry tongue). Inspect for stigmata of chronic liver disease (see Box 20.3). Although sensitive, features of chronic liver disease are non-specific (de Bruy and Graviss, 2001).

Box 20.3	**Stigmata of chronic liver disease**

Clubbing
White nails
Palmar erythema
Spider naevus
Facial telangectasia
Gynaecomastia
Parotidomegaly
Testicular atrophy
Hepatic encephalopathy
Ascites
Irregular liver surface
Tender liver edge
Splenomegaly
Caput medusa

Listen (ausculate)

Occasionally a venous hum or arterial bruit can be heard over the liver in patients with cirrhosis or hepatocellular carcinoma. Bowel sounds will be normal.

Feel (palpate)

Splenomegaly is a key feature. Although is present in many conditions, it is highly suggestive of cirrhosis in the presence of liver disease. Feel for a liver edge. Is it thickened or irregular? Note the presence of ascites by testing for shifting dullness (see Box 20.4).

Box 20.4	**How to test for shifting dullness**

— Place the patient flat and relaxed, with arms by the side. Let any fluid settle in the flanks and explain to the patient what you are doing.
— Percuss in the mid-line of the abdomen. The note should be resonant.
— Move laterally, percussing continuously until a dull note is reached. Mark this spot.
— Move the patient through 90° so they are lying on their side. The spot that was dull should now become resonant (i.e. the dull spot has moved with the fluid).
— Confirm the result by repeating the process in reverse, starting with the patient on their side.

The presence of shifting dullness confirms the presence of fluid (normally ascites) in the abdomen.

Monitoring

Although there is no agreed way of monitoring liver patients in the setting of an acute bleed there is a need for close supervision.

- **Every 15 minutes:** pulse, blood pressure, oxygen saturation monitoring.
- **Every hour:** temperature, central venous pressure, urine output.

Once the patient is stabilised and the bleeding has stopped then all the above measurements can be taken every hour. When in liver failure the patient is at risk of hypoglycaemia so capillary blood glucose should also be monitored.

Fluids

In the acute setting it is not uncommon for the patient to be intravascularly depleted while the extravascular compartment is grossly overloaded. In this situation, central pressure monitoring can be useful (see Chapter 38 on central venous catheters). Initially the patient will have lost blood and so is likely to require blood transfusion. Variceal bleeds often involve large blood loss and so many units of packed red cells may be needed, further depleting clotting factors and platelets. Each hospital should have a protocol for massive blood transfusions to guide them on replacement of clotting factors and platelets. Advice from a haematologist can be invaluable in these situations.

N.B. There is some suggestion that raising the portal pressure with over transfusion may contribute to varices continuing to bleed (McCormick et al., 1999; Duggan, 2001).

Drugs in the acute setting

Terlipressin and somatostatin analogues

These are used initially to lower portal pressure and, therefore, control haemorrhage. They can be used as an adjunct to endoscopic therapy and should be continued for 72 hours. The drug of choice is terlipressin because it has the additional effect of protecting against hepatorenal failure (Nevens, 2004).

Broad-spectrum antibiotics

A large number of cirrhotic patients presenting with upper gastrointestinal haemorrhage have concurrent infection precipitating their bleed (Thalheimer *et al.*, 2005). Early treatment with antibiotics has been shown to reduce mortality.

Other drugs

The value of laxatives and prokinetics in the acute phase is limited. Using these would necessitate discussion with a specialist.

Specialist help

Early help from a gastroenterologist can be helpful. Most are very keen to hear about patients with a variceal bleed and they can assist in the management using the following techniques.

Endoscopy

The first consideration of endoscopy is the loss of protection of the airway. When the patient is starved for endoscopy this is not a problem, but in acute haematemesis the stomach is full and aspiration is a real concern. Prior to endoscopy the patient can be given intravenous erythromycin to improve gastric emptying (Coffin *et al.*, 2002; Frossard, 2002). Intubation to protect the airway should be considered when considering endoscopy in the setting of upper gastrointestinal bleeding. Endoscopy is diagnostic in most cases. During the endoscopy, elastic bands can be placed on the veins in a sequential fashion to stop the bleeding. Varices can also be injected with agents that induce sclerosis and obliteration of the varices (Dib *et al.*, 2006). More recently covered oesophageal stents have been developed to compress acutely bleeding varices.

Tamponade

Once the patient's airway is protected, a Sengstaken–Blakemore tube can be placed. This is a specialised catheter with a large balloon at the end that is passed into the stomach and then inflated. Traction on the catheter pulls on the varices and stems the bleeding. It is not always necessary to inflate the oesophageal balloon. Prolonged use of the balloon can lead to pressure necrosis and so is often a bridge to other therapy (Dib *et al.*, 2006). The patient is better placed in the intensive care unit for this treatment, particularly because then they are better intubated and ventilated to reduce the high possibility of aspiration.

Shunting

In specialist centres shunts may be available. These connect the portal and systemic circulation, reducing the portal pressure that causes the bleeding. Surgical shunts (such as the Le Veen and Denver) were used to reduce the portal pressure in the past. Now the same effect can be achieved without the need for surgery, using a transjugular intrahepatic portosystemic shunt (TIPSS). This metal shunt is placed via the internal jugular, under screening. It is placed along the hepatic vein and pushed through to the portal vein, effectively forming a liver bypass, and lowering the portal pressure. However, bypassing the liver may precipitate hepatic encephalopathy or right heart failure, and there are other problems related to the stent (Dib *et al.*, 2006).

Transplant

One final option is to perform a liver transplant, if the patient meets the necessary criteria. It can be considered by your local centre (Devlin, 2000).

Conclusions

Oesophageal varices present some very specific challenges. Issues concerning immediate resuscitation should be borne in mind when treating these patients. Central monitoring, early use of terlipressin, avoiding sodium, and physical interventions such as endoscopy and transjugular intrahepatic portasystemic stent shunt (TIPSS) all have a role.

References and further reading

Coffin, B., Pocard, M., Panis, Y., *et al.* (2002). Erythromycin improves the quality of EGD in patients with acute upper GI bleeding: A randomized controlled study. *Gastrointestinal Endoscopy*, **56**(2), 174–49.

Cox, C. (ed.) (2004). *Physical Assessment for Nurses*. Oxford, Blackwell Publishing.

De Bruyn, G. and Graviss, E.A. (2001). A systematic review of the diagnostic accuracy of physical examination for the detection of cirrhosis. *BMC Medical Informatics and Decision Making*, **1**(6).

Devlin, J. and O'Grady, J. (2000). *Indications for Referral and Assessment in Adult Liver Transplantation: A Clinical Guideline*. Available at: http//www.bsg.org.uk (last accessed November 2009).

Dib, N., Oberti, F., and Calès, P. (2006). Current management of the complications of portal hypertension: Variceal bleeding and ascites. *Canadian Medical Association Journal*, **174**(10), 1433–43.

Duggan, J.M. (2001). Transfusion in gastrointestinal haemorrhage. If, when and how much? *Alimentary Pharmacology and Therapeutics*, **15**, 1109–13.

Frossard, J.L., Spahr, L., Queneau, P.E., *et al.* (2002). Erythromycin intravenous bolus infusion in acute upper gastrointestinal bleeding: a randomized, controlled, double-blind trial. *Gastroenterology*, **123**(1), 17–23.

Gines, P., Cardenas, A., Arroyo, V. and Rodes, J. (2004). Current concepts: Management of cirrhosis and ascites. *New England Journal of Medicine*, **350**(16), 1646–54.

McCormick, P.A., Jenkins, S.A., McIntyre, N., *et al.* (1995). Why portal hypertensive varices bleed and bleed: A hypothesis. *Gut*, **36**, 100–03.

Murray, E.E. and White, B.S. (1999). *Critical Care Assessment Handbook.* Philadelphia, WB Saunders.

Nevens, F. (2004). Critical comparison of drug therapies in currently used therapeutic strategies for variceal haemorrhage. *Alimentary Pharmacology and Therapeutics*, **20**(Suppl.3), 18–22.

Schuppan, D. and Afdhal. N.H. (2008). Liver cirrhosis. *The Lancet*, **371**, 883–51.

Thalheimer, U., Triantos, C.K., Samonakis, D.N., Patch, D. and Burroughs, A.K. (2005). Infection, coagulation and variceal bleeding in cirrhosis. *Gut*, **54**(4), 556–63.

Wolf, D. (2007). Encephalopathy – Hepatic. Available at: www.emedicine.com/med/topic3185.htm (last accessed June 2009).

Useful websites

British Society of Gastroenterology
www.bsg.org.uk

National Library for Health Gastroenterology and Liver Diseases Specialist Library
www.library.nhs.uk/gastroliver

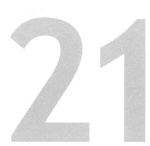

Electrolytes

Philip Woodrow

This chapter outlines some of the more significant electrolytes in the body – what they do, the significance of abnormally high or low levels, and common treatments. It also discusses the metabolite glucose and the pathophysiology of diabetic ketoacidosis.

Using information from this chapter, readers should be able to recognise abnormalities in their patients, to understand the likely causes and to know what actions are probably required. After reading this chapter you should be able to:

- list common acute electrolyte abnormalities
- identify likely causes for acute electrolyte abnormalities in your patients
- identify which of these abnormalities should be treated
- suggest the most appropriate way to treat these abnormalities.

Background and definitions

Electrolytes are elements or compounds that, in solution, dissociate into ions, making them capable of conducting electrical currents. Electrolytes therefore affect skeletal and cardiac muscle conduction and contraction. Electrolytes also regulate movement of substances between plasma, interstitial fluid and intracellular fluid. Electrolyte imbalances can cause:

- cardiac dysfunction
- skeletal muscle dysfunction
- fluid imbalances.

In healthy people, normal daily body intake and production of electrolytes balances any losses. Illness may disrupt this normal balance, either through abnormal intake or absorption or because of abnormal losses. Restoring and maintaining electrolyte balance is fundamental to health. The electrolytes discussed in this chapter are:

- sodium
- potassium
- calcium

- magnesium
- phosphate
- the metabolite glucose.

With the single exception of sodium, plasma levels of all electrolytes are relatively low. Higher levels are found elsewhere in the body, often in the intracellular fluid. Low levels are caused by one or more of the following:

- dilution
- loss
- failure of supply or production.

High levels are caused by one or more of the following:

- dehydration (haemoconcentration)
- excessive intake or production
- failure to clear.

Electrolytes can be divided into two main groups: cations and anions. *Cations* are positively charged, so their symbols have one or more positive ($^+$) signs (e.g. potassium K$^+$). All the electrolytes discussed in this chapter are cations. Some *anions* (negatively charged ions) are involved in acid–base balance which is beyond the scope of this chapter.

> **HOT TIPS**
>
> It is suggested that you refer to an anatomy and physiology textbook or website to examine the following terms: body fluid compartments, intracellular fluids, extracellular fluids (blood, plasma, lymphatic), interstitial fluids, membrane permeability, diffusion, osmosis, facilitated diffusion and active transport.

Sodium (Na$^+$)

Sodium is the main extracellular cation. Bound to chloride as salt, it creates an osmotic pull – 'where salt goes, water follows'. Hormones regulate renal sodium loss – aldosterone (from the adrenal gland) and natriuretic peptides (from the brain and heart). Normally, nearly all filtered sodium is reabsorbed. Except during adrenal disease (e.g. Addison disease and Cushing's syndrome), the quantity of blood sodium is usually stable, but its concentration is affected by water.

Normal range of sodium

The normal range of sodium is 135–145 mmol/L (Chernecky et al., 2002).

Case Scenario

A woman is admitted to the medical assessment unit with a diagnosis of diabetic ketoacidosis. Laboratory blood results show widespread abnormalities, including:

Glucose	43.2 g/dL
Sodium	127 mmol/L
Potassium	5.3 mmol/L
Magnesium	0.65 mmol/L
Phosphate	0.6 mmol/L

She is polyuric (passing large volumes of urine). An intravenous infusion of 1 litre normal saline is in progress, replacing the previous hour's urine output + 150 mL, and an insulin infusion (prescribed on a sliding scale) is in progress.

After reading this chapter, identify the likely cause and significance of her electrolyte abnormalities.

Hypernatraemia

High sodium is usually caused by dehydration, whereby there is haemoconcentration of sodium (Fisher and MacNaughton, 2006; Reynolds *et al.*, 2006). Dehydration should be treated by rehydration. Provided that cardiac and renal function are adequate, water should be given (e.g. intravenous 5% glucose).

Hyponatraemia

Low sodium can be caused by:

- water overload (especially with renal failure)
- fluid shifts (causing loss of sodium to cells or gaining water into blood plasma)
- salt deficiency or excessive loss.

In acutely ill patients, hyponatraemia is usually caused by haemodilution with excess water (Sargent, 2005; Reynolds *et al.*, 2006). This may be caused by failure to excrete water, or excessive shifts of intracellular fluid into blood. Intracellular fluid is potassium-rich but sodium-poor (about 15 mmol/litre), so it dilutes plasma sodium. Very low hyponatraemia (< 120 mmol/litre) may cause encephalopathy.

HOT TIPS

Persistent hyperkalaemia and hyponatraemia, in the context of large cumulative fluid balance deficits, is likely to be caused by fluid shifts.

Hyponatraemia may be treated by:

- giving salt (e.g. normal saline infusion; healthy kidneys will conserve salt while excreting excess water)
- fluid restriction (e.g. 1500 mL).

Causes of hyponatraemia should be carefully assessed to identify appropriate treatment. Fluid restricting an already dehydrated patient is likely to cause further deterioration and renal failure (Sargent, 2005).

Potassium (K$^+$)

Most potassium loss (90% of it) is in urine. The remainder is lost in stools. Abnormal urine output (oliguria or polyuria, including that due to furosemide) is the most common cause of potassium imbalance in hospitalised patients. Except for furosemide, most diuretics either spare potassium or have potassium added.

Potassium is used for muscle contraction, including that of the myocardium. Hyperkalaemia can cause over-excitability, while hypokalaemia can cause under-excitability. Either may cause dysrhythmias, ectopic beats and infarction. Slightly raised levels are safer than slight deficiencies, so if patients are at risk of cardiac dysfunction, target serum potassium levels are usually 4–5 mmol/litre (most critical care units will aim for this level).

When patients are receiving intravenous hydration, potassium imbalance can often be prevented by including solutions containing 20 or 40 mmol of potassium per litre.

Normal range of potassium

The normal range of potassium is 3.5–5.0 mmol/litre (Chernecky *et al.*, 2002).

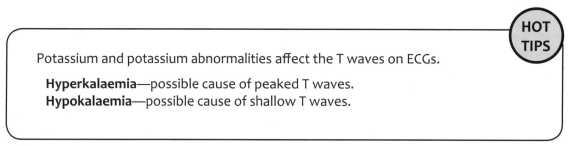

HOT TIPS

Potassium and potassium abnormalities affect the T waves on ECGs.

Hyperkalaemia—possible cause of peaked T waves.
Hypokalaemia—possible cause of shallow T waves.

Hyperkalaemia

High potassium can be life-threatening, causing cardiac arrest. Intracellular fluid is potassium-rich (unlike plasma), normally containing about 155 mmol/litre (Mackenzie, 2002). Therefore trauma, injury or fluid shifts may cause hyperkalaemia as potassium moves from the intracellular compartment. Intracellular fluid shifts usually occur as a result of dehydration (including fluid restrictions). See Box 20.1 for the main causes of hyperkalaemia.

Box 20.1   Main causes of hyperkalaemia

— Oliguria
— Major trauma/massive injury
— Fluid shifts
— Large blood transfusion
— Excessive intake/infusion
— Constipation

Storage of blood for transfusion causes potassium release and, after 35 days, plasma levels in stored blood can reach 30 mmol/litre (Hillman and Bishop, 2004). Because furosemide is usually given concurrently with blood transfusions, this potassium infusion is matched by increased renal loss of potassium.

> **HOT TIPS**
>
> Erythrocyte recovery may cause *rebound* hypokalaemia within 24 hours (Isbister, 2003) so blood levels of potassium should be checked the day following transfusion.

Hyperkalaemia should be treated by removing potassium from the plasma. If urgent (i.e. plasma levels of > 6 mmol/litre) then intravenous insulin and glucose is usually used (50 IU of Actrapid insulin in 50 mL of 50% glucose, infused over 1 hour). Glucose and insulin transports plasma potassium into the intracellular fluid, and therefore averts the immediate risks of cardiac arrest. However, the potassium remains in the body, and may later return into the plasma. Calcium gluconate or calcium chloride is often given concurrently with insulin and glucose to stabilise cardiac conduction. Intravenous calcium can precipitate dysrhythmias in patients taking digoxin.

Less severe hyperkalaemia (< 6 mmol/litre) is usually treated by oral or rectal calcium resonium (Humphreys, 2002). However, calcium resonium reduces serum potassium relatively slowly (2–3 hours). Failure to spontaneously evacuate rectal calcium resonium usually necessitates manual evacuation, which should be performed according to local hospital policy.

Note that evidence for salbutamol reducing hyperkalaemia is mainly based on a few small-scale paediatric studies – it is not proven for adults.

Haemofiltration in the intensive care unit will remove the potassium from the body if the hyperkalaemia remains life threatening. Therefore it is important to get senior critical help with this problem.

Hypokalaemia

Low potassium is usually caused by polyuria, although some drugs, including salbutamol, interfere with plasma and intracellular potassium balance (Arias-Reyes *et al.*, 1989; Kemper *et al.*, 1996). See Box 20.2 for the main causes.

Box 21.2   Main causes of hypokalaemia

— Polyuria
— Malnutrition
— Drugs (insulin, salbutamol)
— Excessive vomiting or diarrhoea

Mild hypokalaemia (> 3 mmol/litre) can be reversed by giving oral or nasogastric potassium (e.g. Kay-Cee-L™; Sando-K™). Potassium supplements often taste bitter so many patients prefer them dissolved in a strongly flavoured drink.

If patients are unable to take or absorb oral or nasogastric drugs, or if their hypokalaemia is severe (< 3 mmol/litre), intravenous potassium is used because hypokalaemia can lead to cardiac arrest. Various concentrations of intravenous potassium are currently produced, but strong potassium concentrations (e.g. 40 mmol in 100 mL; 20 mmol in 10 mL) should *only* be used in critical care areas (National Patient Safety Agency, 2002) and should be administered via a central venous line. Where these are used:

- 20 mmol ampoules should be further diluted before use
- patients should have their ECG continuously monitored
- sufficient staff should be available, with sufficient knowledge of ECG monitoring, to detect promptly significant cardiac changes
- quick access to a blood gas analyser or another means of measuring serum potassium is advisable
- practice should conform to NPSA guidelines (2002) or any subsequent policies.

For most clinical areas, intravenous potassium infusions are restricted to 20 or 40 mmol/litre. Because oliguria reduces potassium excretion, potassium should be replaced cautiously in oliguric patients.

Calcium (Ca^{2+})

Most body calcium (99%) is in bone. The bone–blood balance is regulated by the hormones calcitonin and parathyroid hormone. Calcium is excreted in the urine. Plasma calcium enables contraction of cardiac and skeletal muscle, as well as clotting and nerve conduction. Normally about half of the plasma calcium is protein bound, and is therefore inactive. Only the ionised – or free – calcium is physiologically active.

Protein binding is affected by various factors, including the amount of protein available (usually measured by albumin levels) and by acid–base balance, whereby acidosis reduces protein binding. Laboratories normally measure total blood calcium, but blood gas analysers measure ionised calcium. Because abnormal blood protein concentrations affect the normal total (ionised) balance, laboratories may also correct blood calcium measurements, adjusting them to measure protein concentrations that reflect physiological activity from ionised calcium.

Normal range of calcium

The normal range of total calcium is 2.25–2.75 mmol/litre.
The normal ionised level 1.13–1.32 mmol/litre.

Hypercalcaemia

High calcium is usually caused by hyperparathyroidism, especially from tumours (Walsh, 2003). Hypercalcaemia can cause dysrhythmias (especially supraventricular tachycardias), cardiac arrest and muscle spasticity. Hyperparathyroidism usually necessitates parathyroidectomy.

Hypocalcaemia

Low calcium occurs when calcium plasma loss (either through the kidneys or into bone) exceeds calcium intake. It occurs in conditions such as:

- malnutrition
- polyuria (including drug-induced)
- sepsis (Goldhill, 1997)
- pancreatitis (Goldhill, 1997)
- hypothyroidism.

Hypocalcaemia can cause under-excitable cardiac and skeletal muscle conduction, resulting in dysrhythmias (especially blocks and escape ectopics and rhythms) and muscle weakness. Severe hypocalcaemia may cause tetany. Where sufficient calcium cannot be obtained through the diet, calcium may be given through various oral or intravenous preparations.

> **HOT TIPS**
>
> Frequent ectopic beats and dysrhythmias may be caused by potassium or calcium imbalances.

Magnesium (Mg^{2+})

Only about 1% of body magnesium is in plasma (James, 1991). Although filtered renally, most magnesium is normally reabsorbed (98%), renal losses being regulated by parathyroid hormone (Chalmers, 2002). Physiologically, plasma magnesium acts as a calcium antagonist, stabilising cell membranes.

Sometimes it is called 'nature's tranquilliser' because it relaxes smooth muscle, causing vasodilatation (reducing blood pressure) and bronchodilatation. Magnesium is used intra-cellularly for adenosine triphosphate (ATP) storage and production.

Normal range of magnesium

The normal range of magnesium is 0.75–1.0 mmol/litre.

Hypermagnesiumaemia

High magnesium is relatively rare, but plasma levels above 3 mmol/litre can cause bradypnoea, potentially precipitating respiratory arrest. High levels in acute illness are usually caused by renal failure (Astle, 2005).

Hypomagnesiumaemia

Low magnesium is relatively common among hospitalised patients. The risk factors for hypo-magnesiumaemia include:

- poor diet (including nil by mouth)
- polyuria (including drug-induced)
- critical illness
- alcoholism.

Hypomagnesiumaemia may cause tachydysrhythmias, hypertension and muscle weakness (Astle, 2005). Magnesium is the first-line drug for torsades de pointes (a form of ventricular fibrillation), but its value for other dysrhythmias is less certain (Dubé and Granry, 2003). Its place in treating migraine, alcohol withdrawal, delirium or seizures remains unclear (Kaye and O'Sullivan, 2002).

Phosphate (PO_4^{3-})

Most body phosphate is found in the bones (85%). Phosphate is the main intracellular buffer, so it is crucial for intracellular acid–base balance. It also regulates intracellular production of adenosine triphosphate (ATP), the form of energy produced in and used by cells. In erythrocytes, phosphate regulates 2,3-diphosphoglycerate (2,3-DPG), a chemical that affects oxygen dissociation from haemoglobin. Freely filtered by kidneys, most phosphate is reabsorbed, and regulated by parathyroid hormone. Phosphate loss is increased with polyuria, including furosemide-induced loss (Taylor *et al.*, 2004).

Normal range of phosphate

The normal range of phosphate is 0.8–1.5 mmol/litre

Hyperphosphataemia (high phosphate)

Hyperphosphataemia is extremely rare, and seldom problematic.

Hypophosphataemia (low phosphate)

Hypophosphataemia can cause muscle weakness, dysrhythmias and other problems. In hospitalised patients, hypophosphataemia usually occurs with chronic alcoholism, recovery from diabetic ketoacidosis, and re-feeding malnourished patients (Edwards *et al.*, 1998). It can be treated by giving phosphate, either orally (e.g. Phosphate-Sandoz™) or intravenously (e.g. Addiphos™, polyfusor). Phosphate has no known compatibility with any other intravenous drug, so should be infused through a dedicated line.

> **HOT TIPS**
>
> Phosphate and magnesium affect muscle strength, so before mobilising or rehabilitating patients, check their levels are normal.

Glucose ($C_6H_{12}O_6$)

Glucose is a metabolite – not an electrolyte. It is the main source of cell energy. Transported from blood into cells by insulin, mitochondria metabolise glucose aerobically to produce adenosine triphosphate (ATP).

Normal range of glucose

The normal range of glucose is 4.4–6.1 mmol/litre.

Hypoglycaemia (low glucose)

Low glucose usually occurs when diabetics take medication but insufficient sugar in their diet. Blood glucose below 2 mmol/litre is a medical emergency (Keays, 2003). Mild hypoglycaemia may be reversed with diet or oral glucose (e.g. Hypostop™ or glucagon), but severe hypoglycaemia requires 20 mL of intravenous 50% glucose (follow your local policy guidelines for teatment of hypoglycaemia).

Hyperglycaemia (high glucose)

In health, insulin production varies to maintain normoglycaemia. Hyperglycaemia occurs if insufficient insulin is produced to achieve this. It may be caused by a relative deficiency of insulin production or excessive resistance to insulin function. Although diabetes is usually a chronic condition, transient hyperglycaemia frequently occurs during critical illness (Cely *et al.*, 2004) due to stress responses, and can be caused by drugs (especially cardiac drugs).

Tight glycaemic control reduces mortality and complications from critical illness (van den Berghe *et al.*, 2001), severe trauma (Jeschke *et al.*, 2003) and diabetes (Diabetes Control and Complications Trial Research Group, 1999; Malmberg, 1999; UK Prospective Diabetes Study Group, 1998). Therefore, the importance of tight glucose control within the clinical setting has been emphasised recently.

Diabetic ketoacidosis (DKA)

Diabetic ketoacidosis is also-called diabetic coma, and it causes 14% of all diabetic-related hospital admissions (Palmer, 2004); these admissions are often previously undiagnosed type I diabetics. DKA can occur with blood glucose levels of 14 mmol/L (Keays, 2003) but levels are usually considerably higher.

Insufficient insulin causes hyperglycaemia, depriving cells of their normal main energy source. Without glucose, cells resort to alternative energy sources, especially fat. Fat metabolism releases free fatty acids, including ketones, so excessive fat metabolism causes (metabolic) ketoacidosis, with pH of < 7.3 and bicarbonate of < 15 mmol/litre (Keays, 2003).

Blood glucose of > 10 mmol/litre exceeds the renal reabsorption threshold, resulting in glycosuria. Glucose and ketones both exert high osmotic pressures, causing polyuria, dehydration, hypoperfusion and electrolyte imbalances. The main problems of diabetic ketoacidosis are therefore:

- hyperglycaemia
- metabolic acidosis
- polyuria
- hypovolaemia
- electrolyte imbalances (especially potassium)
- confusion or coma.

Ketones and glucose will be present in urine, and can be detected through ward urinalysis. Priorities of care should be to:

- reduce blood glucose with an insulin infusion
- rehydrate (reperfuse) initially with normal saline
- reverse the acidosis
- restore electrolytes, especially potassium and phosphate.

Rehydration should continue until urine is ketone-free (Charalambous et al., 1999). Once blood glucose is below 13 mmol/litre, 5% glucose should be used (Charalambous et al., 1999). However, each hospital should have a policy on the management of diabetic ketoacidosis, which should be referred to in order to guide practice.

Diabetic ketoacidosis necessitates close monitoring of vital signs, blood glucose, fluid balance, electrolytes and neurological state. During crises, large volumes of intracellular fluid may shift into the bloodstream, causing hyperkalaemia and hyponatraemia. With recovery, intracellular rehydration may cause hypokalaemia. Hypomagnesiumaemia also commonly occurs, secondary to diuresis (Keays, 2003).

Conclusions

Although plasma concentrations of all electrolytes, except sodium, are low, they have important – often vital – functions. Abnormalities can cause significant and often life-threatening complications. Most electrolytes discussed here are measured by analysis of urea and electrolytes (U&Es).

Staff caring for sicker patients should therefore be able to interpret such results in the context of their patients, identifying the likely cause of any abnormalities and what implications they may have for the individual patient. They should also recognise whether these abnormalities should be treated and the most appropriate method for treating them.

References and further reading

Arias-Reyes, J.A., Matos-Martinez, M., Velasquez-Jones, L. and Dubey-Ortega, L.A. (1989). Correction of hyperkalaemia with intravenous salbutamol in children with chronic renal insufficiency. *Boletin Medico del Hospital Infantil de Mexico*, **46**(9), 603–06.

Astle, S.M. (2005). Restoring electrolyte balance. *The Registered Nurse*, **68**(5), 34–39.

Cely, C.M., Arora, P., Quartrin, A.A., Kett, D.H. and Schein, R.M.H. (2004). Relationship of baseline glucose homeostasis to hyperglycaemia during medical critical illness. *Chest*, **126**(3), 879–87.

Chalmers, C.A. (2002). Applied anatomy and physiology and the renal disease process. In: N. Thomas (ed.) *Renal Nursing*, 2nd edn. Edinburgh, Baillière Tindall, pp. 27–74.

Charalambous, C., Schofield, I. and Malik, R. (1999). Acute diabetic emergencies and their management. *Care of the Critically Ill*, **15**(4), 132–35.

Chernecky, C., Macklin, D. and Murphy-Ende, K. (2002). *Fluids and Electrolytes. Real World Nursing Survival Guide Series*. Philadelphia, WB Saunders.

Diabetes Control and Complications Trial Research Group (1993). The effect of intensive treatment of diabetes on the development and progression of long-term complications in insulin-dependent diabetes mellitus. *New England Journal of Medicine*, **329**(14), 997–86.

Dubé, L. and Granry, J.-C. (2003). The therapeutic use of magnesium in anesthesiology, intensive care and emergency medicine: A review. *Canadian Journal of Anesthesia*, **50**(7), 732–46.

Edwards, R., Mitchell, M. and Twaddle, S. (1998). Hypophosphataemia in the critically ill patient – aetiology and management. *Care of the Critically Ill*, **14**(8), 267–70.

Fisher, L. and MacNaughton, P. (2006). Electrolyte and metabolic disturbances in the critically ill. *Anaesthesia and Intensive Care Medicine*, **7**(5), 151–54.

Goldhill, D.R. (1997). Calcium and magnesium. *Care of the Critically Ill*, **13**(3), 112–15.

Hillman, K. and Bishop, G. (2004). *Clinical Intensive Care*, 2nd edn. Cambridge, Cambridge University Press.

Humphreys, M. (2002). Hyperkalaemia: A dangerous electrolyte disturbance. *Connect*, **2**(1), 28–30.

Isbister, J.P. (2003). Blood transfusion. In: A.D. Bersten and N. Soni (eds) *Intensive Care Manual*, 5th edn. Edinburgh, Butterworth-Heinemann, pp. 915–26.

James, M.F.M. (1991). Magnesium in critical care medicine. *Care of the Critically Ill*, **7**(6), 233–37.

Jeschke, M.G., Klein, D. and Herndon, D.N. (2003). Insulin treatment improves the systemic inflammatory reaction to severe trauma. *Annals of Surgery*, **239**(4), 553–60.

Kaye, P. and O'Sullivan, I. (2002). The role of magnesium in the emergency department. *Emergency Medical Journal*, **19**(4), 288–91.

Keays R. (2003). Diabetic emergencies. In: A.D. Bersten, N. Soni (eds) *Intensive Care Manual*. 5th edn. Edinburgh. Butterworth-Heinemann, pp. 551–58.

Kemper, M.J., Harps, E. and Muller-Wiefel, D.E. (1996). Hyperkalaemia: therapeutic options in acute and chronic renal failure. *Clinical Nephrology*, **46**(1), 67–69.

Mackenzie, I. (2002). Assessment and management of fluid and electrolyte balance. *Surgery*, **20**(6), 121–26.

Malmberg, K. (1997). Prospective randomised study of intensive insulin treatment on long-term survival after acute myocardial infarction in patients with diabetes mellitus. *British Medical Journal*, **314**(7093), 1512–15.

National Patient Safety Agency (2002). *Patient Safety Alert. Ref PSA 01*. London, NPSA.

Palmer, R. (2004). An overview of diabetic ketoacidosis. *Nursing Standard*, **19**(10), 42–44.

Reynolds, R.M., Padfield, P.L. and Seckl, J.R. (2006). Disorders of sodium balance. *British Medical Journal*, **332**(7543), 702–05.

Sargent, S. (2005). The aetiology, management and complications of alcoholic hepatitis. *British Journal of Nursing*, **14**(10), 556–62.

Taylor, B., Huey, W.Y., Buchman, T.G., Boyle, W.A. and Coopersmith, C.M. (2004). Treatment of hypophosphatemia using a protocol based on patient weight and serum phosphorus level in a surgical intensive care unit. *Journal of the American College of Surgeons*, **198**(2), 198–204.

UK Prospective Diabetes Study (UKPDS) Group. (1998). Intensive blood-glucose control with sulphonylureas or insulin compared with conventional treatment and risk of complications in patients with type 2 diabetes (UKPDS 33). *Lancet* **352**(9131), 873–53.

van den Berghe, G., Wouters, P., Weekers, F., *et al.* (2001). Intensive insulin therapy in critically ill patients. *New England Journal of Medicine*, **345**(19), 1359–67.

Walsh, J. (2003). Disorders of calcium homeostasis. *Geriatric Medicine*, **33**(1), 27–30.

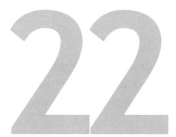

22 Neurological compromise secondary to electrolyte imbalance

Amanda Sudan and Sally A. Smith

This chapter discusses the case of rapid correction of low sodium levels (hyponatraemia) resulting in neurological compromise (central pontine myelinolysis) in a previously fit and well 45-year-old man. It should be read in conjunction with Chapter 21 and also the *Disability* section of the book.

Hyponatraemia is a common electrolyte imbalance found in the hospital setting. It occurs from sodium loss, water gain or inadequate sodium intake. Common causes include loss of electrolytes from the gut through diarrhoea and vomiting, water excess from over infusion of 5% dextrose or over use of diuretics. Medical conditions resulting in hyponatraemia include kidney disease, severe cardiac failure and liver cirrhosis (Kumar and Clark, 2002).

Central pontine myelinolysis (CPM) is a recognised complication of hyponatraemia and its overly rapid correction (Tosaka and Kohga, 1998; Chalela and Kattah, 1999; Seiser *et al.*, 1999; Afsari and Posin, 2002). It is a condition that does not occur spontaneously; rather it is a complication of treatment for other conditions.

Given its iatrogenic tendencies, therefore, it is imperative that nursing and medical staff are able to recognise, assess and prevent its onset, which requires them to be competent in neurological assessment and fluid management care for their patients. This chapter covers the management of a patient with hyponatraemia and suggests appropriate correction methods. At the end of this chapter you should:

- have an understanding of the aetiology and management of low sodium levels
- have sufficient knowledge to assess, monitor and manage a patient
- be able to recognise potentially life-threatening complications.

Background and definitions

Normal serum sodium level is 135–455 mmol/L (Longmore *et al.*, 2001). Therefore hyponatraemia is defined as a sodium level below 135 mmol/L (Mattson Porth, 2006). The clinical context in which hyponatraemia develops may be helpful in differentiating acute from chronic hyponatraemia, which is relevant to its treatment (Decaux and Soupart, 2003). The functions of sodium in the body are explained in Chapter 21.

A 45-year-old man was admitted to a medical ward with a history of diarrhoea and vomiting. On admission all physical examination findings were unremarkable, but his blood sodium concentration was 109 mmol/L. He was admitted for rehydration and correction of hyponatraemia with intravenous fluids (mainly normal saline).

The following day he suffered several grand mal seizures. Arterial blood gases taken at the time showed pH 7.0, pCO_2 3.7 kPa, HCO_3 6.8 mmol/L, base deficit −24.8 (severe metabolic acidosis) and a serum sodium increased of 132 mmol/L.

Over the next day he received a large amount of normal saline rapidly and 150 mL 8.4% sodium bicarbonate to correct his acidosis. An intravenous phenytoin infusion was commenced. The following day his condition remained stable and medical management was oral fluid restriction, continuation of intravenous fluids, and measurement of electrolytes. He then suffered two further seizures with a diagnosis of seizures secondary to rapid sodium correction and a severe metabolic acidosis of unknown cause.

The critical care outreach team was called to review the patient due to his decreased conscious level. Intensive care intervention was requested and a diagnosis of central pontine myelinolysis was assumed. Blood test results were obtained for this patient over the previous day:

TIME	23:15	00:05	01:55
pH	7.0	7.05	7.38
pCO_2	3.7	2.5	4.05
HCO_3	6.8	5.1	17.6
Base excess	− 24.8	− 25.7	− 5.9
Sodium	132	–	130
Lactate	–	–	1.8

Physiology of hyponatraemia

The principal site of sodium regulation in the body is the kidney. Sodium balance is closely related to extracellular fluid volume and sodium depletion is closely associated with hypovolaemia. Disorders of sodium concentration are best thought of as disorders of *body water* content. Sodium content of the blood is regulated by volume receptors and water content is adjusted to maintain normal osmolality. Osmolality is osmotic pressure measured in osmoles per kg of solvent (water). Salt-deficient hyponatraemia, as occurred in the case scenario, is due to salt loss in excess of water. This is commonly due to diarrhoea and vomiting.

Antidiuretic hormone (ADH) is initially suppressed, therefore the urine is more dilute with blood sodium levels being maintained. As volume is lost, osmoreceptors stimulate thirst and the release of antidiuretic hormone. ADH concentrates urine as more water is reabsorbed in the collecting tubules, so that circulating volume is restored at the expense of serum osmolality.

With normal kidneys, urinary excretion of sodium falls in response to volume depletion and water excretion. This results in concentrated urine with a sodium of < 10 mmol/L. If hyponatraemia has developed slowly the brain will have adapted by decreasing intracellular osmolality. A rapid rise in extracellular (serum) sodium will result in severe shrinking of brain cells and central pontine myelinolysis. This is due to the osmotic shift of water from a low solute concentration to a high solute concentration (Kumar and Clark, 2002).

Physiology of central pontine myelinolysis (CPM)

This condition is characterised by nerve damage caused by the destruction of the covering layer (myelin sheath) of nerve cells in the brainstem (pons). The destruction of the myelin sheath that coats nerves inhibits impulse conduction within the cell and thus decreases its ability to communicate with other cells.

The mechanisms for the condition are relatively unknown (Tosaka and Kohga, 1998). One proposed mechanism of demyelination has involved osmotic shifts with harmful metabolic consequences. Another is that demyelination is caused by vasogenic oedema developing from osmotic opening of the endothelial blood–brain barrier (Tosaka and Kohga, 1998).

CPM usually presents with spastic tetraparesis (complete or partial loss of all movement and/or sensation from the neck downward) and pseudobulbar palsy. Examination may indicate involvement of all four extremities or weakness of the face, arms and legs (upper motor neuron syndromes). Reflexes may be abnormal, and eye examination may show loss of control of the eye muscles, particularly cranial nerve VI paralysis. Symptoms include weakness and muscle spasm, reduced and/or double vision, reduced alertness, and poor enunciation. Unusual clinical presentation may include extrapyramidal syndromes, ataxia and neurobehavioural syndromes such as pathological laughing and crying (Chalela and Kattah, 1999). Psychiatric manifestations such as confusion and delirium have been reported in the literature, along with behavioural changes such as personality changes and disinhibition. Florid signs of brainstem and pyramidal tract dysfunction usually overshadow neuropsychiatric symptoms.

CPM is an emergency disorder with no known cure. Treatment is focused on relieving symptoms, with the prognosis involving persistence of serious chronic disability (Afsari and Posin, 2002). However, there are some reversible causes with acute oedema that subsides and there are reports of remyelination occurring (Tosaka and Kohga, 1998). An MRI scan, which in the early stages may be normal, is the primary diagnostic study. Serum sodium levels are also imperative.

Assessment

On examination the patient in the case scenario was lying on his back with a nasopharyngeal airway in situ and he appeared comatose. He opened his eyes briefly to his name but no other response could be elicited. He was monitored but had no oxygen in situ and he was clammy, sweating.

Immediate care

Airway management is the priority in a patient who has disordered conscious level. This man in the case scenario had his airway maintained with a nasopharyngeal airway. However, because of the initial finding of a Glasgow Coma Score of 5/15, he was placed for his own safety in the left lateral position to ensure absolute protection of his airway despite the nasopharyngeal airway and before any further assessment was carried out. The results of the physical assessment can be found in Box 22.1.

Discussion and implications for practice

The diagnosis of CPM for this man was a grave one. He had received large amounts of supplementary intravenous sodium rapidly to correct his hyponatraemia. He was clearly exhibiting adverse signs and symptoms with great risk to his airway and prognosis. The knowledge and skill base of the nursing and medical staff was key to his management and prevention of the condition. A patient such as this requires a thorough neurological assessment at regular intervals, and timely reporting of any trends and changes.

The nursing care of these patients includes a comprehensive assessment of airway, breathing, circulation, and disability (neurological status). Routinely nursing staff undertake vital sign observations, including an assessment of conscious level, such as AVPU (**A**lert, responds to **V**erbal stimulation or command, responds to **P**ainful stimuli, **U**nresponsive) (NICE, 2007).

In this particular patient, formal neurological observations were not recorded. It was difficult, therefore, to ascertain a trend with regard to his deterioration. An important aspect of managing acutely ill patients is reviewing their response to any treatment and interventions instigated (NICE, 2007). This includes reviewing results and tests and also any trends, not only with respect to vital signs but also fluid management. Correcting this patient's hyponatraemia too rapidly may cause a deterioration in conscious level and the onset of CPM. With chronic hyponatraemia, correction of serum sodium should be no more than 15 mmol/L of sodium per day to minimise the risk of such complications (Longmore *et al.*, 2001). Longmore and colleagues also suggest that in emergency situations like this one, serum sodium should be raised gradually to 125 mmol/L with saline (perhaps also using furosemide). They recommend healthcare professionals observe the patient closely for signs of heart failure and CPM. Expert help should be sought in these situations, and referral to the intensive care unit may be needed for a patient whose conscious level and airway are compromised.

Monitoring includes continuous cardiac and oxygen saturation monitoring. Frequency of vital sign recording needs to be assessed at the time and decided according to the patient's condition. Neurological observations on this patient should have been undertaken every 15 minutes, and reduced to 30 minutes when stabilised. He also required a fluid chart, which was carefully kept in this case.

A diagnosis of CPM was suspected and supported by a specialist neurological unit who were contacted for advice. As a result of supportive management the patient continued to improve and made a recovery to his previous level of health. An MRI scan performed several days later confirmed a diagnosis of CPM.

Box 22.1   Physical assessment of patient in case scenario

Respiratory system

Inspection:
— Patent airway maintained, equal chest expansion
— No peripheral or central cyanosis
— Respiratory rate 24 breaths per minute; deep breathing
— No use of accessory muscles
— Oxygen saturations 98% on air

Palpation:
— Trachea central with symmetrical expansion

Percussion:
— Both lung fields resonant

Auscultation:
— Bilateral vesicular breath sounds, quiet to bases
— No added sounds

Cardiovascular system

Heart rate monitored in sinus tachycardia rate 104 per minute
Blood pressure 140/70 mmHg
Temperature 36.5°C
Patient sweating and clammy
Peripherally warm with capillary refill of 1–2 seconds

Neurological system

Glasgow Coma Scale 5/15 (eyes 3, verbal 1, motor response 1)
Nasopharyngeal airway tolerated
Pupils size 3 and both reactive to light
Phenytoin infusion in progress to control seizures

Summary of remaining relevant assessment

10 mL dilute urine in 3 hours
Urine positive for ketones, blood protein and glucose
No intravenous fluids running
Positive balance of 3 litres from previous day
No oral intake for last 12 hours due to reduced level of consciousness
Blood glucose 10.9 mmol/L
Abdomen soft

Conclusions

This man in the current scenario was clearly exhibiting adverse signs and symptoms with great risk to his airway and prognosis. The knowledge and skill base of the nursing and medical staff was key to his management and to prevent any worsening of his condition. It required thorough neurological assessments at regular intervals and timely reporting of any trends and changes. CPM carries with it a poor prognosis, but while it is not commonly seen in general wards, drowsiness due to a low serum sodium is a common condition and is often overlooked as healthcare professionals search elsewhere for a cause. This chapter has outlined a severe case of hyponatraemia that required urgent intervention by critical care, close monitoring and management of fluid status, electrolytes, neurological care and airway management.

References and further reading

Afsari, K. and Posin, J.P. (2002). Central pontine myelinolysis. *Annals of Internal Medicine*, **137**(6), 553.

Chalela, J. and Kattah, J (1999). Catatonia due to central pontine and extrapontine myelinolysis: Case report. *Journal of Neurology, Neurosurgery, and Psychiatry*, **67**, 692–93.

Decaux, G. and Soupart, A. (2003). Treatment of symptomatic hyponatraemia. *The American Journal of Medical Sciences*, July, 25–30.

Kumar, P. and Clark, M. (2002). *Clinical Medicine*, 5th edn. London, Saunders.

Longmore, M., Wilkinson, I. and Torok, E. (2001). *Oxford Handbook of Clinical Medicine, 5th edn*. Oxford, Oxford University Press.

Mattson Porth, C. (2006). *Essentials of Pathophysiology. Concepts of Altered Health States*. London, Lippincott Williams and Wilkins.

National Institute for Health and Clinical Excellence (2007). *NICE Guideline 50: Acutely ill patients in hospital: Recognition and response to acute illness in adults in hospital*. London, NICE.

Seiser, A., Schwarz, S., Aichinger-Steiner, MM, Funk, G., Schnider, P. and Brainin, M. (1998). Parkinsonism and dystonia in central pontine and extrapontine myeliolysis. *Journal of Neurology, Neurosurgery, and Psychiatry*, **6**(1), 119–21.

Tosaka, M. and Kohga, H. (1998). Extrapontine myelinolysis and behavioural change after transphenoidal pituitary surgery: Case report. *Neurosurgery*, **43**(4), 993–96.

Springhouse, A. (2006). *Fluids and Electrolytes. A 2-in-1 Reference for Nurses*. London, Lippincott, Williams and Wilkins.

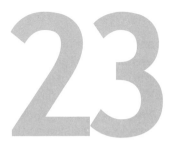

Diabetic ketoacidosis

Russell Canavan

Diabetic ketoacidosis is a true medical emergency that, if managed well, can be rewarding to treat. Early appropriate diagnosis and treatment results in a patient that will get better very quickly. This chapter cannot replace your Trust guidelines, but it can give an insight into the principles of management when dealing with such a patient.

By the end of this chapter you should:

- understand the principles behind the management of diabetic ketoacidosis
- provide insight into management of patients with diabetic ketoacidosis.

Background and definitions

Insulin is an obligatory anabolic steroid that is produced as pre-insulin in the pancreas. There is cleavage of pre-insulin to insulin and C peptide, which is then released into the portal circulation. This then passes via the liver to the systemic circulation where it acts on the insulin receptors (Pessin, 2000).

Diabetes mellitus comprises of a number of conditions related to insulin that lead to a state of chronic hyperglycaemia and subsequent organ damage. The main two types of diabetes are known as type 1 and type 2.

Type 1 diabetes

Type 1 diabetes is an autoimmune condition characterised by destruction of the insulin-secreting pancreatic cells. It occurs at an early age and as the pancreatic cells are destroyed the portal and systemic levels of insulin fall. Insulin drives movement of glucose from the serum into the cell. Extreme low intracellular glucose stimulates production of glucose via lipolysis, where fats are broken down producing ketones and fatty acids.

It is important to note that only a small amount of insulin is needed to avoid ketoacidosis. In type 1 diabetics the absence of insulin means that lipolysis is high, producing large amounts of ketones and leading to diabetic ketoacidosis (DKA).

Type 2 diabetes

Type 2 diabetes is characterised by peripheral insulin resistance. The pancreas is stimulated to produce very high circulating levels of insulin. After many years the pancreas starts to fail and levels of insulin reduce. As there is still circulating insulin, ketoacidosis does not occur. Glucose levels rise much higher and exceed the renal threshold. Glucose in the urine acts as an osmotic diuretic and the patient becomes dehydrated. It continues until the patient becomes hyperosmolar. This is known as hyperosmolar non-ketosis (HONK) or hyperosmolar hyperglycaemic syndrome (HHS).

Diabetic ketoacidosis is a catastrophic metabolic condition, whereby no physiologically significant circulating insulin is present. It results in a metabolic acidosis (pH < 7.3 or bicarbonate < 15 mmol/L), ketonuria and often hyperglycaemia (although this is not a necessary criterion). Approximately half of patients with DKA have an underlying source of infection.

Case Scenario

A 17-year-old girl with known diabetes has a long history of non-attendance and is admitted via the emergency department with abdominal pain and vomiting. You are asked to review her as she is clearly unwell.

A—Airway
She is maintaining her own airway.

B—Breathing
Her respiratory rate is 30 per minute with saturation of 100% on air. Her chest is clear.

C—Circulation
She is cold and clammy to touch but all pulses are present. She has a blood pressure of 95/50 mmHg.

D—Disability
She is drowsy and groaning but responsive to voice. Her capillary blood glucose is noted to be raised at 14 mmol/L.

E—Exposure and Environment
She is covered in vomit.

Physical examination reveals:

—Inspection: As above.
—Palpation: She is guarding over her abdomen.
—Percussion: Her abdomen is tympanic.
—Auscultation: She has a succussion splash (see Box 23.1).

Box 23.1	**Succusion splash**

To test for a succussion splash, explain to the patient what you are about to do. Place your stethoscope over his or her stomach and gently rock the abdomen. If there is a large gastric residual (in this case secondary to gastroparesis/gastric stasis) then a 'splash' will be heard.

HOT TIPS

A high respiratory rate with normal saturations could be a sign of acidaemia.

DKA can rarely present with a normal glucose.

50% of DKA patients have underlying infection.

Only some people can smell ketones.

Diagnosis of diabetic ketoacidosis

Unless this is a first presentation, the patient is a known diabetic. They may have a preceding illness, or may have missed their insulin. The patient can have a wide variety of symptoms such as abdominal pain and vomiting. They are likely to have polyuria and polydypsia.

On examination, patients vary from acutely unwell to unconscious and peri-arrest. The patient's condition is related to the speed of onset of the illness and the severity of the metabolic disturbance. You may smell acetone (pear drops) on their breath. See Box 23.2 for criteria for the diagnosis of DKA.

Box 23.2	**Criteria for the diagnosis of diabetic ketoacidosis (De Beer *et al.*, 2008)**

1. Hyperglycaemia

Serum glucose of > 13.9 mmol/L. It is worth noting that the hyperglycaemia may not be very high. Patients with even mild hyperglycaemia can be in florid ketoacidosis.

2. Ketosis

Often smelt on the breath as pear drops (acetone). A significant proportion of the population cannot smell acetone. A urine dip stick for ketonuria is essential.

3. Acidaemia

On arterial blood, a pH of < 7.3 or serum bicarbonate of < 15 mmol/L. A venous bicarbonate may be reassuring if normal, but the presenting arterial pH indicates the severity of the illness.

See Chapter 41 on interpreting blood gases for more information.

Pathophysiology, aetiology and mechanism of condition and therapy

Diabetes care and support has improved in recent years but some patients find it difficult to accept their condition and comply with their treatment; these issues often complicate their care so it is important to contact the diabetic team for information. Engaging some patients can be challenging and a non-critical approach is essential.

The patient in the case scenario has lost contact with her diabetes service and was likely to be neglecting glycaemic control. It is still possible that she has another underlying medical condition that has precipitated her deterioration. Hyperglycaemia itself causes gastroparesis and abdominal pain so this maybe a manifestation of DKA rather than the primary pathology.

Despite having hyperglycaemic serum, intracellular glucose is low. Insulin signalling is mandatory for transmembrane glucose transport. Soon the intracellular glucose is used up and the body switches to fat metabolism. The metabolism of fat leads to the production of ketones and acidaemia.

Patients with hyperglycaemia often pass glucose into their urine and this acts as an osmotic diuretic, causing excessive loss of water. The patients often feel very thirsty but, if they are unable to drink, they will dehydrate very quickly. Patients can be grossly dehydrated (by up to 10 litres or more) – in both intracellular and extracellular compartments.

Assessment, monitoring and management

Every unit should have its own guidelines on DKA, which should be followed meticulously. Early discussion with a diabetologist should be sought for every patient in DKA. Often they know the patient well or have been looking after them for many years. Early aggressive treatment gives satisfying results but it is not uncommon for a patient to decline or fail to improve if not carefully monitored. A venous line occlusion or insulin pump failure can be left alarming for a few minutes, leading to a decline in the patient's clinical condition. Meticulous monitoring of infusions and serum biochemistry can have the patient well by the next day.

A—Airway

In this scenario the patient is well. If there is any change in conscious level then airway protection is vital. Patients with DKA have a high incidence of gastroparesis and are at high risk of aspiration.

B—Breathing

Patients may seem to have abnormally deep respirations as a way of hyperventilating. This is known as Kussmaul's breathing (Kussmaul, 1874).

C—Circulation

Vital signs should be under regular monitoring (according to local guidelines, usually a minimum of half-hourly in the acute phase) and, if there is cardiovascular comorbidity, a central line should be considered.

Fluid

Insulin and fluid replacement are priorities in a patient with DKA following your **ABCDE** approach. It should be done during the clinical assessment in consultation with the local guidelines. Do not be reassured by a good urine output as this may be the *osmotic diuretic (glucose) effect*.

In the past, a patient could be up to 10 litres dehydrated, but more modern insulins mean that patients lapse into DKA much faster and, therefore, tend not to get quite so dehydrated. Although treatment with fluids is the priority some patients may need central line monitoring if they are at risk of cardiac disease.

Initially the patient should be given 0.9% saline, but 5% dextrose can be given as the blood glucose falls. Initially, fluid resuscitation is the priority, but after the first 2 hours a more considered approach is required. Too much sodium or fluid can lead to neurological sequelae (De Beer *et al.*, 2008).

Bicarbonate is a contentious issue. It is an alkali and, therefore, should increase the pH and relieve the acidaemia by forming H_2CO_3. This is then broken down to CO_2 and H_2O. Sadly HCO_3^- cannot cross the cell membrane and so does not increase the intracellular pH. In the worst case scenario, the CO_2 produced from the bicarbonate could cross the cell membrane and lower the pH further, making intracellular conditions worse. If used at all it should be reserved for those with very low pH.

Insulin

Only a small amount of insulin is needed to switch off fatty acid metabolism. Intravenous insulin (such as Actrapid™) has a half-life of 4–7 minutes; this means that an interruption to the infusion (such as bending of the arm, occlusion of the infusion, or the pump stops) can cause the patient to deteriorate very quickly.

HOT TIPS

There must be no interruption to the insulin pump for any reason. Patients are often being disconnected, taken for imaging, and so on, so everyone needs to be aware of the importance of *not* stopping this insulin infusion.

It is recommended that you follow local hospital guidelines for the insulin regimen. Initially, a continuous insulin infusion can be given until the capillary blood sugar starts to come down. At this point the patient is swapped to a sliding-scale insulin. Sliding scales are adjusted from a retrospective measurement of the hour before and so do not tell you of the patient's requirement in the next hour (for example, if the patient is eating). The amount of insulin needed to maintain normoglycaemia will vary between patients and also depend on insulin resistance. Hence a sliding scale may need to be revised. An example of a sliding scale that is very easy to remember is shown in Table 23.1.

Table 23.1   An easy to remember sliding scale (infusion set up as a 50 units of short-acting insulin (e.g. human Actrapid™) made up to 50 mL with 0.9% saline and infused against fluid)

Capillary glucose (mL per hour)	Rate (units per hour)
0–5	0.5
5–10	2
10–15	4
15 +	6 (Call for a doctor)

A type 1 diabetic *must* always have a small dose of insulin in progress, even if the blood sugar is low or normal. This is because the short half life of intravenous insulin means that, by the next hourly capillary blood glucose, the patient will be ketotic again.

> **HOT TIPS**
>
> Intravenous insulin has a short half-life so any interruption to the infusion can be fatal in a patient who is insulin dependent.

Potassium

The patient is initially acidaemic, dehydrated and insulin depleted; this leads to hyperkalaemia as potassium leaks from intra- to extracellular spaces. As the biochemistry corrects and potassium re-enters the cell, it is not uncommon to see a dramatic drop in the serum potassium – this should be closely monitored (at least every 4 hours initially). Even when the potassium is normal, supplemental potassium should be given according to local guidelines as insulin will continue to push serum potassium intracellularly (see Chapter 21).

Nasogastric tube

A patient with poorly controlled diabetes may have an underlying autonomic neuropathy that leads to gastroparesis. Hyperglycaemia itself can also precipitate this and so patients may well have litres of stomach contents that do not empty. If a patient is drowsy they are at high risk of aspiration. Too avoid needless deaths, patients at risk of aspiration should have their stomach emptied by a large-bore nasogastric tube. In the current case scenario, the patient had already vomited but patients may be asymptomatic until they aspirate.

Infection

There may well be an underlying source infection precipitating the admission. Blood cultures should be taken and, if indicated, a broad-spectrum antibiotic started. This is a clinical decision as the white cell count maybe raised anyway in DKA. In this scenario, the patient is unlikely to have a surgical cause for her abdominal pain and vomiting. Having said this, it is not unreasonable to ask the surgical team for their opinion. She may have, for example, appendicitis precipitating the DKA.

Heparin

Patients with DKA or HHS are hypercoagulable and immobile. It is important that they have prophylactic heparin when in hospital.

Monitoring

This very much depends on the state of the patient. Some patients with DKA improve quickly and ask to leave. If you can convince them to stay, and their bloods are not too far from normal, it would not be unreasonable to monitor them on the ward, making sure there is no interruption to the insulin therapy.

If the patient is hyperkalaemic or significantly acidaemic, cardiac monitoring will be needed. Diabetic patients are at risk of cardiac disease and should be considered for central line monitoring. If the patient is hypotensive, then they may need catheterisation. Monitoring of bloods should be done at least every 4 hours initially. Frequency of blood gases will depend on the patient's condition. If gases are being done regularly, a patient may benefit from an arterial line.

Aftercare

An episode of DKA should never be assumed to be a 'one off' and there are a number of treatment options available to the diabetes team, following an episode of DKA. They may know the patient well and be able to offer physical, social, and psychological support in conjunction with community services. To prevent long-term problems, reduce the chance of readmission, and provide continuity of care, patients should be seen by the diabetes team prior to discharge.

Hyperglycaemic hyperosmolar syndrome (HHS)

HHS is less common than DKA in current western practice. Patients with HHS are usually more elderly, have multiple comorbidities, have a very high glucose, and have a high mortality. Often the deterioration is triggered by sepsis. As the patient is not ketotic, they can progress to more marked hyperglycaemia until their blood becomes more akin to treacle (hyperosmolar). This leads to the patients being more at high risk of ischaemic or thrombotic events (Scott, 2006).

If the serum sodium is high in a hyperglycaemic patient, then this should raise the suspicion of HHS. Sending a serum osmolality as well as a glucose on these patients will confirm the diagnosis. See Box 23.3 for more on the diagnosis of HHS.

Box 23.3 Diagnosis of hyperglycaemic hyperosmolar syndrome (HHS)
Blood glucose   > 35 mmol/L Serum osmolality   > 320 mmol/L

Patients with HHS have a high mortality and care needs to be taken not to fluid overload the patient or correct the biochemistry too fast. The full management of HHS is beyond the scope of this book but most hospitals have guidelines that can be followed for treatment.

Conclusions

DKA is a time consuming medical emergency that requires attention to detail. Careful watch on insulin and fluid infusions, close biochemical monitoring, and airway protection to prevent aspiration are all required. It is quite rewarding to see both the patient and their biochemistry gradually improve as a direct result of your care.

References and further reading

De Beer, K., Michael, S., Thacker, M., *et al.* (2008). Diabetic ketoacidosis and hyperglycaemic hyperosmolar syndrome – Clinical guidelines. *Nursing in Critical Care*, **13**(1), 5–11.

Kussmaul, A. (1874). Zur Lehre vom Diabetes mellitus. Über eine eigenthümliche Todesart bei Diabetischen, über Acetonämie, Glycerin-Behandlung des Diabetes und Einspritzungen von Diastase in's Blut bei dieser Krankheit. *Deutsches Archiv für Klinische Medicin, Leipzig*, **14**, 1–46.

Pessin, E. and Saltiel, A. (2000). Signaling pathways in insulin action: molecular targets of insulin resistance. *Journal of Clinical Investigation*, **106**(2), 165–69.

Scott, A. (2006). Hyperosmolar hyperglycaemic syndrome. *Diabetic Medicine*, **23**(Suppl.3), 22–41.

Useful websites

Diabetes UK
www.diabetes.org.uk

National Library for Health
www.library.nhs.uk/diabetes

Emedicine
www.emedicine.com/emerg/topic135.htm

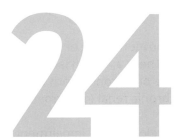

24 Renal failure

Russell Canavan

Renal failure is a common condition (Palevsky, 2006) where the excretory and metabolic function of the kidneys is insufficient to meet the requirement of the body. The nephron is the functional unit of the kidney and has both passive and active functions in the handling of water and electrolytes. The kidney also has a role in blood pressure control, in stimulation of haemoglobin synthesis, and in bone metabolism.

By the end of this chapter you should be able to identify patients at risk of renal impairment and manage those patients in established renal failure.

Case Scenario

A 43-year-old male lorry driver with a history of hypertension is admitted with shortness of breath. He has not been well for some time but has been reluctant to seek help from his GP. He is normally on lisinopril 10 mg once daily but is away from home and has missed a couple of days of medication. On arrival he is slightly agitated and confused.

A—Airway
He is maintaining his own airway.

B—Breathing
His respiratory rate is raised to 24 breaths per minute and his pulse oximeter reads 89% FiO$_2$ 0.21 increasing to 100% FiO$_2$ 0.85. Auscultation of his lungs reveals bi-basal crepitations.

C—Circulation
His pulses are all present but he has a blood pressure of 195/136 mmHg which is repeated and still remains elevated.

D—Disability
He is alert on AVPU (see Box 2.1) but is agitated and slightly confused. Pupils are normal.

E—Exposure and Environment
There is nothing else to note.

Presentation of renal impairment

Often renal impairment is identified in the asymptomatic individual by the monitoring of urea and electrolytes (U&Es) or is noted as low urine output by the ward staff. These are both late signs in renal impairment. Renal impairment can be acute, chronic or acute on chronic. Both acute and chronic renal failure has some preventable underlying causes. Chronic renal impairment is managed by a nephrologist.

It is sometimes possible to anticipate which patients will develop renal impairment, for example in a patient who has overdosed on paracetamol or a patient with prolonged hypotension, ischaemia, or hypoxia. These patients should be adequately hydrated, and drugs that may compromise renal function avoided.

The RIFLE classification of renal impairment is an attempt to classify renal impairment to deliver appropriate care (Box 24.1).

Box 24.1 The RIFLE classification of renal impairment (Bellomo, 2007)	
R (Risk)	Creatinine increased by 1.5 (glomerular filtration rate, GFR, down by 25%) which equates to a urine output of < 0.5 mL/kg/hour for at least 6 hours.
I (Injury)	Creatinine increased by 2 × (GFR down by 50%) which equates to a urine output of < 0.5 mL/kg/hour for 12 hours.
F (Failure)	Creatinine increased by 3 × (GFR down by 75%) which equates to a urine output of ≥ 4 ml/kg/hour or anuria for 12 hours.
L (Loss)	Persistent renal failure for > 4 weeks.
E (Endstage)	Loss of renal function for > 3 months.

Interpretation of data

Low urine output

Firstly check there is not a blockage or leak in the catheter, otherwise the patient may have renal impairment. Complete anuria is a blocked catheter until proved otherwise. Most commonly this is pre-renal (dehydration) but not always. A fluid challenge maybe helpful in assessing whether the patient is dehydrated. Accurate fluid balance charts are crucial and good liaison with ward staff to ensure the quality of the charts is vital in early identification and monitoring of renal failure.

Creatinine

Creatinine (40–80 μmol/L in women; 60–110 μmol/L in men) is produced by the breakdown of creatine in the body and is filtered by the glomerulus. It gives an estimated glomerular filtration rate but there are a number of confounding factors. As a breakdown product of muscle it can be artificially low in thin people. It also follows a logarithmic curve so that a change of 100 to 150 is vital but one of 400 to 450 is less so.

Recently the term eGFR has been introduced; eGFR is the estimated GFR calculated by the equation:

$$186.3 \times (\text{creatinine}) - 1.154 \times (\text{age}) - 0.203 \times (0.742 \text{ if female}) \times (1.210 \text{ if black})$$

This is widely employed, but should be used with caution in the setting of acute kidney injury.

Urea

This is a useful measurement to undertake in patients if it is relatively much higher than the creatinine would indicate. This implies the patient is dehydrated or had a significant upper gastrointestinal bleed.

Potassium

This is a vital anion in cellular signalling. It is nearly all held intracellularly and low levels exist in the plasma. Small rises of plasma potassium can lead to life-threatening arrhythmias (see Chapter 21).

pH

pH is a logarithmic scale of hydrogen ions. Small changes outside the physiological pH lead to inactivation of cellular enzymes. There are a number of buffering systems in the body, which counteract small changes to maintain a stable pH. Consequently acidaemia only occurs in extreme pathological states and is considered a poor prognostic factor in most disorders.

Sodium

Sodium is actively re-absorbed in the nephron. Damage to the nephron (e.g. acute tubular necrosis) results in a high loss of sodium in the urine (urinary sodium > 40 µmols/litre). In pre-renal failure the urinary sodium will be low (< 20 µmols/litre) as the kidney tries to conserve water (see Chapter 21).

Urine osmolality

This is useful for establishing the cause of renal impairment (pre-renal versus renal). In pre-renal failure the urine will be concentrated (> 500 mmol/litre). In intrinsic renal failure the kidney loses its ability to concentrate urine and produces dilute urine (< 350 mmol/litre).

Causes of renal failure

Pre-renal causes

Often it is due to dehydration or renal hypoperfusion but it can be due to renal artery stenosis or secondary to liver failure. Classically small volumes of concentrated urine are produced.

Renal causes

This includes diseases of either the glomerulus or tubules. Acute kidney injury (Bonventre, 2007) is most commonly seen on the ward. Other causes include drugs, glomerulonephritis, myeloma, haemolysis and rhabdomyolysis (see below for further explanation). In these conditions the kidney loses its ability to concentrate urine and often the patient produces dilute urine. In many of the above causes the urine dipstick will show at least significant proteinuria or haematuria.

Post-renal causes

Obstruction to the collecting system can be caused at any level and by renal stones or soft tissues (e.g. tumours, prostate, urethral strictures).

Acute tubular necrosis (ATN)

This is a common condition in the acutely ill patient. Either ischaemia or toxins damage the tubular cells. This leads to a reduction in the ability of the tubules to reabsorb water. The key to avoiding ATN is to avoid prolonged ischaemia or hypoxia and to ensure adequate filling.

Rhabdomyolysis

In acute muscle injury (whether through trauma or acute muscle disease) there can be a large amount of myoglobin in the serum. This is filtered into the urine and can cause damage to the renal tubules. It is characterised by dipstick positive *haemoglobinuria* (it is actually myoglobin) but negative urine microscopy for red cells, in the presence of a marked rise in serum creatinine kinase and renal impairment.

Emergency treatment

According to Thadhani (1996) you should consider the following.

Precipitants

Avoid these. It is not uncommon to find the patient on hypotensive agents, ACE inhibitors, non-steroidal anti-inflammatories, etc. Even if these are not the cause of the renal failure, in the short term you should consider stopping them. Seek senior advice if patient has cardiac problems before stopping the drugs.

Fluid balance

Early recognition is key. If unsure, then a fluid challenge with 250 mL of crystalloid is unlikely to cause much harm and, following re-assessment, may tell you the patient's fluid status. The aid of a central venous line in managing fluid challenges is highly recommended. If the patient is overloaded then loop diuretics may help such as furosemide (Sumnall, 2007). A diuretic-sensitive patient may only need small doses of a loop diuretic to start with, but other people require large doses as a driver. Remember the action of furosemide lasts for 6 hours (hence Lasix™) and then the urine output will tail off again. Patients who are fluid overloaded and resistant to diuretics may require removal of the fluid using renal replacement therapy; referral to the intensive care team will be required.

Potassium

If greater than 6.0 mmol/L treatment is usually recommended. The patient should have cardiac monitoring and their ECG assessed for signs of cardiac involvement. If treatment is indicated then it is generally accepted that 50 mL of 50% glucose with 8 units of Actrapid™ insulin can be given as an infusion, and then check potassium. If there is evidence of cardiac involvement then 10 mL of 10% calcium gluconate is advised to stabilise the myocardium. If this fails, then salbutamol, furosemide or exchange resins may all be useful. If they all fail, then renal replacement may be called for.

pH

Acidaemia is not well tolerated. Sodium bicarbonate can normalise the extracellular pH but can worsen intracellular acidaemia. Appropriate fluid balance and oxygenation are often enough to correct acidaemia.

Renal replacement

The choice of therapy and when to start treatment depends on an overall assessment of the patient (Formica *et al.*, 2007; Himmelfarb, 2007). Most commonly in the UK in the acute setting the chosen therapy is haemofiltration. Generally, if the potassium, acidaemia and fluid overload fail to respond to medical therapy then renal replacement should be considered. There are essentially four main types of renal replacement.

1. *Dialysis:* This is used for chronic renal failure patients. Blood is run past a semipermeable membrane with fluid running on the other side of it. Toxins in the blood pass across the membrane by osmosis. Haemodialysis takes the blood out of the body through a line or fistula and runs it through an external membrane against a very pure water countercurrent with added solutes. Peritoneal dialysis uses the peritoneum as a dialysis membrane. Fluid is placed into the peritoneum via a peritoneal catheter and then washed out again. In both of the above, oncotic pressure is the predominant force. The amount of fluid removed can be determined by the concentration of the dialysate and the time given for fluid to diffuse across the membrane (see Box 24.1).

2. *Filtration:* This is used for acute renal failure patients who have failed to respond to medical therapy. It is a commonly available technique within the intensive care unit. Blood flows past a semipermeable membrane and hydrostatic pressure is used to extract waste products (e.g. water, potassium and hydrogen ions).

3. *Transplant:* When a patient is stable on long-term renal replacement this may be an option. It is used in chronic renal failure and needs specialist referral to a transplant centre.

4. *Haemodiafiltration:* More recently, haemodiafiltration has been developed that is half way between dialysis and haemofiltration. There is a theoretical benefit of being able to combine the advantages of both techniques. Some trials have been hopeful (Page *et al.*, 2005) but more are needed.

> **Box 24.1   Managing patients on haemodialysis and continuous ambulatory peritoneal dialysis**
>
> It is preferable to manage *haemodialysis* patients in their base hospital, but occasionally patients are admitted to a hospital other than their own. Close liaison with the renal unit can help with managing drugs and fluid balance, as well as renal-related problems. With good communication the only problem is logistical. Patients have to be off the ward having dialysis and therefore miss scans, for example, and often have longer stays in hospital.

Patients on *continuous ambulatory peritoneal dialysis* (CAPD) are seen less often by the renal unit and so are often managed in hospitals other than their home unit. Renal teams are still keen to help with their management. Patients are normally independent, normally exchanging one bag of fluid four times per day. Essentially they have a catheter passing through the skin into the peritoneal cavity. The old dialysis solution is passed via the catheter into a waste product bag. The peritoneal cavity is then filled with a fresh bag of fluid for another 5 hours. The amount of fluid dialysed off can be altered by changing the osmolality of the dialysate solution. Solutions of varying strength are colour-coded and patients often mention their 'green' or 'yellow' bags. Again fluid, drugs and diagnosis can be made much easier by liaising with the renal team

Scenario review

This case in the current scenario is likely to represent a hypertensive renal crisis. The diagnosis is confirmed by end-organ damage. The basal crackles represent pulmonary oedema (cardiac failure), the agitation and confusion represent leukoencephalopathy (brain failure), and the creatinine was elevated with a positive urine dipstick for protein (renal failure). Further examination by fundoscopy showed severe hypertensive retinopathy. The patient was oliguric. Following CT head (confirming leukoencephalopathy), an ultrasound Doppler of the renal arteries confirmed there was renal artery stenosis. This was angioplastied and within 24 hours the blood pressure was settled. Over the next few days the creatinine fell and returned to almost normal. In the outpatient clinic, the patient was noted to have made a full recovery.

Conclusions

Acute renal failure (now called acute kidney injury) is a common problem in the acutely unwell patient and is often a result of the presenting illness. Early identification, fluid balance and consideration of the underlying problems can prevent deterioration of renal function. Existing renal patients can be managed away from their home unit with close cooperation with the renal team.

References and further reading

Bellomo, R., Kellum, J.A. and Ronco, C. (2007). Defining and classifying acute renal failure: from advocacy to consensus and validation of the RIFLE criteria. *Intensive Care Medicine*, **33**(3), 409–13.

Bonventre, J.V. (2007). Pathophysiology of acute kidney injury: roles of potential inhibitors of inflammation. *Contributions to Nephrology*, **156**, 39–46.

Formica, M., Inguaggiato, P., Bainotti, S., Gigliola, G. and Canepari, G. (2007). Acute renal failure in critically ill patients: indications for and choice of extracorporeal treatment. *Journal of Nephrology*, **20**(1), 15–20.

Himmelfarb, J. (2007). Continuous renal replacement therapy in the treatment of acute renal failure: critical assessment is required. *Clinical Journal of the American Society of Nephrology*, **2**(2), 385–89.

Page, B., Vieillard-Baron, A., Chergui K., *et al.* (2005). Early veno-venous haemodiafiltration for sepsis-related multiple organ failure. *Critical Care*, **9**, 755–63.

Palevsky, P.M. (2006). Epidemiology of acute renal failure: the tip of the iceberg. *Clinical Journal of the American Society of Nephrology*, **1**(1), 43–51.

Sumnall, R. (2007). Fluid management and diuretic therapy in acute renal failure. *Nursing in Critical Care*, **12**(1), 27–33.

Thadhani, R., Pascual, M. and Bonventre, J.V. (1996). Acute renal failure. *New England Journal of Medicine*, **334**, 1448–60.

Useful websites

Renal Association
www.renal.org

National Library for Health
www.library.nhs.uk/kidney

• A B C (D) E •

Disability

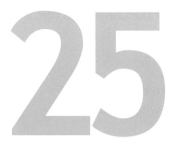

Severe acute pain in the acutely unwell patient

Jane Donn

For a number of reasons the relief of acute pain is often poorly managed. A general lack of understanding of the pharmacology and pharmacokinetics of analgesia, compounded by inappropriate attitudes and organisational barriers, has left the acutely ill patient exposed to the harmful side effects of unresolved pain.

At the end of this chapter you will:

- be able to identify the patient in acute pain
- have a working knowledge of the harmful effects of unresolved acute pain
- be able to direct logical prescribing of the most commonly used analgesics
- have an awareness of the potential barriers to effective pain management
- understand the role of patient-controlled and epidural analgesia in the acutely unwell patient.

Understanding pain

The International Association for the Study of Pain describes pain as 'an unpleasant sensory and emotional experience associated with actual or potential tissue damage, or described in terms of such damage' (Merskey and Bogduk, 1994). Acute pain is defined as 'pain of recent onset and probable limited duration. It usually has an identifiable temporal and causal relationship to injury or disease' (Ready and Edwards, 1992).

The ability to detect noxious and potentially tissue-damaging stimuli is an important protective mechanism that involves both central and peripheral mechanisms. Pain may be classified by inferred physiology into two major types: *nociceptive* pain in which stimuli arise from somatic and visceral structures and *neuropathic* pain whereby stimuli are abnormally processed by the nervous system. In the acute setting, nociceptive pain is most often encountered.

The four basic processes of pain transmission are:

- **Transduction:** This process occurs in the periphery when a noxious stimulus causes tissue damage. The damaged cell releases sensitising substances that cause an action potential.

- **Transmission:** The action potential is transmitted from the site of the damage to the spinal cord and on to the higher centres.

- **Perception of pain:** This is the conscious experience of pain.

- **Modulation:** The neurons originating in the brainstem descend to the spinal cord and release endogenous opioids, serotonin and norepinephrine which inhibit the transmission of nociceptive impulses (Pasero *et al.*, 1999).

In addition, the perception and experience of pain is overlaid with psychological, cultural and environmental factors (Linton, 2005; Pavlin *et al.*, 2005).

Harmful effects of unresolved pain

The presence of trauma, surgical insult, or the pain of disease triggers a number of physiological responses. This is called the *stress response* and the purpose of this response is to activate the sympathetic nervous system and alert the body to impending or existing harm. If left unmanaged this response can lead to a number of harmful effects (Desborough, 2000) as outlined in Table 25.1.

In addition to these potentially life-threatening physiological effects, there is a basic humanitarian imperative to prevent suffering of a fellow human being. This philosophy is supported by Liebskind and Melzack, cited by Harmer (2007), who believe that by any standard, freedom from pain should be a basic human right. Its limitations should only be our current evidence and knowledge regarding treatment.

Case Scenario

A 29-year-old man attends A&E with a history of upper abdominal pain. He describes it as severe, deep and gnawing. It travels from left of the midline through to his back. He rates the severity as 10 out of 10. The pain is reduced when he leans forward. He is sweaty and distressed.

He has been vomiting, complains of breathlessness and has a fever. His vital signs are BP 102/56 mmHg, temperature 38.2°C, heart rate 119 b.p.m. and oxygen saturation is 92% on air. He has decreased breath sounds. Bowel sounds are sluggish.

Blood tests show an amylase of 938 U/L, white blood cell count of 11.2×10^9/L, sodium 141 mmol/L, potassium 3.1 mmol/L and blood glucose of 10.3 mmol/L.

He gives a history of attending a stag weekend in Scotland and becoming unwell on the journey home. He admits to drinking large quantities of alcohol over 2 days. He has no allergies.

On catheterisation his urine is dark and concentrated and there is a residual volume of 110 mL.

Table 25.1   The effects of pain on the body (adapted from Pasero *et al.*, 1999)

System	Physiological changes	Effect on the body
Endocrine	Increased ACTH, cortisol, ADH, epinephrine, glucagon, renin, angiotensin II, catecholamines Decreased insulin, testosterone	Excess production of hormones
Metabolic	Hyperglycaemia Insulin resistance Muscle protein catabolism	Raised blood sugar
Cardiovascular	Increased heart rate, myocardial oxygen consumption, SVR Hypercoagulation	Hypertension, DVT Myocardial ischaemia Tachycardia
Respiratory	Decreased tidal volume, cough Splinting Increased respiratory rate	Sputum retention Chest infection Hypoxaemia
Genitourinary	Increased release of hormones regulating urinary output	Urinary output down Urinary retention Hypokalaemia Fluid overload
Gastrointestinal	Decreased gastric and bowel activity	Delay in return to function
Musculoskeletal	Fatigue Immobility	Pressure damage DVT Chest infection
Immune	Depression of immune system	Pneumonia Wound infection Sepsis

ACTH, adrenocorticotrophic hormone; ADH, antidiuretic hormone; DVT, deep vein thrombosis; SVR, systemic vascular resistance.

Assessing pain

The starting point of any successful pain management plan must be assessment. Because pain is a subjective experience, the gold standard is the patient's self-report of pain (McCaffery and Pasero, 1999). This approach may cause concern for those who fear being duped, but what should be remembered is that malingerers are rare. Although accepting every patient report of pain may result in being fooled by the few, the alternative to this is to doubt every patient and risking 'under-analgesing' the vast majority. If a patient is successful in duping a healthcare professional the responsibility for this rests with that patient.

Different types of validated pain assessment tools are available to the clinician and it is important to choose the right tool for the clinical situation (Bird, 2003). For the unwell patient in acute pain there are two main elements of the assessment – how *much* does it hurt and *where* does it hurt?

How much does it hurt?

The unwell patient does not want to be bothered with charts and diagrams – he or she just wants to quickly get over to you how bad things are. To this end the most useful tool is a numerical pain scale. The most commonly used scale is a scale from 0 to 10, where 0 is no pain on movement and 10 is the worst pain imaginable, but others can be used. The important factor is that the same scale is used throughout the patient's journey to ensure consistency. The patient in this case study rated his pain as 10/10.

Once the pain is better under control and the patient's condition has been stabilised, a more detailed pain history can be taken. While nociceptive pain is more frequently seen in the acute setting, misdiagnosing neuropathic pain may lead to delay in appropriate treatment. Features that may suggest neuropathic pain include:

- pain described as burning, shooting or stabbing
- hyperalgesia (a heightened response to normally painful stimuli)
- allodynia (abnormal response to a stimulus that does not normally cause pain (e.g. light stroking)
- abnormal or unpleasant sensations such as crawling, numbness or tingling (Stacey, 2005).

While neuropathic pain may be partially responsive to opioids, the ongoing management can be complex and the clinician is advised to obtain advice from the hospital pain team, or the team responsible for pain management of the patient.

Where does it hurt?

As well as ascertaining how bad the pain is, it is important to regularly check *where* the pain is. Patients do not always think to mention that the pain is now in their chest or other leg and changes in the clinical condition may be missed. This is particularly important to remember if the patient is self-administering their analgesia. Any acute change in the severity or nature of the pain in a patient whose pain has previously been well managed must result in a full re-assessment.

An inability to communicate does not mean that the patient is not experiencing pain. In the absence of a patient self-report a common-sense approach should be adopted. If a broken leg would reasonably give you pain then it will be giving your patient pain too. In addition behavioural responses such as a particular facial expression or a reluctance to use a limb, or physiological responses such as a tachycardia or raised blood pressure can indicate that your patient is in pain (Davies *et al.*, 2004). Patients with special needs or communication difficulties may need additional help to express their pain. A carer and close relative or friend may be familiar with how the patient is responding and know how to elicit a pain assessment with the staff caring for them.

The management plan

Once a pain management plan has been formulated pain assessment needs to be ongoing to enable evaluation of that plan. Further uncontrolled pain should be a trigger to a re-assessment of the diagnosis or alert to developing complications.

Having identified your patient is in pain, action needs to be swift, especially if the patient is also unwell. The healthcare professional has access to effective analgesics but they are often not used effectively. Keeping things simple and using these analgesics well will improve pain management for 99% of patients.

Step 1

Exclude any medications that the patient is allergic to or that are contraindicated (e.g. non-steroidal anti-inflammatory drugs in poor renal function, clotting abnormality and gastric ulceration). Ensure the patient is reporting an allergy and not a side effect that can be managed (e.g. nausea with opioids). Also consider what analgesics have already been tried and how the pain responded to them.

Caution is required if using opioids in patients with major organ failure by starting with less than the usual recommended dose and titrating gradually upward. All opioids are metabolised to some extent by the liver and in patients with liver disease adverse effects may be seen from higher than expected plasma concentrations. The metabolism of morphine and methadone is not significantly altered in liver disease, so these drugs are well tolerated (Portenoy, 1996).

Caution and close monitoring is recommended when using morphine in a patient with renal insufficiency. Synthetic opioids such as hydromorphone or oxycodone may be better tolerated (Portenoy, 1996).

There is no rationale for delaying the appropriate administration of an opioid to the patient presenting with an acute abdomen. There is good evidence that opioids can be safely given before assessment and diagnosis without increasing the risk of errors in diagnosis or treatment (National Institute for Clinical Studies, 2008).

For the patient in the case history, non-steroidal anti-inflammatory analgesics are contraindicated due to poor renal function.

Step 2

After allergies and contraindications have been taken into account the next step is to choose an analgesic of an appropriate strength. This is easier said than done. There are many myths and misconceptions about the relative efficacy of analgesics amongst healthcare professionals. This has led to mass under-dosing of patients and inappropriate preparations being used. Thankfully researchers have developed league tables that can enable logical progression of prescribing. Analgesics at different strengths and by different routes are allocated a number needed to treat

(NNT). The NNT is calculated from the proportion of patients with at least 50% pain relief over 4–6 hours compared with placebo (in randomised, double-blind, single-dose studies in patients with moderate to severe pain). The lower the NNT the more effective that drug or dose is likely to be. Although this may vary in individual patients, it is a good place to start!

The following is a short version of the full NNT table (Table 25.2) that is available from the Oxford Pain Research Unit (2008). Remember that relative strength may be dose related. A summary of available analgesics is given in Box 25.1.

Table 25.2   League table of analgesic efficacy and number needed to treat (Oxford Pain Research Unit)

Analgesic	No. of patients in comparison	Percent with at least 50% pain relief	Number needed to treat (NNT)
Ibuprofen 800 mg	76	100	1.6
Diclofenac 100 mg	411	67	1.8
Paracetamol 1000 mg + codeine 60 mg	197	57	2.2
Diclofenac 50 mg	738	63	2.3
Ibuprofen 600 mg	203	79	2.4
Ibuprofen 400 mg	4703	56	2.4
Morphine 10 mg (intramuscular)	946	50	2.9
Ibuprofen 200 mg	1414	45	2.7
Paracetamol 1000 mg	2759	46	3.8
Tramadol 100 mg	882	30	4.8
Tramadol 50 mg	770	19	8.3
Dihydrocodeine 30 mg	–	–	9.8
Codeine 60 mg	1305	15	16.7
Placebo	> 10,000	18	N/A

In the current case study, John requires an easily titratable analgesic suitable for severe pain. Opioids are the group of choice. Non-steroidal anti-inflammatory analgesics can be very effective for severe pain, but were contraindicated in this case.

Step 3

Having decided what you are not going to give your patient and which analgesics are likely to be effective, the available routes of administration need to be considered (Box 25.2). Does the patient have intravenous access? Is the oral route appropriate? Can the rectal route be utilised?

Step 4

Another and sometimes unsatisfactory consideration is when the patient asks what is available to me? Different institutions have different formularies and this may unfortunately play a part in your decision making. Short-acting preparations are the most appropriate for quick titration of analgesia.

Box 25.1   **Overview of available analgesics**

Non-steroidal analgesics—These are very effective for most patients (as Table 25.2 indicates) but are often the most troublesome, in terms of side effects, for the acutely unwell patient. Some analgesics are limited in use due to a maximum safe daily dose (e.g. paracetamol). Opioids, at doses that are not causing over-sedation or respiratory depression, do not have a maximum daily dose and therefore are major players in the management of severe acute pain.

Codeine—Codeine alone has limited use in the management of severe pain. Once absorbed it is metabolised in the liver to morphine, its active form (Reisine and Pasternak, 1996). However up to 8% of Caucasians cannot metabolise codeine (Kroemer and Eichelbaum, 1995).

Pethidine—Pethidine is arguably the most inappropriately used opioid for moderate to severe acute pain and therefore has deliberately not been included in this short table. Pethidine is very short acting and therefore the patient is likely to be exposed to periods of unmanaged pain. In addition (and probably more significantly) pethidine has a toxic metabolite – norpethidine. When allowed to accumulate, this acts on the central nervous system and ultimately causes convulsions, especially (but not exclusively) in patients with renal dysfunction. There is no rationale for its choice over morphine in patients with biliary colic as has previously been suggested (Nagle and McQuay, 1990).

HOT TIPS

In acutely unwell patients, remember:

— The intravenous route is the preferred choice.
— The intramuscular route is not recommended.
— Transdermal preparations play no part in acute pain management.

Step 5

The next step is to ensure that your ongoing analgesic regimen is balanced. Reliance on a single analgesic may necessitate its use at high doses and is therefore likely to be more troublesome. As a general rule, choose one analgesic from each group and use them together (e.g. paracetamol and diclofenac and morphine) but not two from the same group.

   Box 25.3 shows all the analgesic groups.   The patient in our case scenario should be administered up to 10 mg morphine intravenously and 1 g paracetamol intravenously. He should be assessed for effect after 5 and 15 minutes. The initial dose of morphine is the start dose only. Be prepared to adjust. There is no correlation between weight and analgesic requirements. Age, on the other hand, is a valid consideration (Gnjidic *et al.*, 2008). Doses should be adjusted for people at the extremes of age (Macintyre and Jarvis, 1996).

> **Box 25.2   Routes of administration**
>
> For the relief of severe acute pain, speed is of the essence and therefore the intravenous route is the preferred choice. Fine titration of dose is achievable by this route.
>
> Although commonly used, the intramuscular route of administration is *not* recommended. This route has numerous disadvantages, the key one being unreliable absorption with a 30–60 minute delay to peak effect (Austin *et al.*, 1980).
>
> Transdermal preparations play no part in acute pain management.
>
> The route of choice in the case scenario is the intravenous route. It allows rapid onset of effect and careful titration of dose.

Barriers to effective pain management

Acute pain management continues to be poorly understood and the effects of unresolved pain discounted. It is important that healthcare professionals examine their own practice and deal with any education deficits or attitude issues they have (Clarke *et al.*, 1996). The challenge for educational institutions is to ensure that pain management education is high on their list of priorities (Twycross, 2000).

It is worth noting that patients attending hospitals with 'self-inflicted' illnesses are often exposed to high levels of prejudice and negative attitude. Healthcare professionals have the same duty of care to these patients and should indeed take the opportunity to exert a positive influence. While nurses and doctors are often keen to promote smoking cessation advice, discussions about alcohol and illicit drug taking are often avoided. When the patient in the current scenario has recovered from this acute episode, the opportunity to provide health education should be taken.

Patients themselves present barriers to successful pain management. Fear of the use of opioids because of the risk of addiction is commonplace and health professionals often do nothing to correct this misunderstanding. Large studies have estimated an iatrogenic addiction rate of less than 1% (Porter and Jick, 1980). The elderly, who are also the most vulnerable, do not like to trouble nursing or medical staff and will suffer in silence. A cultural disposition may also encourage the 'stiff upper lip' approach (Davidhizar and Giger, 2004).

Hospital staff encourage the patient to endure mismanaged pain by being positive towards patients who do not request analgesia and negative towards those who do (Carr and Thomas, 1997). The correct approach is to actively encourage the patient to report pain and to simply prescribe analgesia regularly and not on an 'as and when' basis.

Organisational barriers to effective pain management also exist (Mann and Redwood, 2000; Schafheutle *et al.*, 2001). For example, it is not a legal requirement to double-check controlled drugs, but in some institutions it remains a local policy. Double-checking has not prevented error or diversion of drugs but it has been found to cause delay in analgesia administration. These risks need to be weighed up within a culture of patient safety and patient need.

Box 25.3	Analgesic groups
NSAIDs	Ibuprofen Diclofenac Aspirin Ketorolac Celecoxib
Others	Paracetamol
Opioids (weak)	Codeine Dihydrocodeine Tramadol
Opioids (strong)	Morphine Oxycodone Fentanyl Diamorphine
Adjuvants	Amitriptyline Gabapentin Diazepam
Anaesthetics	Entonox Local anaesthetics

Maintaining analgesia

Once severe escalating pain has been brought under control a plan for ongoing management is required. There are several options for this. Sticking to the principle of keeping things simple, the oral route is the preferred route but it may not be available for the acutely unwell patient if, for example, regular (as opposed to 'as and when') prescribing is likely to be most effective. Long-acting opioid preparations are available, but when dealing with acute escalating pain short-acting, quickly titratable preparations are required.

Patient-controlled analgesia

The concept of patient-controlled analgesia (PCA) allows very small doses of analgesia to be administered frequently, from a syringe pump with a timing device, on the patient's demand. Thus the patient can titrate his or her own analgesic dose within certain limits. PCA may be considered, but it is not suitable for use until pain is under control. It should be used as 'top up' rather than a 'catch up'. Patients report positively on its use (Hudcova *et al.*, 2005) although it does have disadvantages. It has been effectively used in patients with severe pain from pancreatitis (Di Vadi *et al.*, 1999).

Some patients report that nursing staff spend less time with them. Also sleep can be difficult because they are woken by pain and it may take some time before enough doses can be taken from the machine to get it back under control. One study using subcutaneous diamorphine for PCA has shown better results for night-time pain relief (Dawson *et al.*, 1999).

Continuous infusions of opioids are an alternative but if patients are not suitably observed they may cause more over-sedation because the infusion will continue even if the patient does not require analgesia at that time.

Epidural analgesia

Epidural analgesia is an effective technique for postoperative or trauma pain. The infusion of local anaesthetics and opioids into the epidural space causes blockade of afferent impulses to the brain. It has the potential to provide complete analgesia while the infusion is running. It has one major advantage over other techniques in that it can attenuate the stress response to trauma and surgery as discussed at the beginning of this chapter (Kehlet and Holte, 2001; Fotiadis *et al.*, 2004). This is a valuable effect to remember.

The use of epidural analgesia is contraindicated in patients:

- who refuse the technique
- who have local infection around the potential insertion site
- who have systemic infection or sepsis
- who have raised intracranial pressure
- who have some allergy or sensitivity to local anaesthetics
- with uncontrolled coagulation disorders.

There are several benefits of epidural analgesia:

- By limiting systemic opioid use and by blocking nociceptive and sympathetic reflexes, reduction of the duration of postoperative ileus can allow for earlier enteral feeding.
- There is a reduction in the incidence of atelectasis and chest infection.
- There is a reduction in the incidence of myocardial infarction.
- The hypercoagulable response to surgery is attenuated.

Many institutions run a ward-based epidural service and if staff are adequately trained and supervised it is a very safe technique to employ in the general ward area.

Conclusions

This chapter has aimed to guide a logical and systematic approach to developing an effective pain management plan for the acutely unwell patient. The benefits of adequate pain management have been outlined, and considerations when assessing and deciding on pain relief have been discussed. The case scenario has shown, in a practicable sense, how the pain in an acutely unwell person may be managed.

References and further reading

Austin, K., Stapleton, J. and Mather, L. (1980). Multiple intramuscular injections: a major source of variability in analgesic response to meperidine. *Pain*, **8**, 47–62.

Bird, J. (2003). Selection of pain measurement tools. *Nursing Standard*, **18**(13), 33–39.

Carr, E.C. and Thomas, V.J. (1997). Anticipating and experiencing postoperative pain: the patient's perspective. *Journal of Clinical Nursing*, **6**(3), 191–201.

Clarke, E., French, B., Bilodeau, M., Capasso, V. and Edwards, A. (1996). Pain management knowledge, attitudes and clinical practice: The impact of nurses' characteristics and education. *Journal of Pain and Symptom Management*, **11**(1), 18–31.

Davies, E., Male, M., Reimer, V. and Turner, M. (2004). Pain assessment and cognitive impairment: Part 2. *Nursing Standard*, **19**(13), 33–40.

Davidhizar, R. and Giger, J. (2004). A review of the literature on care of clients in pain who are culturally diverse. *International Nursing Review*, **51**(1), 47–55.

Dawson, L., Brockbank, K., Carr, E. and Barrett, F. (1999). Improving patient's postoperative sleep: a randomised control study comparing subcutaneous with intravenous patient-controlled analgesia. *Journal of Advanced Nursing*, **30**(4), 875–81.

Desborough, J.P. (2000). The stress response to trauma and surgery. *British Journal of Anaesthesia*, **85**(1), 109–17.

Di Vadi, P., Schnepel, B., Bunton, T., Luffingham, N., Condon, D. and Lanigan, C. (1999). The use of patient-controlled analgesia in acute and chronic relapsing pancreatitis. *The Pain Clinic*, **11**(4), 345–48.

Fotiadis, R., Badvie, S., Weston, M. and Allen-Mersh, T. (2004). Epidural analgesia in gastrointestinal surgery. *British Journal of Surgery*, **91**(7), 828–41.

Gnjidic, D., Murnion, B. and Hilmer, S. (2008). Age and opioid analgesia in an acute hospital population. *Age and Aging*, **37**(6), 699–702.

Harmer, M. (2007). Postoperative pain relief – Time to take our heads out of the sand? *Anaesthesia* **46**(3), 167–68.

Hudcova, J., McNicol, E., Quah, C., Lau, J. and Carr, D. (2005). Patient-controlled intravenous opioid analgesia versus conventional opioid analgesia for postoperative pain control: A quantitative systematic review. *Acute Pain*, **7**, 115–32.

Kehlet, H. and Holte, K. (2001). Effect of postoperative analgesia on surgical outcome. *British Journal of Anaesthesia*, 87 (1), 62–72.

Kroemer, H.K. and Eichelbaum, H.K. (1995). 'It's the genes, stupid'. The molecular bases and clinical consequences of genetic cystochrome P450 2D6. *Polymorphism, Life Sciences*, **46**(26), 2285–98.

Linton, S.J. (2000). A review of psychological risk factors in back and neck pain. *Spine*, **25**, 1148–56.

Macintyre, P.E. and Jarvis, D.A. (1996). Age is the best predictor of postoperative morphine requirements. *Pain*, **64**, 357–64.

Mann, E. and Redwood, S. (2000). Improving pain management: breaking down the invisible barrier. *British Journal of Nursing*, **9**(19), 2067–72.

McCaffery, M. and Pasero, C. (1999). Assessment. Underlying complexities, misconceptions and practical tools. In: M. McCaffery and C. Pasero (eds) *Pain: Clinical Manual*, 2nd edn. St Louis, Mosby.

Merskey, H. and Bogduk, N. (1994). Pain terms: a current list with definitions and notes on usage. *Classification of Chronic Pain*, 2nd edn. Seattle, IASP.

Nagle, K. and McQuay, H. (1990). Opioid receptors: Their role in effect and side-effect. *Current Anaesthesia and Critical Care*, **1**, 247–52.

National Institute for Clinical Studies (2008). *Pain Medication for Acute Abdominal Pain. A Summary of Best Available Evidence and Information on Current Clinical Practice*. Canberra, National Health and Medical Research Council.

Oxford Pain Research Unit (2008). *The Oxford League Table of Analgesic Efficacy*. Available at: jr2.ox.ac.uk/bandolier/booth/painpag/ (accessed June 2009).

Pasero, C., Paice, J.A. and McCaffery, M. (1999). Basic mechanisms underlying the causes and effects of pain. In: M. McCaffery and C. Pasero (eds) *Pain: Clinical Manual*, 2nd edn. St Louis, Mosby.

Pavlin, J.D., Sullivan, M.J.L., Freund, P. and Roesen, K. (2005). Catastrophizing: A risk factor for post-surgical pain. *Clinical Journal of Pain*, **21**, 83–90.

Portenoy, R.K. (1996). Opioid analgesics. In: R.K. Portenoy and R.M. Kramer (eds) *Pain Management Theory and Practice*. Phildadelphia, PA: FA Davis, pp. 249–76.

Porter, J. and Jick, H. (1980). Addiction rare in patients treated with narcotics. *New England Journal of Medicine*, **302**, 123.

Ready, L.B. and Edwards, W.T. (1992). Management of acute pain: A practical guide. *Taskforce on Acute Pain*. Seattle: IASP.

Reisine, T. and Pasternak, G. (1996). Opioid analgesics and antagonists. *The Pharmacological Basis of Therapeutics*, **9**, 521–55.

Schafheutle, E., Cantrill, J. and Noyce, P. (2001). Why is pain management suboptimal on surgical wards? *Journal of Advanced Nursing*, **33**(6):728–37.

Stacey, B.R. (2005). Management of peripheral neuropathic pain. *American Journal of Physical Medicine and Rehabilitation*, **84**, S4–16.

Twycross, A. (2000). Education about pain: a neglected area. *Nurse Education Today*, **20**, 244–53.

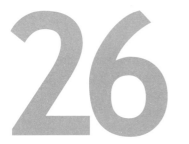

Compartment syndrome

Ann M. Price

Compartment syndrome usually occurs when an injury leads to increased pressure within a certain body space that affects the circulation and tissues (**Singh** *et al.*, **2004**). The decrease in circulation and damage to tissues can lead to deformity of the affected area, renal failure and amputation, and in severe cases death. The commonest area affected is the lower limb (**Singh** *et al.*, **2004; Sahjian and Frakes, 2007**) but compartment syndrome can occur in any space within the body and the significance of abdominal compartment syndrome is becoming more widely recognised.

Background and definitions

Matsen *et al.* (1980) defined the compartment syndrome as 'a condition in which increased pressure within a limited space compromises the circulation and function of the tissues within that space' (p. 286). Kostler *et al.* (2004) stated that most cases of compartment syndrome occurred after a traumatic injury. Kostler *et al.* (2004) identified the following causes as leading to compartment syndrome:

- **Orthopaedic causes:** both traumatic fractures and orthopaedic surgery can be implicated.
- **Vascular causes:** arterial and venous injuries, whether traumatic or secondary to surgery. Reperfusion injury and haemorrhage can deprive muscles and tissues of oxygen, thus leading to tissue swelling.
- **Soft tissue damage:** conditions such as crush injury, burns and prolonged limb compression.
- **Iatrogenic causes:** accidental puncture in anticoagulated patients, use of pneumatic antishock garments and constricting casts or dressings.
- **Rare causes:** snakebites and overuse of muscles.
- **Abdominal causes:** usually associated with severe abdominal injury or extensive surgery where the abdominal contents swell leading to tissue damage.

Early recognition of the signs and symptoms of compartment syndrome is vital to prevent and reduce the possible serious effects on the patient.

Case Scenario

A 48-year-old man was admitted after a motorcycle accident in which he sustained an open fracture of the tibia and fibula of his left leg. Surgery was undertaken and an external fixator frame inserted to support the bones while healing occurred. His calf became swollen and more painful over the following day and his toes became cool. Pedal pulses were difficult to palpate.

A diagnosis of compartment syndrome was made and a fasciotomy was performed to release the tissue pressure.

Pathophysiology, aetiology and mechanism of condition and therapy

Three possible mechanisms have been suggested for the development of compartment syndrome (Singh *et al.*, 2004):

- The tissue swelling from the injury causes the arterioles to go into spasm and reduces blood flow.

- The tissue swelling causes the arterioles to collapse and, thus, reduces blood flow.

- The tissue swelling causes the venioles to collapse; as pressure rises in the venous system from the arterial system the veins re-open, but pressure is increased. This affects the pressure gradient from veins to tissues so that oxygen delivery is affected.

All three mechanisms lead to restricted oxygen delivery to the affected area and causes tissue hypoxia. The affected tissue and muscles develop increased permeability, so allowing more fluid shifts within the compartment and increasing swelling further; thus, it is a cycle of tissue damage that can be difficult to break (Singh *et al.*, 2004).

Compartment syndrome is a medical emergency and needs to be treated quickly to prevent serious and long-term effects such as contractures, amputation and disability. Clinical diagnosis can be difficult as the initial injury can mask the early signs. The 'Five Ps' have been suggested as indicative of compartment syndrome (Singh *et al.*, 2004), namely:

- *P*—Pain
- *P*—Pallor
- *P*—Paraesthesia
- *P*—Paralysis
- *P*—Pulselessness.

However, pulselessness is a late sign and pain and pallor can be mistakenlyrelated to the initial injury. Dincer (2008) noted that these signs are not evident in the unconscious patient and suggests using addition tests such as serum creatinine, phosphakinase, serum and urine myoglobulin levels to identify injury. Doppler and ultrasound can also be used to assess the extremity for poor blood flow (Dincer, 2008). Mamaril *et al.* (2007) suggest a sixth 'P':

- *P*—Pressure.

Methods are available for measuring intracompartment pressure (ICP) such as tanometers; the normal pressure is 0–15 mmHg and pressures above 30 mmHg, in conjunction with clinical signs, are diagnostic of compartment syndrome (Dincer, 2008). However, ICP measurements are not always reliable or easily available and they do not necessarily show a true picture of the pressure throughout the compartment, thus clinical signs are vital and ICP measurement aids diagnosis, particularly in unconscious patients.

Monitoring and management of compartment syndrome

As already noted, early detection and treatment of compartment syndrome are vital to reduce complications. Patients who are at risk of compartment syndrome should be monitored in a variety of ways depending on the compartment or compartments likely to be affected.

- **Limbs:** at least hourly recording of temperature of the limb, pain, movement, feeling and pulses. Increasing pain, cooling of the limb, reduction in movement, feeling or pulses should be quickly reported to the relevant senior clinician.

- **Abdominal:** the Five Ps are difficult to apply to this compartment and measuring girth is an unreliable indicator of abdominal pressure. Therefore abdominal pressure is usually measured using a urethral catheter and manometer device (Sahjian and Frakes, 2007). However, in practice this is difficult to use on all susceptible patients and is generally confined to the intensive care patient.

Early decompression of the affected compartment is considered to be the treatment of choice (Singh *et al.*, 2004) usually by using a fasciotomy – although this does add to the risk of infection. The abdomen is often left open with a sterile protective cover until swelling has reduced. The affected limb should be left at heart level to aid circulation and prevent further swelling (Mamaril *et al.*, 2007) and any constricting casts, traction or bandages should be loosened or removed (Mamaril *et al.*, 2007).

Conclusions

This chapter has provided an overview of the care of patients with compartment syndrome. In general wards these patients require close monitoring of their vital signs, their limb (if a limb is affected) and their pain score. Seek expert help quickly if deterioration occurs and ensure the hospital's pain team or anaesthetists are involved in their care.

References and further reading

Dincer, H.E. (2008). Acute compartment syndrome: are we close to making an early diagnosis? *Critical Care Medicine*, **36**(6), 1962-63.

Kostler, W., Strohm, P.C. and Sudkamp, N.P. (2004). Acute compartment syndrome of the limb injury. *International Journal of the Care of the Injured*, **35**, 1221–27.

Mamaril, M.E., Childs, S.G. and Sortman, S. (2007). Care of the orthopaedic trauma patient. *Journal of Perianesthesia Nursing*, **22**(3), 184–94.

Matsen, F., Winquist, R. and Krugmire, R. (1980). Diagnosis and management of compartmental syndromes. *Journal of Bone and Joint Surgery*, **62**(2), 286–91.

Sahjian, M. and Frakes, M. (2007). Crush injuries: Pathophysiology and current treatment. *The Nurse Practitioner*, **32**(9), 13–18.

Singh, S., Trikhab, S.P. and Lewis, J. (2004). Acute compartment syndrome. *Current Orthopaedics*, **18**, 468–76.

Useful websites

American Academy of Orthopaedic Surgeons
www.orthoinfo.aaos.org/topic.cfm?topic=a00204

Medline Plus
www.nlm.nih.gov/medlineplus/ency/article/001224.htm

Wheeless's Textbook of Orthopaedics
www.wheelessonline.com/ortho/compartment_syndrome

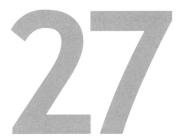

27 Altered level of consciousness and confusion

Ann M. Price

This chapter aims to discuss the significance of altered conscious level, highlighting definitions, possible causes, patient assessment and key actions required. The pathophysiology of altered consciousness will be outlined to enable readers to link theory to practical issues. Altered consciousness and confusion are complex subjects with many factors that affect recovery and treatment; thus, this chapter can only outline key issues for everyday use.

Background and definitions

Consciousness is a mental state in which we are aware of our surroundings and able to interact with the environment (Waterhouse, 2005). Altered consciousness is usually caused by an event that affects the reticular activation system (RAS) within the brain. The RAS is normally involved in the wake–sleep cycle and adverse events can cause disruption of this system (Tortora and Nielsen, 2009). Disturbance of conscious level is usually manifest by difficulty in arousing the patient and possibly coma (unrousable).

Confusion is when a person becomes disorientated to their surroundings. It can be caused by injury to various components of the brain cortex, and it can vary in severity and be specific (e.g. the patient may be disorientated in current time but remember past events). Confusion and altered consciousness can be sudden or slow in onset, depending on whether the disease process is an acute event or a degenerative process. See Table 27.1 for descriptions used to describe altered consciousness and their meanings.

Primary causes

There are *primary* neurological causes of altered consciousness such as head injury, brain tumour, meningitis, electrolyte imbalances, metabolic disturbances (e.g. diabetic ketoacidosis) and cerebrovascular accident (CVA or stroke) that result from a disease process (Haymore, 2004).

Secondary causes

There are also *secondary* causes of neurological dysfunction such as drugs, pain, alcohol, dementia and psychological causes. These can be termed delirium or psychosis and often need to be dealt with differently from the primary causes (Haymore, 2004).

Table 27.1	Description and characteristics of altered states of consciousness (from Haymore, 2004)
Description	**Characteristics**
Normal consciousness	Easily aroused, wakefulness, awareness of environment
Lethargy, obtunded, stupor	These are poorly defined terms, so specific information about the patient's response to verbal and tactile stimuli is more useful
Confusion	Poorly defined term as there are many types and causes of confusion; again more information about the patient's response and specific details about confusion are more useful
Coma	Completely unresponsive even to specific stimuli
Persistent vegetative state	Unaware of self and the environment, but continues to have sleep–wake cycles
'Locked-in' syndrome	Normal consciousness with nearly complete paralysis; can answer questions using (usually) eye movements
Brainstem death (see Chapter 32)	Irreversible loss of brainstem and cortical functions; characterised by no movements, fixed pupils and no respiratory effort, hence ventilated in the intensive care unit

Pathophysiology, aetiology and mechanism of condition and therapy

The reticular activating system (RAS) is an area of specialised cells situated in the brainstem (Tortora and Nielsen, 2009). The RAS has to interact with the brain (cerebral) hemispheres to produce consciousness. Thus damage to the RAS or parts of the cerebral hemispheres can lead to altered conscious level and – in severe cases – to unconsciousness (Geraghty, 2005).

Injury to the brain or brainstem leads to neurological dysfunction. The type and severity of dysfunction depends on the area of the brain affected and the size of the insult, but initial signs may be headache, nausea and vomiting, drowsiness, and seizures that can escalate to unconsciousness.

The Glasgow Coma Score (GCS) is used to assess the level of consciousness (see Chapter 45) (Cree, 2003; Waterhouse, 2005). A normal GCS is 14/15 but a Glasgow coma score of 3–8 is considered to be severe neurological impairment (coma), 9–12 is moderate impairment and 13 is mild impairment (Woodrow, 2006). Limb response and pupil response give additional information about the nature of the neurological dysfunction.

In severe neurological insults or injuries that affect the brainstem, vital functions such as respiration and pulse can be affected. The aim of nursing care and medical treatment is to reduce and limit further damage by controlling intracranial pressure (Hartshorn and Gauthier, 2001).

Intracranial pressure (ICP) is the result of pressure in the skull from the components of brain tissue (the major component), blood and cerebral spinal fluid (about 300 mL) (Woodrow, 2006). In normal people, the ICP will rise transiently (for example, when coughing) but in head-injured patients the brain swells, leading to increasing ICP and reducing blood flow to the brain, so leading to further brain ischaemia (often termed secondary injury). A normal ICP is 0–15 mmHg (Woodrow, 2006) although this can only be measured in specialist areas. Many nerves emanating from the brain cross at the level of the brainstem before travelling to the body. Thus, if an injury occurs on the left side of the brain then the right side of the body's limbs will be affected.

Cerebral vascular accidents (CVA or stroke) are usually caused by bleeding into the brain tissue or reduction in blood flow (ischaemia) to an area of the brain. This is often caused by atherosclerosis (build up of plaque in the arteries) and hypertension which can reduce blood flow to the brain or cause ruptured blood vessels in the brain. People with diabetes or heart disease are at particular risk of stroke.

Case Scenario

A 69-year-old man is admitted to a medical ward with a suspected cerebrovascular accident. His Glasgow Coma Score is 10 (see Chapter 44 for how to undertake a GCS properly). He is:

- opening his eyes to pain
- only moving to pain but localising
- muttering confused words.

He has a left-sided paralysis but his eye pupils are equal and reacting to light.

The incidence of stroke increases with age, is more common in males, if there is a family history of stroke and with ethnicity (Asian, African and Afro–Caribbean) (The Stroke Association, 2008) thus staff should identify patients risk of developing a stroke. Around 150,000 people per year in the UK are affected by stroke. It is the third most common cause of death and the main cause of severe disability (The Stroke Association, 2008).

HOT TIPS

The early signs of stroke are given by FAST:

F—Facial weakness
A—Arm weakness
S—Speech problems
T—Test all of these and call ambulance if they are present (The Stroke Association, 2008).

If the CVA is large it can lead to unconsciousness and death; if it is smaller it leads to other neurological signs such as one-sided limb weakness or paralysis, speech impairment, visual changes and changes in cognitive understanding and abilities (The Stroke Association, 2008). Recovery from CVA is variable; a mild stroke (transient ischaemic attack, or TIA) usually has symptoms lasting only a few hours (less than 24) whereas some patients are permanently and severely disabled (The Stroke Association, 2008). Rehabilitation can improve the patient's functional ability over time (The Stroke Association, 2008).

Monitoring and management based on current evidence

Initial management should ensure that damage to the brain is limited or reduced. For some types of head injury this may mean neurosurgery, but other important aspects are airway/respiratory management, cardiovascular stability and fluid regulation (see Box 27.1). Specific drug treatments will vary with the type of head injury. Box 27.1 details issues pertinent to the care of patients with altered conscious.

Box 27.1   Caring for patients with altered consciousness

Airway
- Consider using recovery position
- Use airway adjuncts (e.g. a Guerdal)
- Watch for signs of obstruction (e.g. gurgling, stridor)
- Inability to cough

Rationale: To ensure there is no airway obstruction that would limit oxygen to the brain and increase ischaemic injury (Cree, 2003). If the patient cannot cough they cannot clear their airway and may need an endotracheal tube (Hartshorn and Gauthier, 2001).

Breathing
- Monitor rate, depth, rhythm and pattern for abnormalities
- Give oxygen therapy
- Monitor oxygen saturations

Rationale: Monitoring respiratory function should pick up difficulties more quickly – report changes in pattern and low/high rates. Giving oxygen reduces risk of further hypoxic brain damage (Geraghty, 2005).

Cardiovascular
- Monitor pulse and blood pressure
- May need treatment for hypotension or hypertension, tachycardia or bradycardia
- Monitor temperature

Rationale: The brain needs an adequate supply of blood to maintain function so a low blood pressure is as bad as a high one (Cree, 2003). High temperature is a rare complication of severe head injury when the hypothalamus is affected. However, elevated temperature has been suggested as having a negative impact on mortality (Greer *et al.*, 2008).

Box 27.1 (*Cont.*)

Conscious level

- Assess GCS, movement for differences in limbs, and pupils for changes in size and reaction
- Usually do GCS half-hourly until stable and then reduce frequency (Waterhouse, 2005)
- Antiplatelet and anticoagulation drugs may be given to stroke patients to reduce risk of further clots in brain (NICE, 2008; The Stroke Association, 2008)

Rationale: After the initial injury there is a risk of extension of damage and early recognition and treatment can improve outcome (NICE, 2007; 2008). Conscious level should slowly improve (for most patients) after the initial insult. Some CVA patients will have a further stroke in the following days and weeks.

Fluid and nutritional intake

- Give intravenous fluids or nasogastric feeding until the patient is able to eat and drink
- Should assess swallowing ability if any concerns (e.g. coughing when drinking) and hospital policy for swallow tests should be adhered to
- Insulin may be needed to control blood sugar (Geraghty, 2005)

Rationale: Depressed conscious level means that the patient will not be able to drink adequate fluids and is at risk of dehydration. Aspiration of fluids into the lungs needs to be avoided as it complicates recovery – and can be fatal (Cree, 2003). Half of stroke patients have swallowing impairment and so a swallow test is vital before freely giving fluids and food orally (The Stroke Association, 2008). A nasogastric tube may be needed for feeding or to prevent aspiration if the patient is vomiting (Cree, 2003). Diabetes is linked to risk of stroke and controlling blood sugars within normal range is necessary.

Bed rest

- Assess for signs of deep vein thrombosis (e.g. swollen and warm calves)
- Anti-embolytic stockings and prophylactic anticoagulation may be ordered (Geraghty, 2005)
- Encourage limb movements (if able) and physiotherapy
- Encourage deep breathing
- Sit patient up at 30°

Rationale: Bed rest is common in the first few days after a CVA to promote recovery, but the complications of bed rest can delay recovery through DVT and pneumonia. Sitting the patient up reduces risk of aspiration and aids intracranial pressure (Cree, 2003).
Note: Anticoagulation therapy may not always be used in haemorrhagic strokes and head injury if there is concern about further brain bleeding.

Unable to maintain hygiene

- Skin care, mouth and eye care

Rationale: Hygiene needs will be individually adjusted to meet the patient's needs and promote independence where possible (Geraghty, 2005).

Box 27.1   (Cont.)

Pressure ulcers

- Assess Waterlow score (or other pressure risk score)
- Use pressure-relieving devices where appropriate
- Promote side lying and position changes
- Assess patient's ability to move self

Rationale: Reduced conscious level often means that the patient cannot or does not move him or her self. One-sided weakness in CVA patients can make it difficult for patients to adjust their position. CVA often affects elderly people with complex health needs that make them more prone to pressure ulcers.

Mobility/risk of falls

- Assess patient's understanding of commands
- Assess movement and strength in limbs
- Use appropriate moving and handling aids (e.g. hoists)
- Assess need for cot-sides
- Physiotherapy regimen

Rationale: Altered conscious level and confusion can affect mobility and put the patient at risk of falling. We do want to promote independence and mobility but this needs to be done carefully to ensure the safety of the patient and others (Geraghty, 2005). Often CVA patients lean to the affected side, making sitting and walking more difficult, and they may have difficulty understanding commands.

Incontinence

- Assess bladder and bowel control
- May need urinary catheter or bowel management regimen
- Risk of constipation (consider laxatives)

Rationale: Bladder and bowel control can be affected in head injury and is particularly a problem in stroke patients. Incontinence adds to the risk of pressure ulcers so measures to limit soiling are needed. Many stroke patients will regain bladder control in time. Constipation often results from prolonged immobility (Geraghty, 2005).

Psychological

- Assess for fear, anxiety, agitation, aggression, mood swings, depression
- Antidepressants may be used in some patients or review by psychologist
- Difficulty in communicating

Rationale: Any brain injury can create huge anxiety and fear for patients about the long-term effects. Stroke patients are particularly at risk of difficulties as they try to cope with changes in mood and physical function and difficulties in mental processing (The Stroke Association, 2008). Observe non-verbal cues as well as speech to aid communication (Geraghty, 2005).

Conclusions

Any brain injury can lead to long-term disability that impacts on the patient and their family. Early recognition and management of the disease can reduce the initial damage and improve the long-term outcome for many people. The rise of modern stroke units and thrombolysis for non-haemorrhagic strokes means that early identification, urgent CT scan and referral of these patients is vital. A great deal of time must be given to the unconscious patient in order to meet his or her needs and to reduce the potential risks (Geraghty, 2005). Very often this is a traumatic time for the relatives and friends of the patient, who require full support and information. Rehabilitation and social support are also needed to ensure that the patient can achieve their maximum potential for recovery. Other relevant information can be found in Chapter 45 (undertaking a Glasgow Coma Score) and Chapter 3 (simple and advanced airway manoeuvres).

References and further reading

Cree, C. (2003). Acquired brain injury: acute management. *Nursing Standard*, **18**(11), 45–56.

Greer, D.M., Funk, S.E., Reaven, N.L., Ouzounelli, M. and Uman, G.C. (2008). Impact of fever on outcome in patients with stroke and neurologic injury: a comprehensive meta-analysis. *Stroke*, **39**, 3029–35.

Geraghty, M. (2005). Nursing the unconscious patient. *Nursing Standard*, **20**(1), 54–64.

Hartshorn, J.C. and Gauthier, D.M. (2001). Nervous system alterations. In: M.L. Sole, M.L. Lamborn and J.C. Hartshorn (eds) *Introduction to Critical Care Nursing*, 3rd edn. London, WB Saunders.

Haymore, J. (2004). A neuron in a haystack: advanced neurological assessment. *AACN Clinical Issues*, **15**(4), 568–81.

National Institute of Health and Clinical Excellence (2007). *Head injury. Triage, assessment, investigation and early management of head injury in infants, children and adults.* Available at: www.nice.org.uk/nicemedia/pdf/CG56QuickRedGuide.pdf (last accessed November 2009).

National Institute of Health and Clinical Excellence (2008). *Stroke. Diagnosis and initial management of acute stroke and transient ischaemic attack (TIA).* Available at: www.nice.org.uk/nicemedia/pdf/CG68QuickRefGuide.pdf (last accessed November 2009).

The Stroke Association (2008). *What is a stroke?* Available at: www.stroke.org.uk/information/what_is_a_stroke/index.html (last accessed November 2009).

Tortora, G.J. and Nielsen, M.T. (2009). *Principles of Human Anatomy*, 11th edn. Chichester: John Wiley & Sons.

Waterhouse, C. (2005). The Glasgow Coma Score and other neurological observations. *Nursing Standard*, **19**(33), 56–64.

Woodrow, P. (2006). *Intensive Care Nursing: A Framework for Practice* 2nd edn. London, Routledge.

Useful websites

Headway: the Brain Injury Association
www.headway.org.uk

National Institute for Health and Clinical Excellence (NICE)
www.nice.org.uk

National Service Framework for Stroke
www.dh.gov.uk/en/Healthcare/NationalServiceFrameworks/Stroke/index.htm

National Service Framework for Long-Term Neurological Conditions
www.dh.gov.uk/en/Healthcare/NationalServiceFrameworks/Long-term
NeurologicalConditionsNSF/index.htm

Scottish Intercollegiate Guidelines Network: Early management of patients with a head injury
www.sign.ac.uk/guidelines/fulltext/46/index.html

The Stroke Association
www.stroke.org.uk

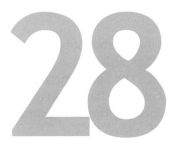
Neurogenic shock

Ann M. Price

Neurogenic shock is most commonly associated with spinal cord injuries. However, the incidence of neurogenic shock is lower than expected. Guly *et al.* (2008) noted that neurogenic shock was a complication in 19% of cases of cervical spinal injury, in 7% of cases of thoracic spinal injury and only in 3% of cases of lumbar spinal injury in the initial emergency phase. Nevertheless, neurogenic shock is a life-threatening complication of spinal cord injury that needs to be recognised and treated promptly.

Definitions

Several terms are used in the literature that have similar causes and some similar manifestations as neurogenic shock. These terms are clarified below.

Neurogenic shock (Dawodu, 2007)

This usually occurs in spinal injuries above T6 level. It is characterised by hypotension, bradycardia and hypothermia due to vasodilation caused by disruption to sympathetic nerve impulses.

Spinal shock (Dawodu, 2007)

Spinal shock is a transient depression of cord reflexes below the level of injury. There is a loss of all sensorimotor functions. Catecholamine release causes an initial increase in blood pressure followed by hypotension and bradycardia. The symptoms, including flaccid paralysis and bowel and bladder dysfunction, last from hours to days until the reflex arcs below the injury level start to function.

Autonomic dysreflexia

This is a syndrome that occurs in spinal cord injury patients where massive reflex sympathetic discharge leads to hypertension, bradycardia, profuse sweating and flushed appearance (Campagnolo, 2006). The syndrome usually occurs in patients where the injury is above the splanchnic sympathetic outflow (T5–T6), and it usually results when reflexes return after a period of spinal shock.

Pathophysiology

The autonomic nervous system contains both sympathetic and parasympathetic motor fibres. These fibres are important in the function of smooth muscle including cardiac muscle. The sympathetic pathways are mainly transported via the spinal cord, whereas the parasympathetic pathways are mainly transported via the vagal nerve (10th cranial nerve) (Ciechanowski *et al.*, 2005). This difference in nerve impulses is the reason why, in spinal injuries, the sympathetic pathways are suppressed and the parasympathetic is dominant (initially at least).

Patients with high spinal cord injuries lack sympathetic stimulation and are prone to bradycardia, hypotension secondary to vascular dilation, and hypothermia due to dilation and heat loss. Other functions that are affected due to the loss of sympathetic input include bowel and bladder function.

Case Scenario

A 23-year-old man was involved in a motorcycle accident earlier today. He has suffered a spinal injury at C5 level and is being cared for on an orthopaedic ward until a specialist opinion is sought. He says he is feeling unwell and observations note hypotension at 80 mmHg systolic blood pressure, a pulse of 60 beats per minute and a temperature of 35°C.

Monitoring and management

Any patient with a spinal injury will initially need close and frequent monitoring to identify neurogenic shock. This includes temperature, blood pressure, respirations and continuous cardiac monitoring via an ECG machine. Patients may require invasive monitoring such as arterial and central venous lines for management.

Treatment of hypotension is initially with fluid challenges; the patient may require large volumes of fluid to compensate for the vasodilation and venous pooling of blood that occurs. Patients who are unresponsive to fluids should be considered for vasopressor drugs such as norepinephrine to induce vasoconstriction. Bradycardia can be limited by the use of atropine, although Bilello *et al.* (2003) noted that a number of patients will require cardiac pacing to treat the bradycardia associated with neurogenic shock. Patients should be kept warm using blankets and other aids but this can induce further hypotension which should be corrected quickly.

Patients who develop neurogenic shock should ideally be managed within a critical care setting until they have stabilised and no longer require intensive treatment.

Conclusions

Several syndromes are associated with spinal injuries with varying time frames for onset. Neurogenic shock is an early and life-threatening complication of spinal injury that needs swift fluid resuscitation and management of bradycardia to compensate for vascular dilation and hypotension.

References and further reading

Bilello, J.F., Davis, J.W., Cunningham, M.A., Groom, T.F., Lemaster, D. and Sue, L.P. (2003). Cervical spinal cord injury and the need for cardiovascular intervention. *Archives of Surgery*, **138**(10), 112.

Campagnolo, D.I. (2006). *Autonomic Dysreflexia in Spinal Cord Injury.* Available at: http://emedicine.medscape.com/article/322809-overview (last accessed November 2009).

Ciechanowski, M., Mower-Wade, D., McLeskey, S.W. and Stout, L. (2005). Anatomy and physiology of the nervous system. In: P.G. Morton, D.K. Fontaine, C.M. Hudak and B.M. Gallo (eds) (2006). *Critical Care Nursing: A Holistic Approach*, 8th edn. Philadelphia, Lippincott Williams and Wilkins.

Dawodu, S.T. (2007). *Spinal Cord Injury: Definition, Epidemiology, Pathophysiology.* Available at: emedicine.medscape.com/article/322480-overview (last accessed November 2009).

Guly, H.R., Bouramra, O. and Lecky, F.E. (2008). The incidence of neurogenic shock in patients with isolated spinal cord injury in the emergency department (on behalf of Trauma Audit and Research Network). *Resuscitation*, **76**(1), 57–62.

Useful websites

Emergency Medicine
www.emergencymed.wordpress.com/2009/03/11/neurogenic-shock/

Bone and Spine Health
www.boneandspine.com

· A B C D (E) ·

Exposure and Environment

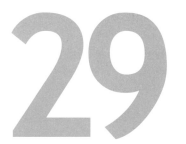

29 The post-ICU patient

Catherine Plowright

Admission to an intensive care or high dependency unit (ICU/HDU) has been described as a traumatic and frightening experience for patients and their families, and many highlight the fear, anxiety and psychological distress induced by critical illness (McGonigal, 1986; Quinn *et al.*, 1996; Viney, 1996; Jones, 2002; Skirrow, 2002) as well as the physiological problems induced by critical illness on leaving the intensive care unit (Jones and Griffiths, 2002; Kennedy *et al.*, 2002; Waldmann, 2002). This phenomenon is defined in a number of ways, for example as transfer anxiety, relocation anxiety and translocation anxiety. It is recognised as a DSM diagnosis (American Psychiatric Association, 1994).

This chapter offers practical guidance on how to care for patients recently relocated to a ward environment from the critical care area, enabling healthcare professionals to care for these patients with understanding. At the end of this chapter you should:

- understand about the physical care needs of patients following a spell in the intensive care or high dependency unit
- understand the psychological effects of critical illness on a patient
- know how to assess and deliver holistic care to this patient group.

Background

Patients who have been critically ill not only suffer from the effects of their critical illness but can also find that the transfer to a ward environment poses problems for them. This is despite the improved health status of the patient (Whittaker and Ball, 2000). Healthcare professional workers need to remember that critical illness will affect all patients differently, regardless of the time they have spent in the intensive care unit. Whether the patient was intubated and ventilated also has a bearing on how they may find the transition.

Handover from intensive care or the high dependency unit

Handover from the intensive care or high dependency unit is of paramount importance. The NICE guidance (National Institute of Health and Clinical Excellence, 2007) states that the handover of care from these areas should include the following:

- A summary of the critical care stay including diagnosis and treatment.
- A monitoring and investigation plan.
- A plan for ongoing treatment including drugs and therapies, nutrition plan, infection status and any agreed limitations of treatment.
- physical and rehabilitation needs.
- Psychological and emotional needs.
- Specific communication and language needs.

The guidance also states that the critical care team and the ward multidisciplinary teams should take shared responsibility for the care of the patient being transferred. The handover should be formal, structured and supported by a written plan. It is important for the critical care teams caring for the patient to ensure that the receiving ward can deliver the agreed plan.

This ensures that continuity of care is maximised and that the ward staff, including nursing, medical and allied healthcare professionals have adequate and relevant information of the patient's condition and needs.

Specific needs of patients

The needs of patients post intensive-care unit fall into two broad categories:

- physical, and
- psychological.

It is advisable for patient safety and continuity of care to ensure that the transfer to a ward from the intensive care unit or high dependency unit takes place before 2200 hours at night and not before 0700 in the morning (National Institute of Health and Clinical Excellence, 2007). This enables the step down to another area to occur when multidisciplinary teams are readily available to care for all of the patient's needs.

This step down can be a difficult time for patients who have been critically ill, and for their visitors. They are moving from a very highly staffed and complex area to a general ward area where there are fewer nurses per patient. Patients who have had a long stay in intensive care sometimes experience a sense of abandonment when transferred to the ward. This is in addition to the other physical and psychological problems they may have.

The physical and psychological problems this creates, and ways to resolve them, are now discussed.

Physical problems

Muscle weakness is probably the most obvious and incapacitating feature of recovery from critical illness that patients and healthcare professionals are presented with. It would have contributed to the overall recovery of the patient while on intensive care, and will continue to do so on return to the ward. Critically ill patients can develop critical illness polyneuropathies, myopathies or a combination of both (Kennedy et al., 2002). They can also develop drug-induced neuropathies or generalised demyelination caused by infections (Kennedy et al., 2002). Whatever the cause, muscle wasting will occur, as well as wastage of lean tissue and skeletal muscle. Critically ill patients can lose 1% of their lean body mass per day of their critical illness (Griffiths, 2002). The consequences of this are often manifested on the intensive care unit, especially if the patient has been intubated and ventilated for any significant period of time, and during what is often a prolonged weaning phase from the ventilator. Prolonged weaning from a ventilator in intensive care is necessary because the diaphragm and other respiratory muscles are among the muscles affected by the wastage. They need to build up strength over the weaning period.

Respiratory problems

Patients who have respiratory muscle weakness often endure prolonged weaning from mechanical ventilation. Less obvious may be their inability to cough and clear secretions adequately because they need to have respiratory muscle power and cough power to perform this simple task. A tracheostomy is often required during admission to intensive care and this will often remain in place when the patient returns to the ward environment, for secretion control (see Chapter 4 on tracheostomies). The multidisciplinary healthcare team (especially physiotherapists and nurses) need to work together with the patient to maintain respiratory function and remove the tracheostomy as soon as possible (see Chapter 12 on physiotherapy). The nurse should encourage the patient to undertake the breathing exercises that the physiotherapist has given them, and to use any adjuncts that they were given (e.g. inspirometers).

Eating and drinking problems

Patients should have received nutrition when on the intensive care or high dependency unit, and yet they will lose weight. The importance of their nutrition must continue when they leave the unit, yet this can be challenging to ward staff (see Chapter 44 on feeding patients). Patients who are recovering from critical illness present a number of challenges that need to be overcome, including the desire, the opportunity and the physical ability to eat and drink. The desire to eat is limited by many factors such as pain, tiredness, psychological issues and taste problems. Changes reported by patients include food tasting metallic or salty, or having no taste at all. Patients who do not experience the desire to eat and drink pose specific challenges to healthcare professionals for whom achieving adequate nutritional status is of paramount importance.

The physical ability to eat and drink can be affected by the general muscle weakness that these patients may have, which limits the use of their arms when bringing food from the plate to their mouths. They also may not be able to sit up or hold their heads up. These problems are easily identified by healthcare professionals as they can be visualised, but the effects of muscle weakness that cannot be seen are often not appreciated, such as difficulty in swallowing and chewing. Eating, drinking and swallowing are complex mechanisms that require control and timing because breathing is interrupted as part of the process. There are a number of swallowing difficulties which can be presented and which healthcare professionals must be aware of. These include aspiration, regurgitation and avoidance of food and drink (Griffiths, 2002). It is important to involve dieticians and speech and language therapists in the care of these patients. This will ensure that they are able to swallow and that all their nutrition needs are being met. Information about nutrition on discharge from hospital may help the patients who are still experiencing some of the difficulties noted above. General advice would consist of having small and frequent meals, and a broad, balanced diet. Healthy eating and exercise should be encouraged to promote muscle growth and fat distribution and improve pulmonary and cardiovascular function (Griffiths, 2002).

Mobility

Mobility is often reduced when patients are discharged from the intensive care or high dependency unit, as a direct result of muscle weakness. The longer the length of stay in critical care areas and the greater the number of days spent ventilated, the higher the chance of mobility problems (Jones and Griffiths, 2002). The extent of the problem is clear when patients have difficulties getting in and out of bed, moving themselves up in the bed, walking to the toilet, and balancing.

Teams need to work together to improve the recovery of these patients, and it is vital that physiotherapists and occupational therapists are involved. Patients need encouragement to mobilise within their limits. By working together with the patient, teams can agree a plan that will enable the patient to recover strength and independence. For example, if the physiotherapist assists the patient to sit out in a chair, the nurse should agree with the patient and the physiotherapist the length of time the patient should remain there. Exercises that the physiotherapist has prescribed for them should also be encouraged.

Caring for patients post intensive care with physical problems

Significant numbers of patients surviving critical illness have continuing physical problems. For many the discharge from intensive care or the high dependency unit is the start of an unknown journey. Rehabilitation of these patients should commence in intensive care and be followed up when they are on a ward, and should continue through to discharge from hospital and into the community (National Institute for Health and Clinical Excellence, 2009). Healthcare professionals in ward environments should continue to ensure that any rehabilitation initiated during the stay on intensive care or the high dependency unit is continued on the ward.

It is essential that all healthcare teams work together to improve the recovery of these patients, and it is vital that nurses, doctors, physiotherapists, speech and language therapists and occupational therapists are involved in the needs of the patients. The physical rehabilitation for these patients must be specific and individualised. There is limited evidence on the clinical effectiveness of rehabilitation strategies when these patients are in ward environments (National Institute for Health and Clinical Excellence, 2008). Jones *et al.* (2003) devised a 6-week structured and supported self-help rehabilitation programme which has been shown to improve the physical recovery of patients. This programme is based on the individual physical and cognitive capacity of patients at different stages in their recovery. The rehabilitation manual includes information on the types of exercise that patients should be undertaking, including leg and arm strengthening exercises, as well as providing information about what to expect during the journey to recovery, about eating and drinking and sex after serious illness. It also includes a diary to maintain.

Psychological problems

There has been increasing awareness of the psychological problems encountered by patients following admission to intensive care or a high dependency unit over recent years. The psychological effects reported include anxiety and depression, hallucinations, sleep disorders, memory disturbances, confusion and cognitive impairment (Jones *et al.*, 2000; Jones *et al.*, 2001; Jones, 2002). It is important for all healthcare professionals caring for patients following discharge from intensive care to understand that they may have psychological problems. Patients often have little or no memory of the time they spent in the critical care area, or of how critically ill they were. Therefore they often have difficulties understanding the slowness of their recovery and feel hopeless, which can lead on to psychological problems (Jones, 2002). These patients often cannot recall the events before their admission to hospital (Jones *et al.*, 2000). There is a view held by some healthcare professionals that not remembering may be helpful, however this is not the case (Griffiths *et al.*, 1996). Staff should ensure that patients have a full understanding of what happened to them and of how ill they were. These patients often have delusional memories such as hallucinations, which they find very frightening and very real, and they often suffer from anxiety and depression and demonstrate the symptoms of post-traumatic stress disorder (Griffiths *et al.*, 1994; Jones and Griffiths 2000; Scragg *et al.*, 2001). Post-traumatic stress is more likely to occur if the only memories that patients have are delusional (Jones *et al.*, 2001). Patients experiencing sleep difficulties often have nightmares and it can be the fear of the nightmares that causes the sleep difficulty. Remember that night sedation may not help the situation as the nightmares will still be present.

Caring for post intensive-care patients with psychological problems

The anxiety and depression experienced by recently discharged intensive care unit patients often resolves with time, but if prolonged psychological problems are evident then formal help must be obtained. You need to talk to these patients, using simple measures such as breathing control to help with any panic attacks, and have an understanding of the experiences that they had while on the unit. If you are unable to do so then perhaps the critical care outreach nurses, intensive care unit nurses or nurse consultants for critical care, if available, will be able to assist you in talking to these patients. In addition, it is essential to seek out whatever specialist help is available within the Trust to assist with this aspect of a patient's care. Although they are alarming, these types of post intensive-care unit problems are not uncommon and should resolve in time with appropriate help.

Some intensive care units use patient diaries as a tool to explain to patients what happened to them when they were so sick that they were not aware of anything (Backman, 2002; Backman and Walther 2005; Coombe 2005). These diaries can assist with any gaps in their memory and give the facts of what happened while the patient was on the unit. There are two types of diaries: prospective and retrospective.

Retrospective diaries involve a healthcare professional examining the patient's health records after discharge from intensive care, and writing a record of the significant events and care and treatment received. Patients can find this type of diary impersonal and difficult to relate to and they are time consuming for staff to complete (Coombe, 2005).

Prospective diaries are written by all healthcare professionals involved in the care of the patient and the family, and are added to on a daily basis, recording the all-important milestones. They might also include photographs (Backman, 2002; Backman and Walther, 2005) and serve to provide a realistic picture to the patient of how ill they were. The diary is then given to the patient following discharge from the unit when it is considered that they are psychologically ready to read about the extent of their illness. It requires time from the critical care nurse to explain about the diary to the patient. In some Trusts this role is shared between the intensive care staff and critical care outreach nurses. The efficacy of this initiative has yet to be robustly evaluated, but testimony from patients and their families is that the diary helps to fill the memory gaps and helps them understand what happened.

Case Scenario

A 30-year-old man is admitted to your ward following a 3-week stay in intensive care and a 4-day stay in the high dependency unit. He was admitted to hospital with pneumococcal meningitis. He was fit and healthy, and is married with two children. You are the registered nurse caring for him.

Describe how you would plan this patient's critical care rehabilitation up to the time of his discharge from hospital. What other healthcare professionals would you involve?

Conclusions

Patients who have been discharged from intensive care may experience significant physical and psychological effects of their critical illness, which will affect their care when on a ward. An understanding of why this occurs enables the healthcare professional to care for these patients in a way that minimises these effects.

The latest National Institute for Health and Clinical Excellence (NICE) clinical guidelines concerning critical care were published on 25 March 2009. These are for critical illness rehabilitation (rehabilitation after critical care). The guidelines look at the care and rehabilitation of patients after critical illness, and they apply to patients in both England and Wales. The full final version of this guideline can be accessed at www.nice.org.uk/Guidance/CG83.

References and further reading

American Psychiatric Association (1994). *Diagnostic and Statistical Manual of Mental Disorders*, 4th edn. Washington DC, American Psychiatric Association.

Backman, C. (2002). Patient diaries in ICU. In: R.D. Griffiths and C. Jones (eds) *Intensive Care Aftercare*. Oxford, Butterworth Heinemann.

Backman, C. and Walther, S.M. (2005). The photo-diary and follow-up appointment on ICU: Giving back time to patients and relatives. In: S. Ridley (ed.) *Critical Care Focus: The Psychological Challenges of Intensive Care*. Oxford, Blackwell Publishing.

Brett, S. (2005). Cognitive impairment and consequences for recovery. In: S. Ridley (ed.) *Critical Care Focus: The Psychological Challenges of Intensive Care*. Oxford, Blackwell Publishing.

Coombe, D. (2005). The use of patient diaries in an intensive care unit. *Nursing in Critical Care*, **10**(1), 3–4.

Griffiths, R.D. (2000). Nutrition after intensive care. In: R.D. Griffiths and C. Jones (eds) *Intensive Care Aftercare*. Oxford, Butterworth Heinemann.

Griffiths, R.D., Jones., C. and Macmillan, R.R. (1996). Where is the harm in not knowing? Care after intensive care. *Clinical Intensive Care*, **7**, 14–45.

Griffiths, R.D., Jones, C., Macmillan, R.R. and Palmer, T.E.A. (1994). Psychological problems occurring after intensive care. *British Journal of Intensive Care*, **4**, 46–53.

Jones, C., Griffiths, R.D. and Humphris, G.M. (2000). Disturbed memory and amnesia related to intensive care. *Memory*, **8**(2), 79–94.

Jones, C., Griffiths, R.D., Humphris, G.M. and Skirrow, P. (2001). Memory, delusions and the development of post-traumatic stress disorder-related symptoms after intensive care. *Critical Care Medicine*, **29**(3), 57–80.

Jones, C. (2002). Acute psychological problems. In: R.D. Griffiths and C. Jones. *Intensive Care Aftercare*. Oxford, Butterworth Heinemann.

Jones, C. and Griffiths, R.D. (2002). Identifying post intensive care patients who may need physical rehabilitation. *Clinical Intensive Care*, **11**, 3–8.

Kennedy, D.D., Coakley, J. and Griffiths, R.D. (2002). Neuromuscular problems and physical weakness. In: R.D. Griffiths and C. Jones. *Intensive Care Aftercare*. Oxford, Butterworth Heinemann.

McGonigal, K.S. (1986). The importance of sleep and the sensory environment to critically ill patients. *Intensive Care Nursing*, **2**(2), 73–83.

National Institute of Health and Clinical Excellence (2007). *Acutely ill patients in hospital: Recognition of and response to acute illness in adults in hospital*. Available at: www.nice.org.uk/nicemedia/pdf/CG50FullGuidance.pdf (last accessed November 2009)

National Institute of Health and Clinical Excellence (2009). Critical illness rehabilitation – rehabilitation after critical care. Available at: guidance.nice.org.uk/CG86/NiceGuidance/CG83/pdf/English (last accessed July 2009).

Quinn, S., Redmond K. and Begley, C. (1996). The needs of relatives visiting adult intensive care units as perceived by relatives and nurses. *Intensive and Critical Care Nursing*, **12**(3), 16–72.

Scragg, P., Jones, A. and Fauvel, N. (2001). Psychological problems following intensive care unit treatment. *Anaesthesia*, **56**, 9–14.

Skirrow, P. (2001). Delusional memories of intensive care unit. In: R.D. Griffiths, C. Jones. *Intensive Care Aftercare*. Oxford, Butterworth Heinemann.

Viney, C. (ed.) (1996). Pain and sedation needs. In: *Nursing the Critically Ill*. London, Bailliere Tindall.

Waldmann, C. (2002). *Sexual problems and their treatments*. In: R.D. Griffiths and C. Jones. *Intensive Care Aftercare*. Oxford, Butterworth Heinemann.

Whittaker, J. and Ball, C. (2000). Discharge from intensive care: a view from the ward. *Intensive and Critical Care Nursing*, **16**(3), 13–43.

Useful websites

National Institute for Health and Clinical Excellence (NICE)
www.nice.org.uk/Guidance/CG83

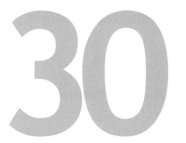

30 Ethics of acute care

Victor Nebbiolo and Sally A. Smith

The ethics of acute care is a vast, controversial and complex topic. With the advancement in medical science over recent years it has has become more so, and the situation is further complicated by the multicultural and ethnic backgrounds of patients, their relatives, and staff who live and work in our society. Today's healthcare system truly knows no cultural or ethnic boundaries for its staff or clients. Access to information via the media, television and internet means people are better informed (accurately or otherwise) about options and alternatives that may be available nationally and internationally. In today's society, expectations of healthcare have changed, and they will continue to do so.

This chapter discusses ethical principles, human rights, decision-making, 'do not resuscitate' decisions, consent and resuscitation in acute care. The chapter aims to help you understand the principles that can be used when thinking about ethical issues, and it will also make you aware of how an individual's personal, social, cultural, ethnic and political background influences the decision-making process.

Background

Today's modern healthcare system has changed and continues to do so. Gone are the days when patients and their relatives do as healthcare professionals tell them because 'they know best'. Today, people are more prepared to challenge decisions about care options, and patients have a legal right to be involved in the decision-making process (British Medical Association, 2004). Decisions taken by doctors are likely to be compliant with the Human Rights Act 1998, which covers issues such as human dignity, communication and consultation, and best interests. All are central to good clinical practice (see Box 30.1).

For all professionals, practice must always entail ethical decision-making within our professional codes of conduct as laid down by our professional bodies, such as the General Medical Council and the Nursing and Midwifery Council.

In addition, caring for patients and decisions made about care must consider the patient's rights within the Mental Capacity Act 2005. This poses particular challenges with the acutely

Box 30.1   Convention rights of the Human Rights Act 1998 with particular relevance to the practice of medicine (British Medical Association, 2004)

Article 2	Right to life
Article 3	Right to freedom from torture or inhuman or degrading treatment or punishment
Article 5	Right to liberty and security
Article 6	Right to a fair trial
Article 8	Right to respect for private and family life
Article 9	Freedom of thought, conscience and religion
Article 10	Freedom of expression
Article 12	Right to marry and found a family
Article 14	Enjoyment of these rights to be secured without discrimination

unwell patient who may not be competent to understand or agree to treatment options. Box 30.2 outlines the five principles that underpin this Act.

In addition, there can be some very challenging situations when there is a difference in the perceived care pathways and likely benefit of this pathway to all concerned. Discussions will include the patient, their relatives, carers and the wider establishment that is charged with providing and managing the resources to provide optimum care to all those concerned.

In order to try and address some of these complex moral and ethical dilemmas, some simple, basic, fundamental rules should be applied to the situations that we may find ourselves in. In idealistic terms we should be doing what the patient wants with an underlying principle of what is best for the patient. In the most simplistic terms, all care pathways should be guided by:

- beneficence
- nonmaleficence and
- respect for autonomy and
- the principle of justice.

Beneficence

This means that the care and decisions made by all concerned should have a benefit for the patient. Not only for their short-term care, but ultimately the holistic management (both physically and psychologically) during the long-term care of their disease process. This in the past has often been perceived as prolonging life to its maximum.

The principle of beneficence relate to the notions of 'do no harm' and 'maximise possible benefits, and minimise possible harms' (National Commission for the Protection of Human Subjects of Biomedical and Behavioural Research, 2003). It is where nurses and doctors do what will benefit the patient 'according to their best judgement'.

In today's modern health service it is sometimes possible to maintain and preserve functionality of a body with no perceived benefit to the person. This philosophy may challenge some religious and cultural values, but we must consider whether they are the values of the patient or of the caregivers.

> **Box 30.2** **Five principles underpinning the Mental Capacity Act 2005 (Department of Health, 2005)**
>
> **1. A presumption of capacity.** Every adult has the right to make his or her own decisions and must be assumed to have capacity to do so unless it is proved otherwise.
>
> **2. Individuals being supported to make their own decisions**. A person must be given all practicable help before anyone treats them as not being able to make their own decisions.
>
> **3. Unwise decisions.** Just because an individual makes what might be seen as an unwise decision, they should not be treated as lacking capacity to make that decision.
>
> **4. Best interests.** An act done or decision made under the Act for or on behalf of a person who lacks capacity must be done in their best interests.
>
> **5. Less restrictive option.** Anything done for or on behalf of a person who lacks capacity should be considerate of options that are less restrictive of their basic rights and freedoms if they are as effective as the proposed option.

Nonmaleficence

This requires all concerned to look at their motives during the decision-making process and ensure they are always following the principle of 'doing the patient no harm' (Seedhouse, 2002).

Respect for autonomy and the principle of justice

Linked with the patient's ability to understand and make decisions as stated in the Mental Capacity Act 2005, these principles require us to respect the patient's choices and to ensure all care prescribed and given is just and fair (Cribb, 2002).

Resuscitation issues

These days, resuscitation no longer means 'blowing and bashing' although this is still a misperception commonly held by the public – and some healthcare professionals. The fact of the matter is that resuscitation today covers a vast array of treatments from some simple oxygen and fluid therapy to full intensive-care unit therapy with its multi-organ support facilities. Any discussion on resuscitation issues about a patient must be very specific to that patient. It must also be very clear exactly what the parameters are for the decisions being made, and it must be an intrinsic part of that patient's care pathway, following the philosophy of beneficence and nonmaleficence. These issues can be expanded to cover some of the legal aspects and practicality of attempting resuscitation. Ideally they should be made ahead of time as part of the overall treatment planning of care (Resuscitation Council 2005, British Medical Association, 2007).

Case Scenario

A 71-year-old man has been admitted to a medical ward with pneumonia. He is very short of breath and requires high-flow oxygen to maintain his oxygen saturations at above 90%. His respiratory rate is 34, his heart rate is 110 and his blood pressure is 98/54 mmHg. He is drowsy and responds to verbal commands by opening his eyes. He appears to be tiring.

His past medical history is that he has chronic obstructive pulmonary disease and uses home oxygen. He can no longer get out of the house and sleeps and stays in his armchair at home. His family care for him by doing his shopping, cooking for him and helping him with his hygiene needs.

His family report that he has requested that he is left to die peacefully should he become unwell. They too do not want him to suffer unduly. Staff on the ward assess his condition as deteriorating and have called the medical team to review him and agree a treatment plan.

Taking into consideration the principles outlined above, the healthcare teams along with the patient and his family will consider the following ethical questions in order to agree this patient's care plan:

1. What does the patient want? If possible, when addressing these issues, it should be with the patient's known or obtainable wishes.

2. What is the likely outcome both in the short and the long term for him? And would that be acceptable to him?

3. What are the legal implications, including the European Courts Human Rights Act 1998 (implemented in the UK in October 2000) 'The right to life and the right to be free from degrading treatment'? Have all reasonable treatments and treatment options been considered with beneficence and nonmaleficence in mind?

When taking the patient's known or obtainable wishes into consideration, some criteria need to be followed. These relate to the Mental Capacity Act 2005 and the principle of promoting patient autonomy. All seem reasonable criteria on first examination. The patient should be:

1. Of sound mind.
2. Free from duress.
3. Fully informed.

Most commonly issues about resuscitation pathways arise when the patient is acutely unwell. That being the case, some serious consideration needs to be given to these basic questions. If they are acutely unwell are they really:

- of sound mind
- free from duress, and
- fully informed (in an unbiased manner)?

With patients like the man in our case scenario, who lacks capacity, which is common in emergency care, it is necessary to determine the patient's best interests and act in accordance with whatever they are deemed to be (British Medical Association, 2004). Discussion with the patient's family about their prior wishes and opinions may help, although this has no standing in law (British Medical Association, 2004). Ultimately the clinician in charge must make the decision, and it would be reasonable to assume that most people would want any intervention likely to save a life or prevent disability (British Medical Association, 2004). In this case scenario, the family were in agreement that escalating the patient's care to support his respiratory function through ventilation, or resuscitating him should he die, were not his wishes nor in his best interests given his comorbidities.

Patient consent

Consent should be sought before starting a patient on an agreed pathway of care. It should include a full explanation of the risks, the benefits and the possible alternatives available. However, in reality, when patients become acutely unwell, the validity and practicality of gaining consent with these criteria fully met is dubious and is certainly open to being challenged. Failure to obtain valid consent could lead to criminal charges of assault or negligence. When formal consent is not available, healthcare professionals may act with implied consent, that being what they think the patient would want and with the patient's best interest in mind, and in the absence of a clear refusal. All consent gained or implied must be clearly documented in the patient's notes – without ambiguity – for future reference. It may be that other professionals may examine these documents with great scrutiny at a later date. It would have been very difficult to gain consent from the patient in the current case scenario. Fortunately his wishes were known and able to be respected. A 'do not resuscitate' order was agreed and a form was completed and filed in his notes.

Do Not Attempt Resuscitation (DNAR) orders

There are a number of terms used for this inaction when a patient has a full cardiac arrest (defined by no breathing and no effective circulation).

- DNAR – Do not attempt resuscitation.
- DNR – Do not resuscitate.
- NFACPR – Not for attempted cardiopulmonary resuscitation.

There is often a misperception of what such a decision means in relation to patient treatment options. It should mean that if a patient stops breathing and their heart does not pump blood around the body with sufficient pressure to provide organ perfusion, artificial ventilation and external cardiac compressions will not be started. This does not mean withholding other forms of resuscitation action such as oxygen and intravenous fluids, or treatments such as inotropic drugs, antibiotics and analgesia. Decisions to withhold some of these might be classified as non-escalation of treatment. Once treatment has been started, removing said treatment might be classified as withdrawal of treatment, sometimes because the patient is improving and no longer requires that treatment, or because the treatment is having no beneficial effect on their recovery.

In order for an NFACPR order to be valid it should, whenever possible, be discussed with the patient using the above criteria. It should be written, signed, and dated and, if possible, witnessed by an independent party. Most, but not all, will have a review date. This is to allow for the patient's condition to improve and also for the patient to change his or her mind. The decision should be clearly documented in all patient notes, and staff involved in the care of the patient should be informed. The patient in the current scenario continued to receive his oxygen, fluids, nutrition, and drugs as the ceiling of his medical treatment. However, it was essential that he was also kept comfortable.

Decision makers

So who has ultimate responsibility for deciding on a patient's care pathway and treatment options? It should be the most senior doctor in charge of that patient's care (British Medical Association, 2004). This would normally be the patient's GP in the community or their consultant if under hospital care. It may be delegated to someone more junior (i.e. a registrar) but ultimate responsibility is with the GP or consultant. When making these decisions the criteria of beneficence, nonmaleficence and 'what the patient wants' should be employed. It is considered best practice to seek input from other members of the team involved in that patient's care, including the relatives if appropriate, but at present there is no legal obligation to do this. Delays and controversies are more likely to arise with a large and diverse group contributing to the decision-making process. All decisions made should be very clearly documented and it should be ensured that all personnel responsible for, or involved in, delivering care to that patient are aware of the specific treatment pathway for that patient. This will prevent confusion and stop inappropriate resuscitation attempts.

Post cardiac arrest

Patients who have survived a cardiac arrest will require some form of acute care. This may range from simple monitoring to full multiorgan support. There have been various studies on survival outcome predictors, but to date none are sufficiently accurate to be relied upon. The available resources and the abilities of the staff in the location of the patient may raise some dilemmas for those involved in managing and providing for that patient's optimum care. In today's stretched healthcare system, the resources available often govern the optimum treatment. Accessing more advanced treatment options may require transfer of the patient, which in itself can be detrimental. Therefore all the options need to be considered and then the optimum for that patient, in that specific situation, can be decided upon. When these suboptimal decisions have to be made they should be clearly documented, stating the exact reason for the decision, with the options explored and reasons given for not choosing these, always using the principles of beneficence and nonmaleficence and ethical decision-making in professional codes of conduct.

Confidentiality

All patients have a right to confidentiality, and this is essential in all forms of clinical consultations. This principle is essential when working in the field of acute care and is governed in law by the European Convention on Human Rights, Respect for Privacy and Family Life (Article 8) Act 1988 (Data Protection Act 1998). Disclosures required by law or made in connection with legal proceedings are exempt from the non-disclosure provisions by virtue of section 35 of the Act. Also, all NHS Trusts and private sector establishments should have some form of policy covering or incorporating aspects on confidentiality. The 1998 Act aims to protect and control the flow of patient information (data) while ensuring that confidentiality is not undermined. More recently the Caldicott Report (2000) addressed concerns about the ease with which data can be disseminated. Patient confidentiality must be maintained and the patient's best interest ensured when sharing and passing on information between professionals. This can be very difficult in the ward environment where care pathways and sometimes highly sensitive decisions may need to be made at the bedside. For discussion and further thought, consider the case scenario below. It may help to discuss this with some of your colleagues.

Case Scenario

A 65-year-old woman has breast cancer and is receiving chemotherapy treatment for this. She is admitted to the accident and emergency department with a history of chest pain and shortness of breath of 1 week's duration and is now in what appears to be a moribund state.

Chest x-ray shows bilateral lower lobe pneumonia, pleural effusion and what appear to be multiple skeletal metastatic growths.

The relatives say that she had been complaining of 'excruciating pain' prior to admission. Her husband says 'I want everything done to save her'. Her daughter says 'Mum wanted to go in her sleep with no pain'.

How would you address this situation?

What concepts of beneficence need to be addressed?

What principles of nonmaleficence need to be considered before planning a care pathway for this patient?

How would you maintain this patient's confidentiality?

Conclusions

Ethical decision-making while caring for the critically ill poses a huge challenge to healthcare professionals. Using the four ethical principles of beneficence, nonmaleficence, justice and autonomy, as well as adhering to professional codes of conduct, the patient's best interests will be kept at the heart of the decision and management plan. Good teamwork, open communication and consideration of the patient's known wishes are central to caring for the sick ward patient.

References and further reading

American Heart Association, Council on Ethical and Judicial Affairs (1991). Guidelines for the appropriate use of Do Not Resuscitate orders. *Journal of the American Medical Association*, **265**, 1968–71.

Berwick, D.M. and Leape, L.L. (1999). Reducing errors in medicine. *British Medical Journal*, **319**, 136–37.

British Medical Association Ethics Department (2004). *Medical Ethics Today*, 2nd edn. London, British Medical Association.

Caldicott Committee (1997). *Report on the review of patient-identifiable information*. London, Department of Health.

Cioffi, J. (2000). Nurses' experience of making decisions to call emergency assistance to their patients. *Journal of Advanced Nursing*, **32**, 108–114.

Cribb, A. (2002). The ethical dimension: Nursing practice, nursing philosophy and nursing ethics. In: J. Tingle and A. Cribb (eds) *Nursing Law and Ethics*, 2nd edn. Oxford, Blackwell Publishing.

Crighton, I.M. (1997). Failure to recognize the need for readmission to an intensive care or high dependency unit. *British Journal of Intensive Care*, **7**, 46–48.

Department of Health (1998). *The Data Protection Act*. London, Department of Health.

Department of Health (2005). *The Mental Capacity Act – A Summary*. Available at: http://www.dh.gov.uk/en/Policyandguidance/SocialCare/Deliveringadultsocialcare/MentalCapacity/MentalCapacityAct2005?DH_064725 (last accessed November 2009).

General Medical Council (2004). *Confidentiality: Protecting and providing information*. Available at: www.gmc.uk/standards/2004 (last accessed November 2009).

Holm, S. and Ekstrom, L. (1992). Ethics and practice of resuscitation. A Statement for the Advanced life Support Working Party of the European Resuscitation Council. *Resuscitation*, **24**, 239–44.

Leary, T. and Ridley, S. (2003). Impact of an outreach team on re-admissions to a critical care unit. *Anaesthesia*, **58**, 328–32.

McCall Smith, A. (1998). Other people's ethics. *Resuscitation*, **4**, 7–8.

National Commission for the Protection of Human Subjects of Biomedical and Behavioural Research (2003). The Belmont Report: Ethical principles and guidelines for the protection of human subjects of research. In: S. Eckstein, *Manual for Research Ethics Committees*, 6th edn. London, Cambridge University Press.

Neale, G. (1998). Risk management in the care of medical emergencies after referral to hospital. *Journal of the Royal College of Physicians*, **2**, 125–29.

Royal College of Nursing Ethics and Nursing Committee (1992). *Resuscitation; Right or Wrong? The Moral and Legal Issues Faced by Healthcare Professionals*. London, Royal College of Nursing Ethics and Nursing Committee.

Seedhouse, D. (2002). An ethical perspective – How to do the right thing. In: J. Tingle and A. Cribb (eds) *Nursing Law and Ethics*, 2nd edn. Oxford, Blackwell Publishing.

Smith, G.B., Osgood, V.M. and Crane, S. (2002). Alert a multiprofessional training course in the care of the acutely ill adult patient *Resuscitation*, **52**; 281–86.

Useful websites

Department of Health (Mental Capacity Act 2005 and includes downloadable training materials)
www.dh.gov.uk/en/SocialCare/Deliveringadultsocialcare/MentalCapacity/
MentalCapacityAct2005/DH_073511

31 Caring for the suddenly bereaved in the acute care setting

Sally A. Smith and Catherine Plowright

The sudden death of a patient in acute care is not uncommon. For healthcare workers this can be challenging on both a professional and a personal level. At these times they may feel out of their depth and inept (Ferrand *et al.*, 2008). It is not uncommon to feel as though there is little to offer the bereaved at this time.

The sudden death of a close person is always traumatic and has the potential to result in many ongoing problems for the bereaved (Li *et al.*, 2002). The significance and importance of some initial interventions after sudden death and their impact on the bereaved cannot be over-emphasised (Antonacci, 1999; McLauchlan, 1990; Hall and Smith, 1999; Li *et al.*, 2002; Department of Health, 2005). It is a time that the relatives will always remember, and if undertaken incompetently it may result in complicated and protracted grief reactions. For this reason knowing how to deal with these situations allows for greater confidence and competence among healthcare workers.

This chapter offers practical guidance, based on current evidence on how to manage the bereavement of a patient who has died suddenly. It outlines some theories of bereavement, describes the special needs and challenges that unexpected death brings. Hopefully it will enable healthcare workers to effectively care for the suddenly bereaved in acute care settings.

At the end of this chapter you should:

- understand the needs of the suddenly bereaved
- have greater confidence in being able to provide care that helps the bereaved to begin to come to terms with the death of a loved one
- know what strategies to use in order to break bad news kindly and effectively
- be able to provide helpful actions when dealing with different reactions the bereaved person may display.

Specific needs with sudden death

Loss is a universal experience, common to all people of all ages, and it is an inevitable part of life. It is painful for the bereaved person, and for some it can be catastrophic and paralysing. Evidence suggests that the impact of a sudden death on relatives is often more pronounced than death after a long illness. It has the capacity to leave people damaged and disabled (Wright,

1996; Kendrick 1997). It involves intense feelings of distress and disorder, creating a feeling of powerlessness, whereby the bereaved person has neither control nor autonomy and is robbed of a preparatory grief time (Wright, 2007). One reason for this is because sudden death gives no one time prior to the death to prepare for it. This lack of preparation can lead to two kinds of grief – firstly, for what is lost, and secondly, for what might have been (Kendrick, 1997). Unfinished business can be difficult to come to terms with for the suddenly bereaved.

The implication, therefore, is that sudden death is more painful than an expected death, and that having time to prepare and begin the grieving process prior to the death of the patient makes the death easier. Certainly, foreknowledge of the death of someone allows for planning, preparation and farewells. However, it could be argued that no matter how well prepared the family is, the death itself is almost always unexpected, and the family may have needs that are not met.

Grief theories

Many responses to grief have been described and argued over time, from the work of Freud (1917) to Parkes (1996) and that of Wright (2007). Bearing in mind the additional difficulties a sudden death may bring, grief can be considered as work – work that needs to be undertaken and completed prior to moving on in one's life (Wright, 2007). Some theorists believe this work can be described as stages or tasks. It is not a passive process but requires the bereaved person to work hard in order to move on. Box 31.1 describes these theories. The diversity of grief responses needs to be respected because reactions vary enormously. The active processes involved need to be understood and supported. Box 31.1 presents responses and stages in a certain order, but people undergoing grief oscillate among the reactions and can go through them in any order. Improved understanding of the grieving process and what influences it helps inform the way health professionals deal with the bereaved. Certainly training, end-of-life protocols and attending to the needs of families have enhanced the perception of staff that the person who died was cared for in an acceptable way (Ferrand *et al.*, 2008).

Grief reactions

Due to the catastrophic nature of sudden bereavement, people in grief are more prone to experience a sense of unreality and helplessness, and heightened feelings of guilt about having failed to avert the death. Some may have a strong need to blame someone in order to make sense of their loss. Reactions are many and varied and may manifest at different times and for varying durations. Common grief reactions (Wright, 1999; 2007) include:

- **Feelings:** shock, disbelief, fear and anxiety, numbness, anger and hostility, denial, guilt, physical symptoms (e.g. chest pain) and regret.
- **Behaviours:** anxiety attacks and panic, crying and sobbing, inappropriate behaviour (e.g. laughing), withdrawing, bargaining, aggression, searching for the deceased.

Box 31.1 **The work of grieving**

A theory of grief and work (Freud, 1917)

'Each single one of the memories and situations of expectancy which demonstrate the libido's attachment to the lost object is met by the verdict of reality that the object no longer exists. When the work of mourning is completed the ego becomes free and uninhibited again.'

Four tasks of grieving (Worden, 1991)
— Accepting the reality of loss
— Experiencing the pain of grief
— Adjusting to an environment without the deceased
— Withdrawing emotional energy and re-investing in another relationship

Recovery tasks (Scrutton, 1995)
— Intellectual acceptance of bereavement
— Emotional acceptance of bereavement
— Adjusting to loss
— Social re-investment

Syndrome of grief (Stroebe *et al.*, 1997)
— Shock
— Protest
— Despair
— Reorganisation

The normal course of grief (Parkes 1996; 1998)
— Numbness
— Pining and anxiety (pangs of grief)
— Disorganisation and despair
— Reorganisation

Therapeutic interventions

Now consider the case scenario overpage. It often feels like there is very little staff can do to help the suddenly bereaved in an acute care setting. They are in shock and a state of disbelief. Their need for hope has been dashed and they often struggle to assimilate any information given to them. Because there has not been an opportunity to build a trusting relationship up with the staff, it can be difficult to assess the needs of family and friends. However, there are many helpful actions that can help bereaved people, even in such a tragic death as in the following case scenario.

> **Case Scenario**
>
> A 55-year-old woman is admitted to accident and emergency having collapsed at home. She had been complaining of feeling 'odd' over the past week, had been to the GP who said she was suffering from stress and that she should rest. She was found by her daughter unconscious on the floor.
>
> On arrival she was intubated and attached to a ventilator. The ambulance crew had assessed her Glasgow Coma Score as 3. She remained unresponsive. Following a CT scan, she was diagnosed as having had an extensive cerebral bleed. Her prognosis was hopeless and the decision was made to withdraw treatment.
>
> Her husband and three children arrived, along with her brother and sister-in-law. Her children were aged 20, 15 and 10. Her disabled father was telephoned and collected.
>
> The sister-in-law was weepy, but remained calm and in control throughout. She seemed to have accepted that death was imminent. The husband and the youngest son (aged 10) were very withdrawn, not responding and remaining silent. The 20-year-old son was crying, hugging his mother and calling her to wake up. The middle child, the 15-year-old daughter displayed a range of reactions from denial and bargaining (with the accident and emergency and critical care outreach staff to make her better and do anything to ensure this), to hysteria (screaming, running round the carpark shouting) and anger (directed at the GP) as well as sobbing and guilt (for not making her mother go back to the GP).

The goals of care include enabling the bereaved person to understand events so that they can begin the grieving process in as healthy a way as is possible. Bereaved families and healthcare providers have identified a number of helpful actions such as:

- providing privacy to bereaved family members
- offering them emotional support
- allowing them to verbalise their anxieties and concerns
- letting them know that all appropriate treatment had been given to their loved one
- providing them with the opportunity to view the deceased's body (Li *et al.*, 2002) and allowing them to be with the deceased.

Clear, unambiguous, honest information at the earliest available moment at least allows relatives to begin to come to terms with the death. Townsend (1995) states that relatives who are aware that the death will occur, even within hours, may have time to collect their thoughts and memories together in order to prepare themselves. This may help them cope better than having no warning. Lautrette *et al.* (2007) evaluated the use of an information booklet for bereaved relatives and showed a significant reduction in signs of depression after the death.

The family in the current case scenario did not respond well to the news of the imminent death. They continued to display a range of distressing grief reactions to the news, which was painful for them as well as for the team to witness.

Breaking bad news

Suddenly bereaved people are often so overwhelmed that they are for a time incapable of the level of functioning required for grief work; mourning is simply postponed. The efforts of healthcare professionals will relate to enhancing the perception, reality and understanding of the event. In the acute setting we cannot be responsible for their long-term care, so our aims (Wright, 1999) are to:

- give the facts
- confirm reality
- acknowledge feelings
- Identify support.

Supporting and comforting the bereaved

Staff sometimes perceive a difficulty in developing a rapport with relatives. This has been cited as affecting their perception of the quality of care delivered (Ferrand *et al.*, 2008). Researchers found that a close relationship can be developed in a short time span if the nurses showed understanding and support towards the relatives (Jackson, 1998). This is particularly so if the same nurse caring for the patient also deals with the relatives.

An essential aspect to supporting and comforting the bereaved is knowing how to manage their emotional responses. Wright (1996) studied 100 sudden deaths and found that it was the bereaved person who became withdrawn that posed the most difficulty for nurses. Crying, sobbing, weeping and acceptance were the easiest for them to manage. Whatever the profession, caring for the suddenly bereaved can quickly leave someone feeling as if they are not in control and are ineffective in their care. Training and education on how best to deal with emotional responses are imperative. Guidance regarding this is available in the literature and should be integral in the knowledge and skill acquisition training that healthcare professionals undertake. Some of this evidence is described below with respect to enabling staff to care for themselves, while caring for the bereaved.

There may be a tendency, given the helplessness and overwhelming pain the healthcare worker witnesses (and sometimes experience themselves) to 'rush in' and attempt to comfort (Bowman, 1999). When people are shocked and disorientated, it can be destabilising. The goal should be to focus on helping them accept that the death has occurred and to foster and promote autonomy and control. Sometimes it is necessary to guide the relatives because they may not know how to grieve (Wright, 1996). Anticipating their needs and implementing a proactive approach is important. This may involve simply providing certain conditions for the relatives, such as refreshments, or more complex issues like creating a safe open environment in which they are able to ask questions and responding or making suggestions about what may be helpful to do. This helps to promote a sense of control and choice. A useful tool for actively caring for the bereaved is the 'Four Es' (Box 31.2).

Box 31.2   **The four Es (McLaughlan, 1990)**
E—**E**mpathise E—**E**nable relatives to accept reality and to experience the pain E—**E**ncourage in an appropriate way, offering help for example E—**E**ncounter your own feelings and express them later, perhaps as part of a debriefing

Continuous assessment of how each person is coping allows specific interventions and care to be planned and delivered, maximising coping strengths and strategies.

Preparation of the bereaved

Consideration must be given to where the news is to be broken and by whom. The best person to tell the family is someone who is skilled to do so, who knows the patient, who has the correct information, and who is able to answer their questions. The setting needs to be private, peaceful and free from interruption. In the current scenario, the team ensured that the sister-in-law, who appeared to be coping the best, was present with the family and was the main point of liaison for the nurses and doctors. The news was broken in a quiet room away from the main resuscitation room.

Preparation is vital, including ensuring that staff have adequate time. Simple measures like ensuring bleeps and telephones are silenced is important. If there are any communication issues – such as English not being understood, or deafness – these need to be thought through and addressed.

Begin by getting a feel from the family about what they already know and understand – this is a good starting place. Remember all efforts are focused on facts, reality and helping the bereaved to fully understand the situation. Misunderstandings and misinterpretations occur easily with someone who is upset, so avoid euphemisms and instead use the words 'dead' and 'died'. Phrases like 'I am sorry we have lost her' are open to misunderstanding and may feed denial (Wright, 2007). Families value honest direct information. There is an overwhelming need for them to know the 'bottom line'.

Be aware of your posture, and the tone and pace of your voice. Be aware of your facial expressions and the amount of eye contact you make. Consider which of your mannerisms may put people off, but bear in mind that mannerisms are a feature of your personality and that these families will appreciate a glimpse of the real you. Being comfortable with silences is also important, although this can be very challenging.

If the bereaved person becomes very distressed while you are caring for them, remember that it is the information being imparted that is causing the distress – not you personally.

Dealing with grief reactions

The way bereaved people display their grief can be challenging. However there are certain ways staff can manage tricky situations and help them.

Denial

When the reality becomes too much to bear the relative or friend may begin to deny the facts. Some families will ask the same question repeatedly hoping that subsequent answers become more favourable. Try not to be swayed or allow any other member of the family or colleagues to do so either. Continue repeating the same statements of fact in a gentle but assertive way.

Bargaining

Sometimes families may try bargaining with the person breaking the news. Again continue to give the facts, confirming the reality of the death. Sometimes a remark about life being of inestimable value may help them regain insight into what can be realistically achieved.

In our case scenario the teenaged daughter was oscillating between several grief reactions; bargaining with the team was just one. She was able to move on from it by seeing her mother and hearing again that there was nothing that could be done, albeit very painful and distressing for her.

Anger

Anger can pose problems for the doctor or nurse. It can be frightening to witness and sometimes feel threatening. Remembering that anger is a feeling and acknowledging it as such can often help diffuse it.

Withdrawing and isolation

Some people withdraw and just need time to assimilate all the information given to them. Just being with someone who reacts like this may be enough support at this time. Similarly, some bereaved people may feel a great sense of isolation, despite being surrounded by their close family. When they express this the rest of the family can feel rejected. It may be worth pointing out that this is because the bereaved person is concentrating on their specific relationship with the dead person who has gone, leaving them alone. Again, acknowledge this feeling, but ensure that they are not left alone, because the fear this feeling brings will be compounded by the physical reality of being isolated.

The husband in our case scenario displayed these grief reactions. He spent some time with his wife, with a nurse nearby. He did request solitude, during which time he hugged her and sobbed, finally reaching the point where he could accept she was not going to live.

Guilt

Many people feel guilty even when they are not. People who are not guilty will not stop feeling guilty until they have gained insight into the reality. Again, acknowledge the feeling and just listen to them.

Inappropriate behaviour

Inappropriate behaviour, such as telling jokes or laughing, arises because focusing on the death is just too painful for some people (Wright, 1996). It is a common response in children and adolescents who often have little or no experience of grief and have no idea how to react. Remain non-judgemental; the person may well become embarrassed about such responses later on.

Crying

Crying is a very common response and one that healthcare professionals find the easiest to deal with. Bear in mind that men may need permission to cry, and that some people are distressed by a normal early reaction of not being able to cry. Reassurance and comforting often help. Staff who feel they do not know how to react or manage the situation can fall back on basic humanity and on what feels right and natural – these are often helpful.

Resuscitation

On some occasions relatives arrive when resuscitation attempts are still in progress. It is important not to exclude relatives from the proceedings, and regular updates, plus informing them that every effort is being made to save the patient, are sensible stances to take. Some relatives may wish to be present during resuscitation. This does have identified benefits and allows them to be present at the time of death (Wright, 1999; Royal College of Nursing, 2002; Baskett *et al.*, 2005; Fulbrook *et al.*, 2007). Make sure a member of staff stays with the relative who is able to provide support and explain procedures as well as to assess and act if the relative becomes very distressed (and accompany them if they need to leave) (see Chapter 30 on ethics in acute care).

Culture and religion

Religion and culture are important when a person dies. Ensure this aspect of a family's lifestyle is addressed. Consulting them about their wishes and specific requirements so that appropriate religious and cultural interventions are found that are spiritually and culturally acceptable. In certain circumstances organ donation may be discussed, which may provide some comfort or meaning to the death they are experiencing (see Chapter 32 on organ donation).

Closure and viewing the body

Closure is an important aspect of accepting the reality of the death and it should be actively promoted. Viewing the body and taking the opportunity to say goodbye is a positive intervention that staff can encourage, no matter who the relatives are in terms of age or frailty. Reality, although painful, is more manageable than fantasy, which can become intrusive and uncomfortable – especially in children. Telling people what to expect when they see the body will help them. Talking to and touching the dead person allows some of the unfinished business to be addressed. In fact there is little doubt that time and effort spent with the deceased is tremendously valuable. However, because of the disordered thought processes associated with loss, many people are unsure about what is 'allowed' or considered normal. It is therefore helpful if they are told it is all right to touch, hold and speak to their loved one. Family members should be allowed to decide for themselves whether they want to see the dead person or not (Haas, 2003). If they act on someone else's advice, they may risk profound regrets later. Point this out to well-meaning family members who try to decide who should see or not see the body.

Sadly, as previously discussed, suddenly bereaved people remain numb and shocked for some time. Despite their insatiable need for highly detailed information, they may later realise they have not understood or remembered very much. There may be no formal way in which to rectify this. A common perception by families is of abrupt withdrawal of care. Many relatives express a wish to retain contact with staff, and it has been recommended for the use of support programmes for relatives. The benefits are that aftercare can help fulfil the long-term needs of families with respect to obtaining information and clarifying issues surrounding the death of their loved one. They also provide a vehicle through which reassurance and support can be sought, with the opportunity to make referrals to specialist bereavement groups where applicable.

Conclusions

Although it feels like there is nothing one can do to minimise the pain and distress of sudden death when dealing with the bereaved, aiming for simple goals like giving the facts and confirming reality so that the person accepts that the death has happened can be beneficial later, when they begin their journey of grief work. By taking these simple steps, the healthcare professional can ensure that the last moments with a loved one are meaningful and precious. A greater awareness of the grieving process and ways in which the suddenly bereaved can be helped will improve practice; the essence of bereavement care is about intervening in order to facilitate a healthy grieving process.

References and further reading

Antonacci, M. (1990). Sudden death: helping bereaved parents in the PICU. *Critical Care Nurse*, **10**(4), 65–70.

Baskett, P.J.F., Steen, P.A. and Bossaert, L. (2005). European Council Guidelines for resuscitation 2005: Section 8: The ethics of resuscitation and end of life decisions. *Resuscitation*, **67**(Suppl.1), S171–80.

Bowman, T. (1999). Promoting resiliency in those who do bereavement work. *National Association of Bereavement Services*. London, National Association of Bereavement Services.

Chapple, H.S. (1999). Changing the game in the intensive care unit: letting nature take its course. *Critical Care Nurse*, **19**(3), 25–34.

Department of Health (2005). *When a Patient Dies – Advice on Developing Bereavement Services in the NHS*. London, Department of Health.

Ferrand, E., Jabre, P., Vincent-Genod, C., *et al*. (2008). Circumstances of death in hospitalized patients and nurses' perceptions: French multicenter mort a l'hopital survey. *Archives of Internal Medicine*, **168**, 867–75.

Freud, S. (1917). *Mourning and Melancholia. Volume XIV*. London, Hogarth.

Fulbrook, P., Latour, J., Albarran, J., *et al*. (2007). The presence of family members during cardiopulmonary resuscitation: European Federation of Critical Care Nursing Associations, European and Neonatal Intensive Care and European Society of Cardiology Council on Cardiovascular Nursing and Allied Professions Joint position statement. *CONNECT: The World of Critical Care Nursing*, **5**(4), 86–88.

Haas, F. (2003). Bereavement care: Seeing the body. *Nursing Standard*, **17**(28), 33–37.

Hall, S.J. and Smith, G.B. (1999). Breaking bad news to the friends, family and partners of intensive care unit patients: A practical guide. *Care of the Critically Ill*, **15**(3), 101–04.

Jackson, I. (1998). A study of bereavement in an intensive therapy unit. *Nursing in Critical Care*, **3**(3), 141–50.

Kendrick, K. (1997). Sudden death: walking in a moral minefield. *Emergency Nurse*, **5**(1), 17–19.

Kubler-Ross, E. (1969). *On Death and Dying*. New York, Springer.

Lautrette, A., Darmon, M., Megarbane, B., *et al.* (2007). A communication strategy and brochure for relatives of patients dying in the ICU. *New England Journal of Medicine*, **356**, 469–78.

Lewis, C.S. (1961). *A Grief Observed*. London, Faber.

Li, S.P., Chan, C. and Lee, D. (2002). Helpfulness of nursing actions to suddenly bereaved family members in an accident and emergency setting in Hong Kong. *Journal of Advanced Nursing*, **40**(2), 170–80.

McLaughlan, C.A.J. (1990). Handling distressed relatives and breaking bad news. *British Medical Journal*, **301**, 1145–49.

Parkes, C. (1996). *Bereavement: Studies of Grief in Adult Life*, 3rd edn. London, Routledge.

Parkes, C.M. (1998). Coping with loss: Bereavement in adult life. *British Medical Journal*, **316**(7134), 856–59.

Royal College of Nursing (2002). *Witnessing Resuscitation: Guidance for Nursing Staff*. London, Royal College of Nursing.

Russell, P. and Sander, R. (1998). Palliative care: promoting the concept of a healthy death. *British Journal of Nursing*, **7**(5), 255–61.

Scrutton, S. (1995). *Bereavement and Grief: Supporting Older People Through Loss*. London, Edward Arnold.

Stroebe, M.S., Stroebe, W. and Hansson, R.O. (1993). *Handbook of Bereavement: Theory, Research and Intervention*. Cambridge, Cambridge University Press.

Townsend, A. (1995). Sudden death in critical care units. *Care of the Critically Ill*, **11**(3), 126–28.

Weston, R., Martin, T. and Anderson, Y. (1998). *Loss and Bereavement: Managing Change*. Oxford, Blackwell Science.

Worden, J. (1991). *Grief Counselling and Grief Therapy*. London, Tavistock Publications.

Wright, B. (1996). *Sudden Death – A Research Base for Practice. London,* Churchill Livingstone.

Wright, B. (1999). Responding to autonomy and disempowerment at the time of a sudden death. *Accident and Emergency Nursing*, **7**, 154–57.

Wright, B. (2007). *Loss and Grief.* Keswick, M&K Update.

Useful websites

Cruise Bereavement Care
www.cruisebereavementcare.org.uk

Department of Health
www.dh.gov.uk/en/Healthcare/Secondarycare/Bereavement/index.htm

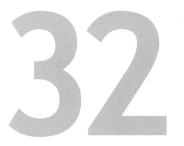

32 Organ and tissue donation

Tim Collins

Organ and tissue transplantation have been proven to be effective treatments for end-stage organ failure and have been shown to significantly improve the quality of life for patients awaiting a tissue transplant. Most organ donations come from patients who have been certified brainstem dead (BSD) whilst in the intensive care unit due to a sudden traumatic brain injury or cerebral insult. Solid organs that can be donated include the kidneys, liver, heart, lungs and pancreas (Human Tissue Authority, 2006).

These organs can be transplanted to replace someone's failing organ and they are often life-saving for the recipients. Solid organs need to have minimal interruptions in perfusion, otherwise the lack of oxygen delivered to the organs in a low-perfusion state will make the organs unviable. This is why solid organs are retrieved from either brainstem dead patients or from non-heart-beating organ donors (NHBOD) where death of the patient has just occurred normally when treatment has been withdrawn in the intensive care or emergency department. Organs can also be obtained from a living donor who could donate a kidney to a relative (Human Tissue Authority, 2006). In addition to organs, tissues can be donated, such as corneas, heart valves, bone, skin and tendons (Human Tissue Authority, 2006). Most people who die can donate at least one tissue but unlike organs these can be retrieved from up to 48 hours after death. Unlike organ donation, tissue donation is not life-saving but it provides recipients with improvements in the quality of their life, for instance, a corneal transplant will restore sight.

Currently there is a mass shortage of organs available for transplantation. The transplant waiting list continues to get longer as demand outstrips supply. Between April 2007 and 2008, 3235 solid organ transplants were undertaken within the UK, which were either life-saving or improved quality of life for the recipients. However, 7655 people were left on the transplant waiting list that year (see the UK Transplant website). A further 2489 people had tissue donations; their sight was restored after transplant of corneas following the death of donor patients. The general yearly trend is that the number of organs becoming available remains static, while the number of patients added to the transplant waiting list increases each year. Therefore it is imperative that healthcare practitioners identify potential organ and tissue donors and approach their families for consent.

The UK Department of Health (Department of Health, 2008) has set up an organ donation task force to look at a number of strategies aiming to increase organ donation by 50% by the next 5 years. This task force has stipulated a number of recommendations including:

- increasing the number of transplant coordinators
- making more financial enhancements to NHS trusts who are involved in donation
- delivering mandatory donation education to staff working in critical care areas
- modernising the transplant service and the development of more local organ donation policies.

After reading this chapter, you should be able to:

- identify what organs and tissues can be donated and the common contraindications for donation
- describe the key concepts related to the organ and tissue donation process
- discuss brainstem death testing (BDT) as well as the concepts of non-heart-beating organ donation
- know how to effectively approach families for donation consent
- analyse the role of the healthcare professional in identifying, managing, supporting and referring organ or tissue donors within the acute environment
- understand the transplant coordination service and the importance of referring potential donor patients.

Differences between organ and tissue donation

Solid organs that can be donated include the heart, lungs, liver, kidneys, pancreas and small bowel. Solid organ retrieval is normally undertaken on brainstem-dead or non-heart-beating patients as the organ cannot suffer from any major ischaemia before transplantation, because the organ may not be salvageable (UK Transplant, 2005). Therefore solid organ retrieval is normally undertaken after BSD certification or just after the patient becomes asystolic (non-heart-beating). The process is often more complicated than tissue donation as the healthcare team have to manage a cardiovascularly unstable patient while trying to ensure maximum organ perfusion prior to retrieval.

In contrast, tissue donation can be undertaken after 24–48 hours following cardiorespiratory cessation (UK Transplant, 2005). Tissues that can be donated following death include corneas, heart valves, skin, tendon and bone (UK Transplant, 2005). Studies have found that the majority of patients who die in hospitals may be eligible for tissue donation, however relatives are infrequently asked for consent because nursing and medical staff are either unaware of tissue donation or inadequately prepared to obtain donation consent (Cantwell and Clifford, 2000; Collins, 2005).

Brainstem death

The management of the brainstem dead patient is one of the most challenging and demanding roles for the healthcare professional. Often these patients are young, having sustained a sudden and catastrophic insult that often means that they and their family have no preparation of them becoming unwell. The current position in UK law is that there is no statutory definition of death (Academy of Medical Royal Colleges, 2008).

The definition of death recommended by the Academy of Medical Royal Colleges (2008) is that 'death is the irreversible loss of essential characteristics which are necessary to the existence of a living human person'. This definition should be regarded as the irreversible loss of the capacity to maintain consciousness, combined with the irreversible loss of capacity to breathe. Therefore death is not confirmed solely by the absence of a palpable pulse because a patient with irreversible damage to the brainstem can be declared dead despite having a palpable pulse and may have a sustained capacity to breathe via a mechanical ventilator.

The brainstem consists of the pons, medulla oblongata and midbrain, and contains vital functions of life like respiratory control. Brainstem death occurs when the brainstem becomes damaged so that it can no longer maintain life. It cannot recover and no treatment can reverse the damage. The patient loses consciousness and the independent capacity to breathe, and is usually intubated and ventilated so the function of breathing is maintained artificially. Excessive raised intracranial pressure compresses the brainstem and subsequently causes ischaemia and hypoxia, causing irreversible damage that is incompatible with life.

The causes (Bersten and Soni, 2003) include:

- intracerebral bleeding (e.g. subarachnoid haemorrhage)
- cerebral infarction
- head trauma
- cerebral hypoxia
- cerebral tumour
- drug overdose
- intracerebral infection and meningitis.

However, if brainstem death occurs and the patient is being mechanically ventilated, the patient's respiratory function will be maintained. Following brainstem testing the patient is certified as dead, and asystole usually occurs within 72 hours (Bersten and Soni, 2003). There are two options for the patient – organ retrieval or discontinuation of mechanical ventilation which will terminate his or her respiration.

Brainstem death testing

Brainstem death testing is undertaken to determine whether the brainstem function is still intact and if the patient is not just suffering from a deep coma. In the UK there are three stages in the diagnosis of brainstem death: preconditions, exclusions and clinical tests. If the patient fails to show any response to the tests, it means the brainstem has been irreversibly damaged and death can be confirmed.

The tests have to be undertaken by two doctors who have been registered for more than 5 years and are conversant with the tests. At least one must be a consultant. Testing should be undertaken together and must be fully completed and successful on two occasions (Academy of Medical Royal Colleges, 2008). The legal time of death is the time of completion of the first set of brainstem death testing. All this needs to be explained to relatives by a practitioner with effective communication skills, who has built up a rapport with the relatives and has appropriate knowledge and understanding of the tests. If it is felt appropriate, consider allowing the relatives to observe the tests themselves. In a small-scale study by Collins (2005), nurses believed the relatives accepted the reality of their loved one's death more readily if they were effectively supported and given clear explanations of the tests being undertaken.

Box 32.1   Criteria for the diagnosis of brainstem death (BSD)

The criteria for the diagnosis of brainstem death from the Academy of Medical Royal Colleges (2008) consist of pre-conditions, exclusions and testing of the brainstem, as follows.

Pre-conditions
— The patient is comatose and mechanically ventilated.
— Diagnosis of structural brain damage has been established or the immediate cause of coma is known.
— It is essential to have a period of observation.

Exclusions
— Drugs are not the cause if coma is present (e.g. barbiturates).
— Neuromuscular blockade has been demonstrably reversed.
— Hypothermia does not exist (> 34°C).
— There is no endocrine or metabolic disturbance.

Testing (using reflexes that involve brainstem function)
— Papillary response to light
— Corneal reflex
— Vestibular ocular reflex
— Motor response to pain
— Gag reflex (to suctioning through endotracheal tube or tracheostomy).
— Apnoea that persists despite a rise in $PaCO_2$ greater than 6.6Kpa against a background of a normal PaO_2.

For further information on BSD testing please refer to the current guidance on brainstem death testing which can be obtained from the intensive care unit or transplant coordinator.

It is now universally accepted that early referral should be made to the transplant coordinators if you suspect a patient is brainstem dead. Transplant coordinators need to be made aware of such patients at the earliest opportunity. Due to the shortage of organs they would rather be called regarding any potential donor even if the patient turns out not to be brainstem dead or the family decline donation. It is also perceived to be best practice to use the collaborative approach for gaining consent from families for their loved one to be an organ donor. The transplant coordinators are experts in the field of donation and provide professional advice

Table 32.1 **Management of the multiorgan donor patient (adapted from Adam and Osborne, 2005)**

Body system	Management goals and treatment aims
Ventilation/ respiratory	Continue with mandatory ventilation Use positive end-expiratory pressure (PEEP) Regular arterial blood gases Adjust FiO_2 and normalise pH CO_2 as required Physiotherapy and suctioning to remove secretions $PaO_2 > 11$ kPa and $PaCO_2$ 4.5–6 kPa Peak ventilation airway pressures < 30 cmH_2O Clear chest x-ray Audible clear bilateral air entry Good respiratory function is maintained
Cardiovascular	Ensure adequate filling; intravenous fluid challenges are required Use inotropes if required (use epinephrine only as a last resort) Maintain mean arterial pressure > 60 mmHg and CVP of 5–10 Urine output > 0.5 mL/kg/hour Maintain good organ perfusion
Temperature	Warm slowly to avoid vasodilation and drops in mean arterial pressure (MAP) Warming blankets, intravenous fluids, warm bladder/nasogastric washouts Maintain temperature between 35°C and 37.8°C Normal temperature is maintained
Electrolyte/ metabolic	Regularly check electrolytes and commence replacement therapy Commence insulin sliding scale to maintain goal glucose levels Check relevant clotting factors (if abnormal and appropriate correct coagulopathy with clotting factors) Maintain sodium 135–155 mmol/L and potassium 3.8–4.5 mmol/L Glucose 4–9 mmol pH 7.35–7.45 Avoid coagulopathy and haemorrhage Electrolyte and metabolic homeostasis is maintained
Elimination/ hydration	Ensure intravenous fluids continue to maintain adequate hydration Continue nasogastric feeding 5% dextrose if required to keep sodium below 155 mmol/L Administer DDAVP™ (desmopressin) 4 µg if evidence of diabetes insipidus with large urine output Ensure adequate fluid hydration, MAP and CVP Ensure maintenance of correct fluid balance and electrolytes Avoid diabetes insipidus and volume depletion Fluid homeostasis is maintained

to both medical and nursing staff, as well as providing invaluable support to patients relatives even if they decide not to give consent to organ donation.

For further information on BSD testing please refer to the current guidance on brainstem death from your hospital's intensive care unit or transplant coordinator.

Non-heart-beating organ donation

Non-heart-beating organ donation (NHBOD) is an option for any patient aged under 65 years where the decision has been made that further medical treatment is futile and there is to be a planned withdrawal of treatment.

The difference between brainstem-dead donation and NHBOD is that the former are already declared dead but are mechanically ventilated and transferred to the operating theatre for donation with a beating heart. NHBOD takes place immediately after the patient has become asystolic; ongoing treatment has been considered futile and the decision has been made to withdraw it. If the patient has no contraindications and meets the inclusion criteria, then NHBOD is a possibility. It is best practice to consider all patients as potential NHBOD when withdrawing treatment and discussions should take place with the transplant coordinators to confirm eligibility.

In order to ensure that the organs do not sustain under-perfusion ischaemia, the patient needs to become asystolic within a short period of time after withdrawal of treatment. This means that long periods of hypotension will exclude the patient from donation because death needs to occur quickly. Withdrawal of treatment often takes place in the anaesthetic room to minimise the delay for the patient entering surgery for organ retrieval. Family members can be present when their loved one's heart actually stops beating (sometimes they want to be present when death occurs, which is not possible with brainstem-dead donors). The patient is then certified dead in the anaesthetic room, the family say their goodbyes and then the patient is moved into the operating theatre for prompt organ retrieval to minimise organ ischaemia time. Currently it is possible for the kidneys, liver, lungs and pancreas (for islet cells) to be donated following NHBOD at the onset of asystole (Bersten and Soni, 2003; Intensive Care Society, 2004). As with brainstem-dead donation, it is imperative that early referral is made to the transplant coordinators to facilitate the process and provide support to the family, as well as to healthcare staff.

General criteria for organ donation

Any patient who meets these criteria should be considered for organ donation and their family should be offered the option:

- If the patient has suffered irreversible brain damage leading to brainstem death or whose condition is such that continuing critical care is considered futile and withdrawal of treatment is being considered.
- If the patient does not test positive for HIV.
- If the patient is not suspected or known to have Creutzfeldt–Jacob disease.

There are no absolute age restrictions to solid organ donation and each potential organ donor should be individually assessed for donation suitability rather than automatic restrictions due to age. Therefore it is imperative that patients should be referred to the transplant coordinators who assess suitability rather than deciding exclusions at a local hospital level.

Tissue donation

Tissue donation is an option for many families following death in hospitals and palliative care settings, however it has been documented that many nursing and medical staff are unaware of this option (Cantwell and Clifford, 2000; Collins, 2005). Patients can donate tissues like corneas, heart valves, skin, bone and tendons, even if they have not been certified as brainstem dead (Human Tissue Authority, 2006). Patients receiving a tissue transplant may not have their lives saved but they will experience significant improvements in the quality of their lives, for example restoration of eye sight from a corneal transplant. It is recommended that healthcare staff routinely assess and approach relatives for consent for tissue donation. This really should be done prior to deterioration of the patient so their wishes can be recorded (Human Tissue Authority, 2006).

General criteria for tissue donation

Tissue donation criteria with respect to age and medical suitability vary depending on the tissue to be donated. Tissues can be retrieved up to 24 hours after circulatory cessation except for heart valves, which can be retrieved up to 48 hours after asystole (Human Tissue Authority, 2006). Individuals suffering from systemic malignancies are contraindicated for donating tissues, except for corneas. There are absolute contraindications for tissue donation which include patients who have:

- tested positive for HIV, hepatitis viruses B and C, human T cell lymphotrophic virus (HTLV) or syphilis (or have high-risk behaviour for contracting these infections)
- suffered from Creutzfeldt–Jacob disease or have a family history of it (Intensive Care Society, 2004)
- a progressive neurological disease of unknown pathophysiology (e.g. multiple sclerosis, Alzheimer's disease, Parkinson's disease or motor neuron disease)
- leukaemia, lymphoma or myeloma
- had a previous transplant requiring immunosuppressive treatment.

In addition to the above, there are contraindications for specific tissues and you are advised to contact your regional transplant coordinator if in doubt and wish to assess patient suitability.

Approaching families for donation consent

Many hospitals in collaboration with their regional transplant coordinators undertake the collaborative approach to asking consent for donations of solid organs. The transplant coordinators are notified early, ideally before undertaking BSD testing, which means a transplant coordinator is present on the intensive care unit to answer questions from both relatives and staff concerning donation. Having a transplant coordinator present during the organ donation process has been shown to significantly improve the chances of relatives offering donation consent. Therefore you are advised to contact the regional transplant coordinator for specialist advice about donation before BSD testing or discussing donation options with relatives (Bersten and Soni, 2003; Intensive Care Society, 2004; Human Tissue Authority, 2006). Due to the number of tissue donation referrals, many regional transplant coordinators do not have sufficient resources to offer the option of a collaborative approach to consent for tissue donation. This is usually undertaken by healthcare staff within the local hospital environment. Healthcare staff often find it difficult to approach families about consent for tissue and organ donation, however following the systematic approach outlined in Box 32.2 will aid the practitioner in this process (Cantwell and Clifford, 2000; Bersten and Soni, 2003).

Points to remember

The situation cannot get any worse for this family so there is no harm in asking; they may even gain some relief in their bereavement by being given the option. If they refuse consent, respect their wishes and just say this was an option open to them to consider. On the other hand, if they do give consent, document this in the medical notes and get one of them to sign consent. Obtain a phone number where they can be reached over the next few hours. A transplant coordinator will ring them to reconfirm consent and follow up any questions they might have. Once they have consented, phone the transplant coordinators (via the hospital switchboard) who will ask you some questions about the patient.

Role of the transplant coordinators

Transplant coordinators are usually specialist nurses who have previously worked in critical care areas and have undergone additional training in organ transplantation. Their role is varied and demanding but they facilitate the organ donation process by:

- organising the donation retrieval
- communicating with and supporting the family before, during and after organ retrieval
- supporting and communicating with healthcare professionals at the donor hospital and liaising between different departments (e.g. theatres)
- ensuring that appropriate medical investigations are undertaken and reviewing medical notes to ensure there are no contraindications that exclude donation
- coordinating the transplant retrieval team and liaising with transplant centres
- providing education and advice for both healthcare professionals and the public on all matters related to donation and transplantation.

These are just some of the duties of a transplant coordinator. They provide a 24-hour service and are always available for advice. Due to the shortage of available organs, they would rather that patients were referred than for potential donors to be missed, so never feel reluctant to contact them if you are unsure about a potential donor. Your hospital switchboard will hold the number for the regional transplant coordinator.

> **Box 32.2** **Key points to consider when approaching a family for tissue donation consent**
>
> **When?**
> — When death is pronounced.
> — When the relatives are informed.
> — When the relatives understand the cause of death.
>
> **Where?**
> — Not at the bedside or in a corridor.
> — In a private and quiet room.
> *Speak at the same level.*
>
> **Who?**
> — A practitioner who is familiar with the family.
> — A practitioner with sensitivity and effective interpersonal skills.
> *It does not have to be a senior person or medical staff member as long as they display the above skills.*
>
> **Phrases that help**
> 'I know this is a very difficult time but I have some important information for you to consider.'
> 'Do you know if {*patient's name*} carried a donor card?'
> 'It may be possible for {*patient's name*} to donate if you think that is what {*he or she*} would have wanted to do.'
> 'Did you ever talk about organ donation as a family?'

Conclusions

Organ and tissue donation is an effective treatment for end-stage organ failure and has been shown to improve the quality of life for patients awaiting tissue transplants. It is imperative that healthcare staff respect the final wishes of their patients and ensure that the organ donation process is followed, otherwise the transplant waiting list will continue to get longer and the last wishes of our patients will be ignored. Regional transplant coordinators are always available to support and assist healthcare staff in this process and should be contacted early, usually via the hospital switchboard, so that a collaborative approach can be used in the management of donor patients and their families.

References and further reading

Academy of Medical Royal Colleges (2008) *Code of Practice for the Diagnosis and Confirmation of Death*. London, Millbank Media.

Adam, S. and Osborne, S. (2005). *Critical Care Nursing*, 2nd edn. London, Oxford University Press.

Bersten, A. and Soni, N. (2003). *Oh's Intensive Care Manual*. London, Butterworth.

Cantwell, M. and Clifford, C. (2000). English nursing and medical students' attitudes towards organ donation. *Journal of Advanced Nursing*, **4**: 961–68.

Collins, T. (2005). Organ and tissue donation: A survey of nurse's knowledge and educational needs in an adult ITU. *Intensive and Critical Care Nursing*, **21**, 226–33.

Department of Health (2008). Organ Donation Task Force Programme Delivery Board. Available at: www.dh.gov.uk/en/Healthcare/Secondarycare/Transplantation/Organdonation/DH_088526 (last accessed October 2009).

Human Tissue Authority (2006). *Code of Practice: Donation of Organs, Tissues and Cells for Transplantation*, 2nd edn. London, Department of Health.

Intensive Care Society (2004). *Guidelines for Adult Organ and Tissue Donations*. London, ICS.

UK Transplant (2005). *Transplant Update* (December 2004). Available at: www.uktransplant.org.uk (last accessed November 2009).

Useful websites

British Transplantation Society
www.bts.org.uk

Intensive Care Standards (for organ and tissue donation with intensive care)
www.ics.ac.uk

UK Transplant
www.uktransplant.org.uk

Family care

Catherine Plowright

Admission to an intensive care unit or high dependency unit has been described as a traumatic and frightening experience for patients and their families, and many highlight the fear, anxiety and psychological distress induced by critical illness (McGonigal, 1986; Quinn *et al.*, 1999; Jones, 2002; Skirrow, 2002), as well as the physiological problems induced by critical illness on leaving the intensive care unit (Cochran, 1984; Chew, 1986; Booth, 1991).

A number of useful websites can be accessed that are designed for families of critically ill patients and which healthcare professionals will find useful in caring for these families. These websites include the Intensive Care Society, DIPex (Database of Individual Patient Experiences) and ICUSteps (Intensive Care Unit Support Team for Ex-Patients). DIPex has a database of audio and video clips and transcript of interviews with patients experiencing a particular illness or health problems which includes a module on intensive care. ICUSteps is a support group set up by former intensive care patients and family members based in Milton Keynes, UK. They hold regular drop-ins and offer support for other ex-patients or family members to come along and talk about their experiences and rehabilitation. The web site includes ex-patients' and family members' own experiences.

The terms family, families and relatives include everyone who is significant to the patient. Families need to be cared for by all healthcare professionals before, during and after their loved one's stay on the intensive care unit. The responsibilities of healthcare professionals extend both before and after admission to intensive care.

By the end of this chapter you will have an understanding of the care that families of patients on the intensive care unit require within the ward environment.

Before admission to intensive care

Many admissions to intensive care are emergencies and cannot, therefore, be planned. It is important that families are informed as soon as possible about the deteriorating condition of their relative. Communication must be timely and appropriate, and delivered by someone who has been trained to deliver bad news (see Chapter 31 on caring for the suddenly bereaved in the acute care setting). If the admission is an elective one, then the families as well as the patient should be involved and fully informed. The effect of good preoperative information is well documented with respect to preparing patients psychologically for operations and providing information (Cochran, 1984; Chew, 1986; Booth, 1991).

Care while in intensive care

Families need to be cared for as much as the critically ill patient when they are on intensive care. They suffer from the physical, social and psychological effects of their loved one's critical illness. Nursing research on the relatives of critically ill patients has generally focused on their self-perceived needs and satisfaction levels around those needs (Molter, 1979; Plowright, 1999; Engstrom and Soderberg 2004; Hughes *et al.*, 2005). The seminal work of Molter (1979) was significant in identifying the needs of relatives of critically ill patients. Molter developed a tool known as the 'critical care family needs inventory' (the CCFNI) which has been used widely over the last two decades for analysing the needs of family members while the patient is in intensive care. Such relatives always have a tendency to prioritise their needs around the patient, rather than themselves (Plowright, 1995) and this can be seen in various studies where they often rank their personal needs as the lowest (Molter 1979; Daley, 1984; Farrell and Frost, 1992; Dyer, 1991). The work over the years clearly identifies the need categories of families when the patient is in intensive care.

The needs of relatives in intensive care

1. The need for relief of anxiety

- To know what the expected outcome may be.
- To know what treatments the patient is receiving.
- To have someone explain the equipment being used.
- To be called at home if the condition changes.
- To know the nurses are giving the best care possible.
- To be told of transfers ahead of time.
- To be told there is hope.

2. The need for information

- To know what is wrong with the patient.
- To talk to a doctor.
- To talk to a nurse.
- To have questions answered honestly.
- To be informed if condition changes.
- To be called at home every morning.
- To have understandable explanations.
- To know the qualifications of the staff caring for the patient.
- To be allowed to call at any time.

3. The need to be with the patient

- To be able to stay with the patient.
- To be able to stay nearby.
- To be allowed to visit at any time.
- To have visiting start on time.
- To be able to have friends visit.

4. The need to be helpful

- To help with the care of the patient.
- To have someone tell them how to help.

5. The need for support

- To be reassured that the patient is doing alright.
- To have the chaplain visit.
- To have friends nearby.
- To be able to talk to others who have a family member in intensive care.
- To talk to the same nurse every day.
- To have a nurse nearby.
- To talk to someone about their feelings.
- To be accepted by staff.

6. Personal needs

- To have a toilet nearby.
- To have food and drinks nearby.
- To be alone.
- To have a private room to sit in.
- To have a place to rest when visiting.
- To have a place to take care of personal needs .

The greatest need that families have when their family member is in an intensive care unit is the need for relief of anxiety. Cultural and spiritual needs for families must also be met when patients are in critical care (Davidson *et al.*, 2007). The American College of Critical Care Medicine have developed clinical practice guidelines for the support of families in the ITU (Davidson *et al.*, 2007).

Although there has been little research on the needs of families following discharge of the patient from intensive care, it follows that their needs may not be very different from what they were when the patient was in intensive care.

After discharge from the intensive care unit

A family's perception of discharge to the ward environment often involves dread and fear. There can be anxiety about transferring to another location, rather than appreciating the improving health status of the patient (Russell, 1999; Jones *et al.*, 1999). Paul *et al.* (2004) identified relatives' information needs around the time of transfer; they designed an information booklet that improved relatives' satisfaction with information and enhanced the communication between intensive care, the wards and families at this stressful time in the patient journey. Diaries written for patients (see Chapter 29 on post intensive care patient support) to help them understand their stay on intensive care and come to terms with their illness, can also help relatives (Roulin *et al.*, 2007).

Physical effects of the critical illness on families

Once patients are discharged from intensive care, families continue to experience difficulties. A study of 2129 families of patients who had been seriously ill, and were no longer in hospital, found that the families experienced burdens of care when the patient was discharged (Covinsky *et al.*, 1994). These burdens included direct physical care of the patient, loss of employment as a result of the care-giving, and financial implications. Studies in cancer patients (Siegel *et al.*, 1991), cardiac patients (Stanley and Frantz, 1998) and paediatric cancer patients (Bodkin *et al.*, 1982) found similar burdens existed in families caring for patients following their illness. If they continue to have these physical burdens of care, then they may be reminded about the seriousness of the illness that the patient experienced, which may have psychological effects.

Even when patients are not discharged from hospital, their family will be experiencing physical burdens of care which, as healthcare professionals, must be recognised and understood. They could be simple things, like the relative who needs to visit outside the ward's usual visiting hours for various reasons – because they cannot afford the taxi to take them home after an evening visiting, because there is no longer a suitable bus service, or because they can only visit when their children are at school. Visiting hours have now been restricted in many hospitals, citing infection control as the reason; this may need to be re-considered when caring for families of critically ill patients who have been in intensive care.

Psychological effects of the critical illness on families

There are also psychological burdens when family members become ill, whether the illness is an acute or chronic one. Studies on the families of patients with a diagnosis of cancer revealed that a substantial number experienced psychological problems up to 12 months after the diagnosis (Ell *et al.*, 1988; Kazak *et al.*, 2004).

Family members of critically ill patients are affected psychologically by the illness; they can clearly recall events that occurred during the time spent in intensive care and they still had a profound effect on them (Russell, 1999; Adamson *et al.*, 2004). As one relative put it: 'it was said in front of me that Kathy was not going to be all right and that we may as well pull the plug … I was sitting beside Kathy' (Russell, 1999; p. 786). Families who have such recall 6 months after the critical care experience are angry and afraid (Jones *et al.*, 1999). However, these studies may have identified the memories that families have, but they did not investigate the effects that these memories were having on them.

Several studies have investigated the psychological state of families of critically ill patients (Jones *et al.*, 1999; Jones *et al.*, 2000a; Azoulay *et al.*, 2001; Pochard *et al.*, 2001; Young *et al.*, 2005). They all used the Hospital Anxiety and Depression Score (HADS) questionnaire and administered it when the families still had patients in the critical care unit or who were recovering within the hospital. All the studies reported that significant numbers of these families had symptoms of anxiety and depression. One study continued their investigation of critical care relatives and found that at 2 months and 6 months post discharge a third of relatives in their sample remained very anxious (Jones *et al.*, 2000b). A study comparing cardiac and critically ill patients and their relatives (Young *et al.*, 2005) collated data from patients and relatives in both groups: all participants completed a HADS questionnaire at a follow-up clinic 3 months after the patients had been discharged home. They found that critical care relatives had a significantly higher number of anxiety symptoms and greater indicators of depression than the relatives of the cardiac surgery relatives; they also had more worrying and life-altering experiences than the relatives of cardiac surgery patients. Critical care relatives have significant memories of what they witnessed when the patient was critically ill, and this may have been traumatic for them.

Transfer anxiety

These families need to be cared for by all members of the healthcare team when the patient is transferred to the ward. It is vital, therefore, that the families are prepared for the patient's transfer. Transfer anxiety can be seen when people display some or all of the following symptoms:

- insecurity
- a lack of trust
- the need for excessive reassurance
- an unfavourable comparison of staff on the ward and on the intensive care unit
- anger or outbursts.

Healthcare professionals caring for relatives and patients following discharge from an intensive care unit may see any of these emotional symptoms displayed by patients or families. The staff in the intensive care unit should therefore prepare the families for the transfer with appropriate planning, explanation and education (Jones and O'Donnell, 1994; Hall-Smith *et al.*, 1997; Coyle, 2001). However, discharge planning often has a low priority in critical care units (Coyle, 2001). If families do not know what to expect when the patient is transferred they will be understandably frightened. Healthcare professionals must remember that although the patient is perceived to be physically ready for discharge to a ward, neither the patient nor their family may be psychologically ready. The patient and the family often perceive the patient as still being critically ill. For the ward staff, the discharged patient may be the sickest patient in their care which adds to the level of anxiety both for the ward staff and the patient and their family.

Preparing families before discharge to a ward is obviously vital, but often patients are discharged quickly to accommodate emergency admissions, often during the night or late evening, or to accommodate planned elective surgery. As a result, many families are not prepared psychologically for the change. Their anxiety may be reduced when there is a follow-up visit from a critical care nurse (Hall-Smith *et al.*, 1997), or if a ward nurse visits the patient and family on the intensive care unit before discharge. If your hospital has a critical care outreach team, their role is not only to facilitate admission to critical care units, but also to enable safe discharge back to the wards (Intensive Care Society, 2002). This can greatly help the discharge process. Many critical care units produce booklets to give to patients and families before or on discharge, which explain the differences between the intensive care unit and wards in terms of staffing, what is to be expected, and what to expect during the patient's recovery.

Conclusions

The families of critically ill patients must be cared for within ward environments – as well as the patients. Their needs must be met because it is the family who will be the main caregivers when the patient is discharged from hospital.

References and further reading

Adamson, H., Murgo, M., Boyle, M., Kerr, S., Crawford, M. and Elliot. D. (2004). Memories of intensive care and experiences of survivors of a critical illness: an interview study. *Intensive and Critical Care Nursing*, **20**, 257–63.

Azoulay, E., Pochard, F., Chevret, S., *et al.* (2001). Meeting the needs of intensive care unit patient families. *American Journal of Respiratory and Critical Care Medicine*, **163**, 135–39.

Bodkin, C.M., Pigott, T.J. and Mann, J.R. (1982). Financial burden of childhood cancer. *British Journal of Medicine*, **284**, 1542–44.

Booth, J. (1991). Preoperative visiting: a step by step guide. *British Journal of Theatre Nursing*, **7**, 30–31.

Chew, S.L. (1986). Psychological reactions of intensive care patients. *Care of the Critically Ill*, **2**, 62–65.

Cochran, T.M. (1984). Psychological preparation of patients for surgical procedures. *Patient Education and Counselling*, **5**, 153–58.

Covinsky, K.E., Goldman, L., Cook, F., *et al.* (1994). The impact of serious illness on patient's families. *Journal of the American Medical Association*, **272**(23), 1839–44.

Coyle, M.A. (2001). Transfer anxiety: preparing to leave intensive care. *Intensive and Critical Care Nursing*, **17**, 138–43.

Daley, L. (1984). The perceived immediate needs of families with relatives in the intensive care unit. *Heart and Lung*, **13**, 231–37.

Davidson. J. E., Powers. K., Hedayat. K.M. *et al.* (2007). Clinical practice guidelines for support of the family in the patient-centred intensive care unit: American College of Critical Care Medicine Task Force 2004–2005. *Critical Care Medicine*, **35**(2), 605–22.

Dyer, I.D. (1991). Meeting the needs of visitors – a practical approach. *Intensive Care Nursing*, **7**, 135–44.

Ell, K., Nishimoto, R., Mantell, J. and Hamovitch, M. (1988). Longitudinal analysis of psychological adaptation among family members of patients with cancer. *Journal of Psychosomatic Research*, **32**, 429–38.

Engstrom, A. and Soderberg, S. (2004). The experiences of partners of critically ill persons in an intensive care unit. *Intensive and Critical Care Nursing*, **20**, 299–08.

Farrell, M.F. and Frost, C. (1992). The most important needs of parents of critically ill children: parents' perception. *Intensive and Critical Care Nursing*, **8**, 130–39.

Hall-Smith, J., Ball, C. and Coakley, J. (1997). Follow-up services and the development of a clinical nurse specialist in intensive care. *Intensive and Critical Care Nursing*, **13**, 243–48.

Hughes, F., Bryan, K. and Robbins, I. (2005). Relatives' experiences of critical care. *Nursing in Critical Care*, **10**, 23–30.

Intensive Care Society (2002). *Guidelines for the Introduction of Outreach Services*. London, Intensive Care Society.

Jones, C. (2002). Acute psychological problems. In: R.D. Griffiths and C. Jones (2002). *Intensive Care Aftercare*. Oxford, Butterworth Heinemann.

Jones, C. and O'Donnell, C. (1994). After intensive care – what then? *Intensive and Critical Care Nursing*, **10**, 89–92.

Jones, C., Griffiths, R.D. and Humphris, G. (1999). Relatives are still very anxious 2 weeks after patient's intensive care discharge. *British Journal of Anaesthesia*, **82**, P797–98.

Jones, C., Griffiths, R.D. and Humphris, G.M. (2000a). Disturbed memory and amnesia related to intensive care. *Memory*, **8**, 79–94

Jones, C., Skirrow, P., Griffiths, R.D., Humphris, G., Dawson, S. and Eddleston, J. (2000b). Predicting intensive care relatives at risk of post traumatic stress disorder. *British Journal of Anaesthesia*, **84**, P666–67.

Kazak, A.E., Alderfer, M., Rourke, M.T., Simms, S., Striesand, R. and Grossman, J.R. (2004). Post-traumatic stress disorder and post-traumatic stress symptoms in families of adolescent childhood cancer survivors. *Journal of Pediatric Psychology*, **29**, 211–19.

McGonigal, K.S. (1986). The importance of sleep and the sensory environment to critically ill patients. *Intensive Care Nursing*, **2**(2), 73–83.

Molter, N.C. (1979). Needs of relatives of critically ill patients: A descriptive study. *Heart and Lung*, **8**, 332–39.

Plowright, C.I. (1995). Needs of visitors in the intensive care unit. *British Journal of Nursing*, **4**, 1081–83.

Paul, F., Hendry, C., Cabrelli, L. (2004). Meeting patient and relatives' information needs upon transfer from an intensive care unit: the development and evaluation of an information booklet. *Journal of Clinical Nursing*, **13**(3), 396–405.

Pochard, F., Azoulay, E., Chevret, S., *et al.* (2001). Symptoms of anxiety and depression in family members of intensive care unit patients: Ethical hypothesis regarding decision-making capacity. *Critical Care Medicine*, **29**, 1893–97.

Quinn, S., Redmond, K. and Begley, C. (1996). The needs of relatives visiting adult intensive care units as perceived by relatives and nurses. *Intensive and Critical Care Nursing*, **12**(3), 168–72.

Roulin. M.J., Hurst. S. and Sririg, R. (2007). Diaries written for ICU patients. *Qualitative Health Research*, **17**(7), 893–901.

Russell, S. (1999). An exploratory study of patient's perceptions, memories and experiences of an intensive care unit. *Journal of Advanced Nursing*, **29**, 783–91.

Siegel, K., Raveis, V.H., Houts, P. and Mor, V. (1991). Caregiver burden and unmet patient needs. *Cancer*, **68**, 1131–40.

Skirrow, P. (2002). Delusional memories of ICU. In: R.D. Griffiths and C. Jones (2002). *Intensive Care Aftercare*. Oxford, Butterworth Heinemann.

Stanley, M. and Frantz, R. (1998). Adjustment problems of spouses of patients undergoing coronary bypass graft surgery during early convalescence. *Heart Lung*, **17**, 677–82.

Thompson, T.L. (1985). Discharge planning for critical care. *Critical Care Nurse*, **5**, 48–51.

Waldmann, C. (2002). Sexual problems and their treatments. In: R.D. Griffiths and C. Jones (eds) *Intensive Care Aftercare*. Oxford, Butterworth Heinemann.

Young, E., Eddleston, J., Ingleby, S., *et al.* (2005). Returning home after intensive care: A comparison of symptoms of anxiety and depression in intensive care unit and elective cardiac surgery patients and their relatives. *Intensive Care Medicine*, **31**, 86–91.

Useful websites

DIPex (Database of Individual Patient Experiences)
www.dipex.org/intensivecare

ICUSteps (Intensive Care Unit Support Team for Ex-Patients)
www.icusteps.com

Intensive Care Society
www.ics.ac.uk/patrel/patrel.asp

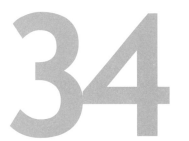

Communication

Julie Cook

This chapter considers the key principles of communication and how they apply when caring for critically ill patients, especially in the ward environment. It critiques a number of ways in which communication takes place and suggests a framework for practice.

At the end of this chapter, you will be able to apply the principles of good communication to your clinical practice.

The importance of effective communication

As a healthcare professional, high-quality communication with patients, their families and the multidisciplinary team (MDT) is not an optional extra; it is not a choice about whether or not you wish to participate. The practice of communication should be considered as a professional tool. In order for the multidisciplinary team to work together effectively it is essential that everyone interacts successfully towards a shared goal. This is particularly important when patients are critically ill and based in a ward environment where additional support is required. There is documented evidence that improved communication and teamwork leads to improved patient outcomes (Dutton *et al.*, 2003; National Patient Safety Agency, 2007). Assessment is essential when caring for critically ill patients, and communication with everyone involved is considered to be vital (Alasad and Ahmad, 2005). Even when patients are sedated or unconscious it may still be possible for them to hear and understand what is being said (Alasad and Ahmad, 2005).

Background and definitions

The topic of communication is vast and includes numerous different aspects. The following will be considered in this chapter in relation to the cases described:

- verbal and non-verbal communication
- active listening
- styles of questioning
- the provision of information
- collaboration

- documentation
- barriers to communication
- the effects of anger and frustration.

A number of factors relevant to the critically ill ward patient can influence communication. These are:

- the variety of individuals involved (including patients, relatives, medical and nursing staff)
- the physical environment (the ward environment can be a very busy and noisy place; just because you pull the curtains around a patient's bed does not mean that nobody else can hear you)
- the high levels of stress and anxiety for everyone involved
- the complexity of the information to be communicated.

Communication in the critical care environment

When patients are critically ill they are exposed to a significant number of clinical investigations that can be both invasive and intimate. Communication (in an accessible format) is therefore essential to reduce anxiety and stress and to ensure that you elicit as much information as possible about your patient and their condition. When communicating with critically ill patients closed questions that elicit a simple 'yes' or 'no' answer may be appropriate because less effort is required to answer them. It is important to acknowledge, however, that closed questions yield less information than open questions. Through the use of semi-structured interviews Sutcliffe *et al.* (2004) investigated the contribution that communication played in adverse clinical events. They found that in 91% of adverse events, failures in communication were either a contributory or an associated factor. They highlighted three themes that affect the effectiveness of communication:

- the hierarchy, power or social structure
- a lack of information
- the mode of communication or misinterpretation.

Because we know that failures in communication adversely affect patient safety and are common when undertaking analysis of adverse events or clinical incidents (National Patient Safety Agency, 2007) it is imperative to ensure effective communication at all times. This is especially important in the care of the acutely unwell patient where the information to be imparted may be complex and detailed, as well as being uncomfortable and difficult to express clearly, gently, appropriately and properly. This relates to communication between teams or with the patient and their visitors.

Communicating with a patient's family and friends

When patients are acutely unwell they may be unable to communicate due to exhaustion, or because of intrusive invasive monitoring or equipment. Where appropriate, communicating with a patient's family and friends can assist in maintaining confidence and helping to clarify a patient's wishes.

Communication by telephone

When patients are critically ill a significant amount of communication and coordination of care takes place over the telephone. This can include keeping members of the multidisciplinary team up to date about any changes in a patient's health. Consider the following scenario in which a nurse calls a doctor about a patient she is worried about.

Case Scenario

Nurse: I'm calling you about Mrs Simpson. Will you come and see her?

Doctor: I'm really tied up with another patient at the moment. Could you tell me a bit more about her?

Nurse: Well, she came into hospital a number of days ago with a chest infection and she does not look right to me.

Doctor: What are her vital signs? What medication is she on?

Nurse: Hang on a minute and I'll go and get her charts.

Doctor: Don't bother. I'll be down when I've finished here.

In this situation it is important to consider the person at the other end of the phone. They may be involved in the care of a number of patients who are acutely unwell. It is important to provide them with enough information to prioritise their workload. At the end of this conversation the nurse is unsure quite when the doctor is going to arrive and the doctor is unaware of just how ill Mrs Simpson really is.

Evidence has shown that medical staff find it more helpful if nurses use concrete information such as trends of observations and say exactly what these vital signs are (Andrews and Waterman, 2005). Indeed, in this scenario it would have helped the doctor if the nurse had been better prepared with the relevant information.

When communicating with colleagues about a critically ill patient over the telephone consider the following points.

- Take a few seconds to think about what you want to say, and what you want. This ensures you include the salient points.
- Be as concise as possible, while including all the relevant information.
- Ensure that you have all the necessary information to hand.
- Consider the people you are communicating with and use jargon appropriately.

Form and style of communication

Regardless of who you are communicating with, it is essential to communicate in a calm and respectful manner. It is not necessarily the person that shouts loudest who gets the most attention – often the complete opposite is true. If you become agitated with someone, the information is often lost amongst the negative messages that you are sending out. Generally the only thing that that person will remember from such an encounter is that they were shouted at – not what they were told! This also occurs when people are afraid to ask for help and can apply to both colleagues and patients. Amon (2002) describes a 'failure to communicate syndrome' whereby other members of the team are reluctant to provide timely updates on a patient's progress. Consider the scenario below.

Case Scenario

Mr Brown has just returned to the ward following an elective total knee replacement. Morphine has been prescribed as part of his postoperative analgesia regimen. Naloxone has also been prescribed with the additional note 'to be given if respirations low'.

During the review the following morning it is noticed that Mr Brown had what the team considered to be a low respiratory rate overnight and the ward staff were asked why the naloxone had not been given.

You cannot expect your colleagues to be mind-readers. When patients are critically ill a number of different healthcare professionals can be involved in their care. In this situation the documentation becomes vital to ensure continuity of care and to keep all members of the multidisciplinary team up to date with appropriate information regarding the patient's progress. Documented information about a patient's care must contain precise information about when further assistance should be sought.

Guidance from the National Institute for Health and Clinical Excellence (2007) on recognising and responding to acute illness in adults in hospital states that this should include 'prescribing' exactly how frequently a patient's vital signs should be taken and what to do if these signs either improve or deteriorate. The following is a typical example of what is commonly seen in a patient's notes:

- Continue with regular observations.
- Contact team if respiratory rate low.

But this information requires further clarification. How frequently are the observations to be recorded? Vital signs could be measured twice a day and still be 'regular'.

Furthermore, just how low is a 'low' respiratory rate? These sorts of instructions place extra stress on the other healthcare professionals involved in the patient's care as they have to 'second guess' precisely what is required. An alternative way to phrase the information might be:

- Continue recording vital signs 4 hourly.
- Contact primary team if respiratory rate less than 8 breaths per minute.

This removes all ambiguity and ensures that everyone involved in the patient's care is aware of what has been requested. It is also important to ensure that sufficient contact details are available, and to meet the standards of the Department of Health (National Institute for Health and Clinical Excellence, 2007; National Patient Safety Agency, 2007). When documenting information about a patient the following details should be considered for inclusion:

- the date and time
- a signature, name and designation
- the frequency of monitoring
- further investigations that are required
- when to contact primary team and how to contact them.

The writing should of course be legible.

Active listening

An important part of communication is listening. It is even more imperative if you are communicating with someone over the telephone. The most effective way to do this is through active listening which involves:

- giving the person that is talking your full attention
- making sure they know you are listening either by giving visual cues (e.g. nodding) or auditory cues (e.g. saying 'Yes' or 'I see')
- repeating the key points of what you have been told.

Boyle *et al.* (2005) stress the importance of active listening and summarising what you have said in their patient-centred communication technique. If you are communicating face to face, this can be facilitated by leaning slightly forward towards the person that is speaking, which shows interest and encourages them to continue talking.

Medical jargon

As healthcare professionals we are all guilty of using 'in-house' jargon to speed up our communication – and in many situations this is a useful and timesaving tool. However, we must beware of using jargon in inappropriate situations, which includes talking to patients and their families or talking to colleagues within earshot of patients. For example, when we say 'Patient X is normotensive and apyrexial' the patient thinks it means 'I am in a very bad way with lots wrong with me ... I may not pull through'. Many patients will not feel confident enough to clarify what you have said, and instead they will sit and draw their own conclusions.

Managing anger and frustration

Experiencing a critical illness can be very stressful for all involved, especially the patients and their relatives. This can manifest itself as anger and frustration. The following is an example of how this situation can be managed in a positive manner. Families and patients may well focus on any comments or aspects of care that appear to be different between healthcare professionals. It is therefore important to ensure consistency between different teams, which can be greatly assisted by thorough documentation. Clearly document all meetings, who the meeting was with, who was present, what was said and what was agreed in the patient's notes.

Case Scenario

Relative: What is happening to {*relative's name*}. They have been waiting for ages to see someone. They just don't seem to be getting any better!

Nurse: I appreciate that this situation must be very distressing for you. If you would like to speak to someone I will contact them for you. In the mean time we are caring for {*relative's name*} in the following way …

The SBAR framework for communication

The National Patient Safety Agency (2007) proposed a simple framework that enables staff to communicate their concerns simply and effectively to each other. Its use and effectiveness have been demonstrated in a variety of different clinical settings (Leonard *et al.*, 2004; Carroll 2006; Denham, 2008). The SBAR tool is based on the principles of ensuring salient points are made and it comprises the following factors:

S—Situation
B—Background
A—Assessment
R—Recommendations.

Box 34.1 explains how each of these factors relates to your practise. It may help to agree with the person you are seeking advice from when you will call them again, and what about, if they gave you telephone instructions to carry out. You could say that if the blood pressure is still below 90 mmHg in 30 minutes time you will call again. They may ask you to inform them in half an hour's time of the patient's progress. Setting these communication parameters helps reduce pressure among staff, and enables planned care to be delivered in a team approach.

Recently a system called RSVP has been devised that is specifically aimed at communicating about patients that are deteriorating while in hospital (Featherstone *et al.*, 2008). RSVP stands for:

R—Reason
S—Story
V—Vital signs
P—Plan.

Box 34.1	SBAR
S—Situation	Describe what is actually happening at the time you are calling. For example, the patient may have become confused and agitated, or aggressive. What is your main concern?
B—Background	Explain briefly what has led to this situation. This may include a summary of why they were admitted and how they have been so far today, or their diagnosis.
A—Assessment	Give an overview of your assessment of the patient, such as their vital signs, and perhaps what you think is wrong with them (if possible).
R—Recommendations	Explain what you wish this person to do, and if possible what you think needs to be done. It may be that they need to review the patient or need to prescribe something, or they need to come and speak with the family.

The RSVP acronym may be easier to remember than the SBAR. The method is becoming more popular in addition to the current tools available for staff to use. How it relates to your practise is shown in Box 34.2.

Box 34.2	RSVP
R—Reason	The nurse calling usually has an overview of the patient and can explain the reason for the call. They should say who they are and why they are calling for help.
S—Story	The nurse usually knows the story about the patient and then should relate the events that have led to their concerns.
V—Vital signs	The vital signs are important for the person receiving the call along with any other pertinent information, such as the patient's track and trigger score.
P—Plan	The nurse may describe their plan or what actions they have undertaken so far, or they may request that the recipient comes and helps to develop a plan of care for the patient following their review of the patient's condition.

The power of timing

Finally it is worthwhile remembering that a mis-timed comment regarding a patient or their condition can significantly affect their care or others' perceptions of that patient.

Conclusions

When communication works well it is a tool that allows all members of the multidisciplinary team, the patient and the patient's relatives to cooperate in the effective provision and acceptance of care given to that patient. It acts to seamlessly glue together the various elements that must work together if the best quality care is to be given. But getting it wrong causes problems. People begin to argue about the manner in which they are being communicated to – rather than taking on board the message that is being given – and that can only lead to a reduction in the quality of care provided, and an increase in the anxiety levels of all concerned. Using a structured communication tool such as the SBAR or RSVP may aid communication among teams as well as among patients and their families.

References and further reading

Alasad, A. and Ahmad, M. (2005). Communication with critically ill patients. *Journal of Advanced Nursing*, **50**, 356–62.

Amon, E. (2002). A guest editorial: Communication strategies for reducing hospital error and professional liability. *Obstetrical and Gynaecological Survey*, **57**, 713–14.

Andrews, T. and Waterman, H. (2005). Packaging: a grounded theory of how to report physiological deterioration effectively. *Journal of Advanced Nursing*, **52**(5), 473–81.

Boyle, D., Dwinnell, B. and Platt, F. (2005). Invite, listen, and summarize: A patient-centered communication technique. *Academic Medicine*, **80**, 29–32.

Carroll, T.L. (2006). SBAR and nurse physician communication: pilot testing an educational intervention. *Nursing Administration Quarterly*, **30**(3), 295–99.

Denham, C.R. (2008). SBAR for patients. *Journal of Patient Safety*, **4**(1), 38–48.

Dutton, R.P., Cooper, C., Jones, A., Leone, S., Kramer, M.E. and Scalea, T.M. (2003). Daily multidisciplinary rounds shorten length of stay for trauma patients. *The Journal of Trauma, Infection, and Critical Care*, **55**, 913–19.

Featherstone, P., Chalmers, T. and Smith, G.B. (2008). RSVP: a system for communication of deterioration in hospital patients. *British Journal of Nursing*, **17**(13), 860–64.

Leonard, M., Graham, S. and Bonacum, D. (2004). The human factor: the critical importance of effective teamwork and communication in providing safe care. *Quality and Safety in Health Care*, **13**, i85–90.

National Institute for Health and Clinical Excellence (2007). *Guideline 50. Acutely ill patients in hospital: Recognition and response to acute illness in adults in hospital*. London, NICE.

National Patient Safety Agency (2007). Safer care for the acutely ill patient: Learning from serious incidents. *Fifth Report from the Patient Safety Observatory*. London, National Patient Safety Agency.

Sutcliffe, K.M., Lewton, E. and Rosenthal, M.M. (2004). Communication failures: an insidious contributor to medical mishaps. *Academic Medicine*, **79**, 186–94.

35 Patient transport

Alistair Challiner

The transfer of an acutely unwell patient out of their ward is a common occurrence in hospital. It is a task that is fraught with potential dangers, and requires meticulous planning, even if ostensibly the journey may appear quite straightforward and may be short (Smith, 2003).

A patient may need to be moved around the hospital for various reasons, for example to go to:

- theatre (for an operation)
- the high dependency unit (for an escalated level of care)
- the radiology department (for x-rays or a CT scan)
- a ward (from the high dependency unit when improved)
- a specialist ward.

The transfer of critically ill patients either in hospital or between hospitals requires the involvement of a specialist team, including an anaesthetist or intensive care doctor and an intensive care unit trained nurse as well as specialist equipment, such as a ventilator (hence they are not discussed here). At the other end of the spectrum, a porter may perform the movement of a well patient, perhaps seated in a chair.

The aim of this chapter is to discuss the transfer of an unwell patient who is not unstable enough to need an intensive care unit team, but who has complex needs due to their acuity. The chapter offers practical guidance for ward staff to undertake the task safely and competently.

Considerations when moving an unwell patient

The first decision is whether or not the patient needs to be moved. If the patient needs an operation then they will need to go to theatre. If the patient is seriously unwell on a ward, requiring maximal oxygen and with inotropes running via a central line, then they need to go to the high dependency unit because additional monitoring is needed and escalation of care is likely. Think about these situations as you review the following list of considerations.

- Stabilisation of the patient (including treatment and monitoring).
- The person in charge of the transfer.
- Communication.

- Resources and level of expertise.
- Categorisation of the patient.
- Packaging the patient.

Each point will be discussed in turn.

Stabilisation of the patient

The principle of patient transfer is to minimise risk. An unstable patient should never be moved without being stabilised first, unless they have a non-compressible haemorrhage requiring immediate surgery, such as a ruptured aortic aneurysm or a bleeding ectopic pregnancy (Intensive Care Society, 2002). Think about the relative risk to the patient who is unstable in a ward area – with space, available staff and readily available oxygen and suction – in comparison to the risks involved for a patient in a corridor or lift when there is a sudden deterioration. Therefore the patient must be stabilised using the principles covered in this book *before* transfer. It is vital if the patient is being monitored on the ward, that the same level of monitoring must be maintained during transfer. This includes at least ECG, pulse oximetry and non-invasive blood monitoring.

The person in charge

Someone has to take charge and organise and delegate all the tasks required. Most importantly, they need to check everything has been done. This should be the most senior and experienced person.

Communication with the destination staff

First of all, consider where the patient is going. Does the receiving location know they are coming? It is very important to telephone the destination before the patient is moved so that they are ready to receive him or her. This avoids waiting around in a corridor because another patient is in the scan room, or the theatre is not ready, or no bed is available. It is also wise to check that the destination has the right equipment; for example, if a patient going for an x-ray requires high-flow oxygen, check that the x-ray department has a full cylinder ready for use, and easily accessible electrical sockets so that the monitor or infusion pumps can be plugged in on arrival, to save battery use. This enhances safety for the patient in an area that is frequently not familiar to the transfer staff, and sometimes quite remote from the main ward areas, such as scanning rooms. Remember to let relatives know of any move, as well as the admitting team, especially if it is where the patient will remain. If other resources are required then skilled help and equipment must be sought including porters.

Type of transfer

In-hospital transfers usually require a trolley that must be appropriately equipped with a full cylinder of oxygen and suction. Someone must check that they are present and working before the transfer takes place. Out-of-hospital transfers necessitate communication with the ambulance service. Most of these transfers will require a hospital nurse to attend with the patient, but will include at least an ambulance technician to help in the back of the vehicle. Many hospital staff are unfamiliar with the equipment found in the back of an ambulance but the ambulance personnel are very helpful in this regard. The equipment includes ECG, pulse oximetry and non-invasive blood pressure monitors, usually combined with a defibrillator. There are strict regulations about carrying loose heavy equipment in an ambulance, which may become flying projectiles in case of accidents. Many hospitals have designated trolleys to use when transferring acutely unwell and critically ill patients in an ambulance. Seek advice about this with your own accident and emergency and critical care teams. For higher-risk patients the nurse should be trained in advanced life support (ALS) or a doctor may need to go as well. For intensive care patients a critical care team should be sent from the intensive care unit.

Resources during transfer

Oxygen and suction have already been mentioned. The worst thing that could happen during a transfer is a cardiac arrest. Therefore at least a bag–valve mask and defibrillator should be provided, as well as fluids and drugs and someone who is trained in ALS (if an ambulance transfer). Calculate the amount of oxygen you need according to what the patient is using. For example, if the patient is receiving 40% oxygen that is being delivered at 12 litres per minute, you know for a journey of 30 minutes you will use 360 litres of oxygen. It is prudent to double the requirement to be on the safe side, in case of hold ups such as lift failure or an unforeseen wait, so make sure you have a cylinder that is full. Ensure any electronic medical devices have charged batteries, or take an extra device if possible – again just in case. Plug everything in on arrival. If you have communicated effectively with the destination department, they will be prepared and helpful when you arrive and need time to ensure patient safety.

Categorising the patient

It is important to classify the personnel and equipment required for the transfer. The following are definitions of such categories:

- *Critical* – extremely ill and at risk of deteriorating (usually requiring rapid transfer plus medical and nursing staff with advanced life support skills).

- *Intensive* – requiring organ support and should be in intensive care (requiring an intensive care unit team in attendance; the speed of transfer is outweighed by invasive monitoring and advanced treatment).

- *Ill and unstable* – such as acute myocardial infarction, post convulsion or severe asthma (requiring at least a skilled nurse with advanced life support skills plus a doctor).

- *Ill and stable* – such as postoperative patients or a stable myocardial infarction (requiring at least a nurse with basic life support skills).

Packaging the patient

This includes preparation of the staff as well as the equipment.

Staff

For in-hospital transfers there is a system for calling for help. If help is required before the transfer, then get extra help from the critical care outreach team (if there is one) or medical staff before commencing the transfer. Otherwise utilise the cardiac arrest call telephones in the hospital if urgent help needed. The most important factor is to plan your route. Use the porter's knowledge about the lifts that work and corridors that are unlocked at night. For ambulance transfers ensure you have a mobile phone and a number to call for advice (before you go). Also bear in mind that the ambulance may break down. Consider what you are wearing; is it safe to be on the road in, and is it warm? Ideally fluorescent yellow waterproof jackets should be provided. Footwear must be appropriate. Remember the ambulance may not be able to bring you home so take money or make arrangements for a taxi before you go. Always be clear about where you are going (e.g. precisely which inner-city hospital you are going to and via which entrance) and check that the ambulance crew has the same information.

Equipment

Consider the following ABC principles outlined throughout this book as well as specifics for the individual patient. Make sure electronic equipment such as monitors, defibrillators and pumps are fully charged and ideally have spare batteries. When at your destination (such as CT scan) plug everything in to save the batteries for the return trip. Remember also about oxygen, ensure there are full cylinders, suction equipment, spare catheters and Yankauer suckers, for example. A bag–valve mask is invaluable as it can work without an oxygen supply and is truly portable. The same equipment is usually required for most transfers hence keeping the equipment in a bag is very useful. It must be checked and replenished after every transfer and staff should be familiar with its contents.

The patient must be transferred on to a trolley for the transfer. This is best achieved using a device such as a pat-slide to avoid injury by lifting. All equipment must be secure and accounted for before moving the patient so that nothing gets pulled out. If the patient is on oxygen then this must be continued at all times, switching to the trolley supply only when ready to move to conserve it. All intravenous lines must be secured well.

For any patient worse than 'ill stable' then at least two intravenous lines should be placed in case of emergency. Chest drains should be well secured to the patient and the bottles kept below the patient. The drains should not be clamped because of the risk of tension pneumothorax, especially if the clamp gets forgotten. If the bottle has to be lifted up level with or above the patient transiently on moving then there is a risk of fluid going back into the thorax (but it will drain out again as soon as the bottle is placed below the patient). The bottles can be tied under the trolley for transfer. It is good practice to check all around the patient before sliding them on or off the trolley to ensure nothing gets caught and pulled out. Keeping the patient warm during transfer along corridors is important and can be achieved by wrapping warm blankets around the patient (make sure there is easy access to cannula sites). If it is very cold, consider providing a hat of some kind for the patient as the scalp blood vessels do not vasoconstrict and lose heat easily.

Preventing problems on transfer

Before setting off, check *everything* following an **ABCDE** approach. Think about the common things that may occur (Box 35.1).

Box 35.1   **Potential problems during transfer**

Something may run out
     e.g. oxygen, fluids, drug infusions, battery power

Something may happen
     e.g. ABCD problems, cardiac arrest, respiratory arrest, convulsions
     Do you have the skills and equipment to deal with a predictable event or an unfortuitous event?

Something may be forgotten
     e.g. notes, x-rays, equipment
     Do you have a special transfer bag that is checked regularly?

Something may stop working
     e.g. monitors, drips
     Have you got a spare or backup?

Monitoring during transfer

This should follow the same standards as before the transfer. For in-hospital transfers, vital signs should at least should be measured immediately before the journey and immediately afterwards at the destination. For longer journeys, they should be taken at least every 10 minutes, to ensure any deterioration is picked up early.

Handover

The person performing the transfer needs to hand over the patient at the destination if the patient is to be left there. This should be a familiar practice but in the case of transfers it is important to hand over all notes and x-rays, as well as to retrieve any equipment.

Documentation

Many critical care networks have devised a specific form to be used for transfers. It includes space for observations and various checklists. Such forms provide a useful basis for audit of transfers. Document all vital sign recordings that have been taken, and document in the notes any interventions or events, or changes in the patient's condition, as you would if they were residing in a ward.

Training of staff for transfers

It is important to delegate the job of transferring patients to experienced staff who ideally have had some training. For inter-hospital transfers where the team is remote from the hospital, ALS training is a good start, but in-house training or courses such as the STAR (safe retrieval and transfer) are appropriate. Intensive care transfers should always be performed by doctors and nurses who are trained in intensive care unit or anaesthetics.

HOT TIPS

Preparation—Preparation is key – to fail to prepare is to prepare to fail!

Safety—Maintain patient safety.

Equipment—Check all emergency equipment before moving the patient. Check all medical devices and their battery life before moving the patient. Calculate and ensure oxygen supplies are adequate. Do not remove monitoring – if it is on already, they need it!

People—Ensure you have the right people and the right equipment (and enough of them both). Communicate with key personnel.

Conclusions

The movement of a patient is potentially a dangerous task. By following the guidance outlined in this chapter the risks of moving sick patients can be minimised. Considering unforeseen events and being prepared to deal with them is an essential part of the process. Patient safety must be paramount when it comes to the transfer of unwell ward patients.

References and further reading

Intensive Care Society (2002). *Transport.* London, Intensive Care Society.

Smith, G. (2003). *Acute life-threatening events recognition and treatment: A multiprofessional course in the care of the acutely ill patient.* Portsmouth, University of Portsmouth.

■ Practical Skills ■

36

Changing a tracheostomy tube

Alistair Challiner and Sally A. Smith

Tracheostomy tubes with an inner cannula should be changed every 28 days or according to the manufacturer's recommendations. The decision to change a tracheostomy tube should be made by the attending physician in conjunction with experienced personnel and the physiotherapy team. A physician or anaesthetist should perform the tracheostomy tube changes, unless individual departments have expanded nurse role procedures in place. The person carrying out the procedure must be suitably skilled and competent.

Equipment required

- Dressing pack.
- Correctly sized tracheostomy tube (a spare tracheostomy tube one size smaller should be within easy reach).
- Tube holder.
- 10 mL syringe (for cuffed tubes).
- Sachet or clean tube of water-soluble lubricant.
- Sachet of normal saline 0.9%.
- Tracheostomy dressing.
- Sterile gloves.
- Protective eye wear.
- Tracheal dilators.

Procedure

Step 1

Explain the procedure to the patient with rationale for the tracheostomy tube change. The patient should give consent for the procedure (unless he or she is sedated, unconscious or the tracheostomy change is an emergency). It is safer to perform the procedure when an anaesthetist is available to deal with difficulties; therefore, planned tracheostomy changes (not urgent ones) should take place during 'normal' working hours.

Step 2

It is recommended that patients are 'nil by mouth' for 3–4 hours prior to the tracheostomy change and nasogastric feeding should be stopped. If a nasogastric tube is in situ this should be aspirated prior to the procedure. The airway is unprotected when the tracheostomy tube is removed. Starving the patient or aspirating the nasogastric tube will reduce the risk of aspiration during the procedure.

Step 3

Position the patient in bed in a semi-recumbent position, ensuring that the neck is extended and the patient is comfortable. Extending the neck allows for easier removal and insertion of the tracheostomy tube. The patient should feel as relaxed and comfortable as possible for the procedure.

Step 4

Wash your hands and prepare the dressing trolley.

Step 5

Pre-oxygenate the patient (if they are receiving oxygen) with 100% concentration for at least 2 minutes. Take care with patients with chronic obstructive pulmonary disorder; it may be more appropriate to increase their inspired oxygen by 20% rather than delivering 100%. During the tracheostomy change the patient will not receive oxygen and may be at risk of hypoxia.

Step 6

Two skilled practitioners should perform the procedure, one to remove the old tracheostomy tube and one to insert the new tube. This means the procedure is as clean and swift as possible. Both should wear eye protection. The first person should open the new tracheostomy tube onto the opened dressing pack and apply sterile gloves.

Step 7

If the tracheostomy is cuffed, check for air leaks in the cuff of the new tube by inflating it and deflating it using the 10 mL syringe.

Step 8

Lubricate the tracheostomy tube sparingly with water-soluble lubricant.

Step 9

Remove the old dressing and clean around the tracheostomy site.

Step 10

The second person (if necessary) suctions to remove secretions. When the patient stops coughing, release the tracheostomy ties. The tube may be more difficult to remove when the patient is coughing because the neck muscles may tense.

Step 11

There are two ways of changing the tube. One is to use the obturator provided with the new tube. The other is to use an airway exchange device that acts as a guide to 'rail road' the new tube over, preventing insertion into tissue instead of the trachea.

- If using the *obturator* (introducer), check that it can be removed ready for the insertion of the new tube. Remove the old tube in an 'out then down' movement on expiration and re-insert the new tube into the stoma using the introducer in the tracheostomy tube lumen. Make sure that the first movement is at 90 degrees to the cervical axis then gently rotate down to allow passage into the trachea. Remove the obturator immediately.

- If using a *airway exchange device*, such as a sterile suction catheter with the suction controller cut off, it should be threaded down the old tracheostomy tube as a guide just beyond the tip of the tracheostomy tube. The old tube can then be removed and the new tube threaded over the guide catheter using an 'up and over' action, preferably on exhalation.

Step 12

Immediately remove the guide catheter (bougie) and observe the patient for signs of respiratory distress. Inflate the cuff and re-administer oxygen. Feel for respiration via the tracheostomy tube and observe the chest movements. Auscultate for equal air entry. The flow of air will be felt via tracheostomy tube if it is in the correct position. Ensure that both lungs are inflating equally.

Step 13

If the tube insertion fails or the patient appears distressed and cyanosed, insert the tracheal dilators, remove the tube and re-insert a smaller tube.

Step 14

If the new tube fails, administer oxygen via the stoma or maintain the patient's airway via the oral route and give oxygen via a mask. If airflow is not felt the tracheostomy tube should be removed and a smaller one inserted (ensuring that it is well lubricated). The track may not have formed or the tracheostomy tube may have been advertently blocked during insertion. An arrest call should be put out in this case.

Step 15

Ensure that the patient is comfortable and breathing without difficulty.

Step 16

Record the tube change in the medical and nursing notes with the time, date, size and type of tube, including complications of the procedure. You will need to stick the sticker in the notes that come with the new tube.

Observe the site for bleeding and, if applicable, ensure the cuff is inflated. Excessive bleeding should be reported to the attending physician. A small amount of bleeding is common due to trauma at the stoma site. An inflated cuff will prevent aspiration of blood. Excessive bleeding may require further treatment.

References and further reading

The Intensive Care Society (2007). *Standards for Care of Adult Patients with Temporary Tracheostomies. Standards and Guidelines.* London, Intensive Care Society.

St George's Healthcare NHS Trust (2005). *Guidelines for the Care of Patients with Tracheostomy Tubes.* Watford Hertfordshire: Smiths Medical.

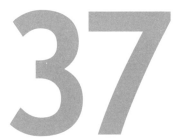

Suctioning a tracheostomy tube

Sally A. Smith

This chapter will describe how to safely and effectively suction a patient's tracheostomy tube. The purpose of suctioning a tracheostomy is to remove any secretions and to maintain patency of the airway. If the tube is not suctioned on a regular basis there is a danger that it may occlude and block the airway, potentially causing a respiratory or cardiac arrest situation for the patient (Intensive Care Society, 2007).

Frequency of suctioning

Tracheal suction must be carried out regularly on patients who have a tracheostomy for several reasons:

- to maintain airway patency
- to prevent collapse of the lung due to small airways becoming blocked by secretions, and prevent potential risk of infections
- to maintain patient comfort.

The frequency of suction will depend on the patient's needs and should be assessed and charted accordingly. Factors that should be assessed are:

- the patient's ability to cough and clear their own secretions
- the amount and consistency of secretions
- the patient's oxygen saturation and arterial blood gases
- the presence of any infection
- selection of the correctly sized suction catheter.

Essential bedside equipment

The following safety equipment should be kept beside the patient who has a tracheostomy. Some of the items can be kept in a small plastic box within easy reach just in case a problem occurs. Such boxes for tracheostomy care are easily ordered from NHS supplies departments.

The bedside equipment should comprise:

- Oxygen supply (tested and functioning) with appropriate adapters.
- Suction (tested and functioning) with pressure range 13.5–20 kPa (120–150 mmHg).
- Correct size suction catheters (see calculation below).
- Yankauer suction catheter.
- Bottled sterile water (labelled and dated).
- Gloves (non-sterile and disposable) and aprons.
- Eye protection or full-face protection (if available).
- Humidification equipment (e.g. tracheostomy mask, T-piece, Swedish nose – whichever is in use; all patients must have some form of humidification).
- Anaesthetic face mask, disposable bag–valve device, catheter mount, swivel connector.
- Oxygen saturation monitor.
- Tracheal dilators or Cottell's nasal speculums (sterile).
- Spare tracheostomy tubes (one the same size and one a size smaller).
- Spare inner tubes.
- Sterile bowl and sterile water (labelled 'for cleaning inner tubes').
- 10 mL syringe, water-based lubricant, tapes and dressing.
- Patient call bell, communication devices, notepad and pen.

Calculating the suction catheter size

Selection of the correct size suction catheter is important. If it is too large it will occlude the tracheal tube, which may cause hypoxia. It is recommended that the catheter should be no more than half the internal diameter of the tracheal tube (St George's Healthcare NHS Trust, 2005). See Box 37.1.

Box 37.1   Sizing a suction catheter

If the tracheostomy tube size is 8, deduct 2 from the size (8 in this case) and multiply the result by 2. Like this:

$$8 - 2 = 6$$
$$6 \times 2 = 12$$

Therefore for a size 8 tube, the suction catheter size should be 12 (French gauge).

N.B. Minitracheostomies should use maximum size 10 FG suction catheter.

Essential suctioning equipment

The equipment required for suctioning a tracheostomy is:

- Functional suction unit with suction set at 13.5–20 kPa (120–150 mmHg).
- Sterile suction catheters (size determined as above).
- Gloves and aprons.
- Bottled sterile water (labelled 'for cleaning suction tubing'; include date when opened and change water every 24 hours).
- Sterile 0.9% saline and syringe (in case they are needed).
- Oxygen therapy, wall flowmeter, tracheal mask.
- Yankauer suction catheter.
- Protective eyewear (goggles or visor).
- Sputum trap if required.
- Correct coloured bag for disposal of waste.

Procedure

Step 1

Firstly prepare the patient for the procedure, explaining what you are going to do and why. Ensure the privacy of the patient. Ensure you have the equipment you need ready. This enables the patient to give verbal or non-verbal consent to the procedure and allows them to feel reassured. It is important to maintain the patient's dignity.

Step 2

Wash your hands. Wear a disposable apron, gloves and protective eyewear.

Step 3

It is advisable to monitor the patient's oxygen saturations during the procedure to check for hypoxia or any changes. You may need to increase the amount of oxygen they are receiving if they desaturate when receiving suction.

Step 4

If the patient has a fenestrated tube in situ, it is advisable to change the fenestrated inner tube to a non-fenestrated tube prior to suctioning. Suctioning with a fenestrated inner tube in situ may cause mucosal damage. The outside of the tracheostomy tube should be held firmly while the inner cannula is removed and the replacement inner cannula inserted. Holding the outside stabilises the tracheostomy tube to reduce the risk of displacement and maintains patient comfort.

Step 5

Turn on the suction apparatus and attach a sterile suction catheter. Ensure that the pressure is checked prior to use. It should be 13.5–20 kPa (120–150 mmHg). High pressures may cause mucosal damage. Put a glove on the dominant hand and *only* touch the sterile suction catheter with this hand. Introduce the suction catheter into the tracheostomy tube. Do not apply suction at this point. Gently but quickly insert it to 0.5–1.0 cm beyond the tip of the tracheostomy tube or until the patient coughs. Then withdraw the catheter approximately 0.5 cm and apply suction. Withdraw the catheter slowly, applying suction continuously. This should take no longer than 15 seconds.

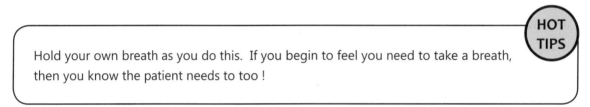

HOT TIPS

Hold your own breath as you do this. If you begin to feel you need to take a breath, then you know the patient needs to too !

Step 6

Gentleness is essential. Damage to the mucosal area can cause trauma and infection. The catheter should go no further than the carina. Continuous suction is most effective in clearing secretions, but the catheter must be kept moving. Prolonged suction will result in hypoxia.

Step 7

Release the suction, remove the catheter and glove and discard, and re-apply the patient's oxygen supply immediately.

Step 8

Observe the patient throughout the procedure for any signs of distress or discomfort. This will also enable you to assess their response to suction therapy and how well they tolerate it.

Step 9

Rinse the suction tubing through with water. It is prudent to change the bottle of water for this use daily and to also change the suction tubing every day. This reduces the risk of bacterial growth. Ensure that the suction reservoir is not full, and change when required.

Step 10

Using a fresh clean glove and sterile catheter repeat the procedure until secretions are cleared and the patient is breathing comfortably. Allow the patient sufficient time to recover between suction, especially if the oxygen saturation is low (ensure pre-oxygenation) or if the patient coughs several times.

Step 11

If you feel that the secretions are very tenacious, it may be worth considering saline nebulisers, but most definitely humidification for the patient. Do not forget to refer the patient to the physiotherapist for further care.

Step 12

Report your findings in the patient's notes. A chart such as the one in Fig. 37.1 may be helpful for recording tracheostomy care.

Patient name: _____

Hospital number: _____

Date: _____

Ward: _____

Time	Respiratory rate	Oxygen		Suction frequency	Secretions colour/ viscosity	Check/ change dressing	Check inner tube	Check water level	Sign
		%	Sats						
0800									
0900									
1000									
1100									
1200									
1300									
1400									
1500									
1600									
1700									
1800									
1900									
2000									
2100									
2200									
2300									
2400									
0100									
0200									
0300									
0400									
0500									
0600									
0700									

Secretion viscosity may be normal, thick, frothy or watery.
Secretion colour may be clear, creamy, brown, yellow, green, pink or blood-stained.

Figure 37.1 A sample tracheostomy care record chart based on that used by Maidstone and Tunbridge Wells NHS Trust.

References and further reading

Intensive Care Society (2007) *Standards for Care of Adult Patients with Temporary Tracheostomies. Standards and Guidelines*. London, Intensive Care Society.

St George's Healthcare NHS Trust (2005). *Guidelines for the Care of Patients with Tracheostomy Tubes*. Watford Hertfordshire: Smiths Medical Limited.

38 Care of central venous catheters and measuring central venous pressure

Sally A. Smith

A central venous catheter (CVC) is a catheter that is inserted into the inferior or superior vena cava. These two large veins return blood to the right atrium of the heart, and they have the largest blood flow of any veins in the body (Woodrow, 2002). This chapter outlines how to care for a CVC, the indications for a CVC, and how to use one to measure the central venous pressure (CVP).

Indications for a CVC

CVCs are inserted for a number of reasons. In acute care, a common indication is to measure the CVP in order to monitor volume deficits in a shocked patient who may be septic or hypovolaemic. They also give an indication of what is occurring in the patient's heart. There are no valves in the vena cava, so the pressure is a direct indication of the pressure in the right atrium.

CVCs are also used to give fluids, particularly if they are required quickly, and to administer drugs and infusions that are not safe to give peripherally. Drugs such as vasoactive infusions, hypotonic or hypertonic fluids, or high concentrations of potassium are examples. Total parenteral nutrition (TPN) is also often infused via a central line. CVCs are also useful for taking repeated blood samples.

Following the Surviving Sepsis Campaign, central venous blood gases are frequently taken as part of the care bundle in sepsis and the management of fluid resuscitation and oxygenation indications.

Insertion sites

CVCs are most commonly sited in the internal jugular vein where the risk of pneumothorax is less. Other sites include the subclavian vein or femoral vein.

Femoral lines are usually short term; they have a greater risk of infection, and are usually replaced with a neck line within a short time. The ward nurse may be required to assist the doctor with insertion of the line.

Before any CVC that is sited in the neck or subclavian site can be used, its position must be checked by chest x-ray and it must be documented in the notes that it is positioned correctly and that there is no pneumothorax.

Infection control

The Department of Health launched a set of guidelines in 2007 regarding the prevention of central catheter infections. These are known as the *High Impact Interventions* (Department of Health, 2007). The guidelines were developed as care bundles – in other words, a group of interventions that when all delivered offer best practice care based on current evidence. Box 38.1 outlines the elements of the care bundle.

Box 38.1   Care bundle elements for preventing central catheter infections (Department of Health, 2007)

1. Catheter type
— Single lumen (unless indicated otherwise).
— Consider antimicrobial impregnated catheter if duration 1 to 3 weeks and high risk of catheter-related bloodstream infections (CRBSI).

2. Insertion site
— Subclavian or internal jugular vein.

3. Skin preparation
— Preferably with 2% chlorhexidine gluconate in 70% isopropyl alcohol (allow to dry).
— If patient has any sensitivity, use single-use povidone–iodine.

4. Personal protective equipment
— Gloves are single-use items (remove and discard immediately after care activity).
— Use eye/face protection if risk of splashing with blood or body fluids.

5. Hand hygiene
— Decontaminate hands before and after each patient contact.
— Use correct hand hygiene procedure.

6. Aseptic technique
— Use gown, gloves and drapes (as indicated) for insertion of invasive devices.

7. Dressing
— Use sterile, transparent, semipermeable dressing to allow observation of insertion site.

8. Safe disposal of sharps
— Make sure sharps container is available at point of use (should not be overfilled).
— Do not disassemble needle and syringe.
— Do not pass sharps from hand to hand.

9. Documentation
— Record date of insertion in notes.

Box 38.1 *(cont..)*

Ongoing care

1. Hand hygiene
— Decontaminate hands before and after each patient contact and use correct hand hygiene procedure.

2. Catheter site inspection
— Observe regularly for signs of infection (at least daily).

3. Dressing
— Should be intact, dry, adherent and transparent.

4. Catheter access
— Use aseptic technique and swab ports or hub with 2% chlorhexidine gluconate in 70% isopropyl alcohol prior to accessing the line for administering fluids or injections.

5. Administration set replacement
— Following administration of blood, blood products – immediately.
— Following total parenteral nutrition – after 24 hours (72 hours if no lipid).
— With other fluid sets – after 72 hours.

6. No routine catheter replacement.

Measuring the CVP

There are two ways of measuring the CVP. The first is via a water manometer. The second is electronically using a transducer and a haemodynamic monitor.

Using a water manometer

To set up the CVP using this method you will need:

- a bag of normal saline 0.9%
- an intravenous infusion giving set
- a manometer set, including a cmH_2O measure and spirit level.

Step 1
Attach the manometer set to the measure and spirit level.

Step 2
Run the saline through the set, ensuring all of it is primed by using the three-way tap to allow the fluid into the different lines.

Step 3
Attach to the central venous catheter on the distal (brown) port.

Step 4
Ensure that the base of the set is in line with the right atrium, or the mid axilla, at the level of the fourth intercostal space. In order to line it up, place the patient on their back at an angle of no more than 45 degrees. It is lined up when the bubble is in the centre of the spirit level.

Step 5
Turn the three-way tap on to allow the saline to run up the measuring line.

Step 6
Turn the three-way tap to the saline bag off, opening the measuring line to the patient. The fluid will then pulsate; dropping slowly until it stops. This is the CVP measured in cmH_2O. If the fluid fluctuates with the patient's breathing, take the lower measurement (Cole, 2007).

Step 7
Remember to turn off the tap to the manometer when you have finished.

Using a transducer

Wards (as well as critical care areas) often use a transducer system attached to a monitor to display a continuous waveform and reading. Ensure you have had the appropriate training for the monitor you have in your hospital. Equipment for the transducer system includes:

- a pressure bag
- 0.9% saline
- a transducer set
- a transducer pressure cable
- a monitor.

Step 1
The transducer set is primed with the saline and the bag of fluid placed in the pressure bag. It is pumped up to 300 mmHg to ensure a slow flush of 3 mL per hour. This helps keep the line patent and it can also be used for flushing the line.

Step 2
Attach the primed transducer line to the distal (brown) port on the central venous catheter.

Step 3
Attach the pressure cable to the transducer and into the monitor. A waveform should appear on the screen.

Step 4
Turn the three-way tap off to the patient and on to the transducer and atmosphere.

Step 5

Press zero on the monitor and wait while the device 'zeros' the line. The term 'zeroed' or 'zero complete' will appear on the monitor and you will see a '0' displayed.

Step 6

Turn the three-way tap off to the atmosphere. This should show a waveform which is the central venous pressure. Replace the sterile cap.

Step 7

Ensure that the transducer is lined up level with the fourth intercostal space, mid axilla, or phlebostatic axis (Fig. 38.1). Marked on the patient's chest, this is the exact anatomical point of origin where the haemodynamic pressures are measured.

Step 8

Observe the trace and document the measurement in the patient's records.

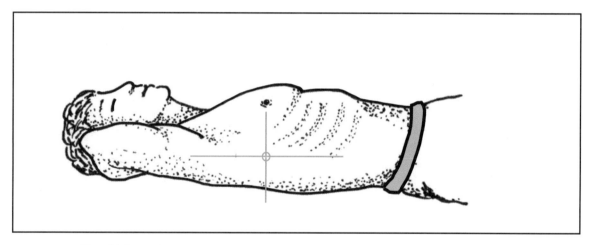

Figure 38.1 The phlebostatic axis.

Interpreting the recordings

The normal range for the CVP is 5–10 cmH$_2$O or 2–6 mmHg when taken from the mid-axillary line, or fourth intercostal space (Cole, 2007).

High CVP

A high CVP may be due to heart failure, pulmonary oedema, fluid overload, a narrowing of the vessels, or an increased intra-thoracic pressure if the patient is receiving, say, non-invasive ventilation or similar. If unusually high, it may be that the line is occluded or kinked, or pressing against the vessel wall. It may simply require a flush.

Low CVP

A low CVP is usually due to hypovolaemia, or vasodilation due to medication or shock (Woodrow, 2002). As part of the ongoing management of a patient with a central venous catheter, goals are usually set with regard to a CVP to aim for. For example, in severe sepsis this may be 8 mmHg to ensure adequate filling and hydration (Rivers *et al.*, 2001). Agree a CVP to aim for and ask the attending physician to prescribe fluid in order to allow you to reach that goal.

Ongoing care of the central venous catheter

Ongoing care of the CVC comprises strict infection control of the site and in the use of any lines used for infusions and drugs or taking blood. The mechanical 'zeroing' should be checked on a shift-by-shift basis. Lining the transducer or manometer up to read a CVP must be done on every occasion.

Taking blood samples

It is advisable to use the distal port that has the flush devices attached for this procedure. Using the central venous catheter means that your patient will not have to endure the discomfort of venopuncture on a regular basis. Also if you are using the sepsis care bundle (Survive Sepsis, 2007) you will need to take a blood gas from this catheter. The procedure must be a sterile one.

Follow your hospital guidelines and the CVC care bundle advice when opening any port or breaking the seal of the line. The aim is to minimise infection risk to the patient. Remove 6–10 mL of fluid from the catheter, then take the blood sample with a fresh syringe to remove fluid from the line (in order to prevent contamination of the blood sample that needs to be taken). After this, flush the line with 0.9% saline or use the attached flush device. Replace the cap with a new sterile one.

Procedure for removing the catheter

When the patient no longer requires the CVC it will need to be removed. This is a simple procedure, but it must be carried out carefully to ensure no air embolus occurs and bleeding is minimised.

Step 1
As with any procedure, explain to the patient what you plan to do and obtain their consent.

Step 2
It is prudent to check the patient's clotting factors and electrolytes in case of bleeding afterwards and any possible risk of arrhythmias during the procedure.

Step 3
Lay the patient as flat as will be tolerated, preferably in the Trendelenberg position (head down and feet up). This is to prevent an air embolus.

Step 4

Use an aseptic technique to remove the dressing and sutures.

Step 5

Ask the patient to perform the Valsalva manoeuvre (holding their nose and breathing against a closed mouth and nose). This also helps prevent air entering when the catheter is removed. At the same time, cover the insertion site with sterile gauze.

Step 6

As you gently press against the site slowly remove the catheter. Pull gently and firmly. Applying pressure during the procedure helps prevent bleeding and air entering, as well as helping vein closure at the insertion site. Maintain pressure on the site for about 5 minutes to enable the wound site to begin to close.

Step 7

At the same time place the tip of the catheter into a sterile specimen pot. You will need an assistant to cut the end off with sterile scissors while you continue to apply pressure to the insertion site. Send the tip to microbiology to check that it is infection free.

Step 7

When the bleeding has stopped, cover with a transparent sterile dressing. Discard the dressing pack following your local infection control procedures.

Conclusions

This chapter outlined the care and management of a central venous catheter. It described how to undertake a central venous pressure measurement, how to take blood from the catheter and how to remove it safely.

References and further reading

Cole, E. (2007). Measuring central venous pressure. *Nursing Standard*, **22**(7), 40–43.

Department of Health (2007). *Saving lives campaign – High-Impact Intervention No. 1: Central Venous Catheter Care Bundle.* London, DH. Available at: http//www.dh.gov.uk/en/Publichealth/Healthprotection/Healthcareacquiredinfection/Healthcareacquiredgeneralinformation/ (last accessed November 2009).

Rivers, E., Nguyen, B., Havstad, S., *et al.* (2001). Early goal-directed therapy in the treatment of severe sepsis and septic shock. *New England Journal of Medicine*, **345**, 1368–1377.

Survive Sepsis (2007). *The Official Training Programme for the Surviving Sepsis Campaign.* Sutton Coldfield, Heart of England Foundation Trust.

Useful websites

Surviving Sepsis Campaign
http//www.survivingsepsis.org

Pleural chest drains

Philip Woodrow

This chapter discusses drains used in the lungs, rather than cardiac chest drains. After finishing this chapter you should be able to describe what pleural chest drains are, why they are used, and how to care for patients with one.

Background and definitions

There are two main body systems in the chest – the heart and lungs. Either of these might require a chest drain. Cardiac chest drains are often used following cardiac surgery, but they are not discussed here. Instead this chapter focuses on chest drains inserted between the pleura of the lungs to drain air (a pneumothorax), blood (a haemothorax), pus (a pyothorax) or fluid exudate (a pleural effusion). Whatever substance needs to be drained, a similar system is used – therefore this chapter will refer throughout to a pneumothorax (air). Drainage occurs by siphoning through sterile water, using either simple gravity or additional low-pressure suction.

Case Scenario

A 30-year-old man with no past medical history, was playing football when he became suddenly breathless. Despite 15 litres of oxygen via a reservoir bag facemask ('100% oxygen') he remained distressed and unable to breathe, with low oxygen saturations.

Following a chest x-ray in accident and emergency, a spontaneous pneumothorax was diagnosed, and a chest drain inserted. He rapidly became less breathless, and his oxygen saturations improved. He has now been transferred to the respiratory ward.

Pathophysiology

Each lung is surrounded by two layers called pleura. Between the inner (visceral or pulmonary) and outer (parietal) pleura is a potential space. This space contains a very small amount of fluid – usually about 10 mL. This thin film of fluid enables the two pleura to slide over each other, preventing friction when breathing. Negative intrathoracic pressure normally ensures the pleura remain adjacent to each other. The negative pressure is lost if the pleural wall ruptures, causing (inward) collapse of the lung wall. Most pneumothoraces are spontaneous, but a minority are caused by trauma.

Spontaneous pneumothoraces

Spontaneous pneumothoraces typically occur in two groups of people (Gallon, 1998; Miller and Harvey, 1999):

- otherwise healthy (usually young) adults
- older people with emphysema or other chronic lung diseases.

Pneumothoraces can be classified into either simple or tension:

- A *simple* pneumothorax is one in which part of the lung has simply collapsed, causing loss of space for ventilation.
- A *tension* pneumothorax is one in which the leak persists, creating a 'one-way valve' that draws more and more air into the pleura on inspiration (Gallon, 1998; Norman and Cook, 2000). As this air cannot escape, a tension pneumothorax causes progressive lung collapse, and often cardiac tamponade, creating life-threatening respiratory and circulatory failure.

Pleural effusions

Pleural effusions, abnormal fluid collections in the pleural space, are usually caused by exudate, but can be caused by transudate.

- *Exudate* may occur with infection, cancer, trauma, surgery or other diseases causing tissue damage to the pleura.
- *Transudate* occurs when fluid is pulled abnormally into the pleural space, which may occur with heart failure, hypoproteinaemia (e.g. liver disease or nephrotic syndrome) or occasionally other conditions creating abnormal osmotic pull (e.g. peritoneal dialysis).

Testing pleural fluid for protein can identify whether fluid is transudate (< 30 g/litre of protein) or exudate (> 30 g/litre protein). Malignant pleural effusions, caused by lung cancer, necessitate repeated chest-drain insertion, often for prolonged periods. Drainage occlusion and pleural infections are relatively common with malignant pleural effusions (Medford and Maskell, 2005).

Treatment

A pneumothorax, or pleural effusion, is usually diagnosed by chest x-ray, although breathlessness, absence of lung sounds and (often) clinical history may indicate diagnosis. Underlying causes (such as infection) should be treated, and system support (e.g. oxygen) is usually needed, but the main treatment for abnormal collections of air, blood, pus or other fluid in the lungs is to remove it. A small (< 20%) pneumothorax may be treated by percutaneous needle aspiration (PCNA) but larger collections are removed with chest drains. A chest drain converts a *tension* pneumothorax into a *simple* pneumothorax (Norman and Cook, 2000). Air is usually removed best by inserting drains higher in the lungs, while fluid is usually removed by placing drains lower.

Chest drains

Larger drains cause more complications, such as empyema. 'Pig-tail' drains are small, 14-Fg catheters connected to a flutter valve or bag (Miller, 1999; Laws *et al.*, 2003). They are usually as effective as larger drains, and enable patients to remain more mobile, so they are commonly used (Henry *et al.*, 2003; Liu *et al.*, 2003). Previously, drain sizes were usually 28 Fg for blood and 24 Fg for air (Hyde *et al.*, 1997). Drains will be connected to an external underwater-seal drainage bottle placed below the patient. The tube draining from the patient's chest will be placed under sterile water, forming a seal that prevents air from re-entering the pleural space. A second tube, above the water, allows air displaced from the collection bottle to escape. This exit tube may be left often to the atmosphere, or connected to low-pressure suction. A typical system is illustrated in Fig. 39.1.

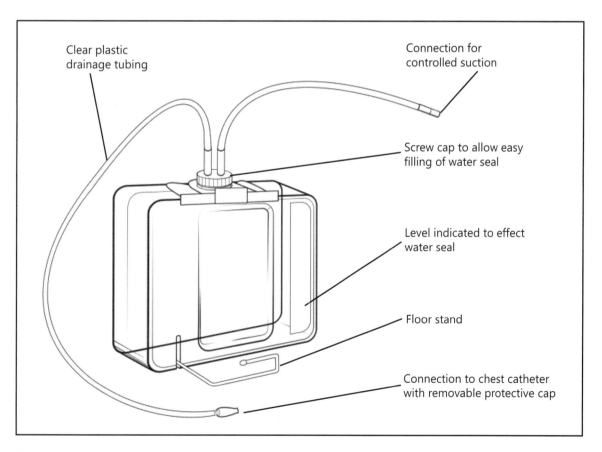

Figure 39.1 An underwater-seal drainage system.

Removing a chest drain

The precise criteria used sometimes vary between different authors and different Trusts. Removing drains causes pain (Owens and Gould, 1999; Gray, 2001) so patients should be given analgesia within sufficient time before drain removal for it to be effective; patients should be warned about this discomfort beforehand. The literature is divided between advising the holding of breath in or out during the removal of drains (Bell *et al.*, 2001); physiologically, neutral intrathoracic pressure (from holding breath out) rather than negative intrathoracic pressure (from holding breath in) would seem more logical.

The small tubes frequently used nowadays do not normally require suture, but an occlusive dressing, such as a hydrocolloid, should be placed over the drain site. Lung re-expansion should then be checked with a chest x-ray, and the patient's respiratory function monitored closely for 24 hours (O'Hanlon-Nichols, 1996) because pneumothoraces can recur.

Conclusions

There is limited evidence regarding most aspects of chest drain management (Charnock and Evans, 2001) which means that there is limited evidence to draw on, hence recommendations tend to vary and are inevitably partly based on individual routines and local preferences.

References and further reading

Allibone, L. (2003). Nursing management of chest drains. *Nursing Standard*, **17**(22), 45–54.

Bell, R.L., Ovadia, P., Abdullah, F., Spector, S. and Rabinovici, R. (2001). Chest tube removal; end-inspiration or end-expiration? *Journal of Trauma*, **50**(4), 674–77.

Carroll, P. (2002). A guide to mobile chest drains. *Registered Nurse,* **65**(5), 156–60.

Charnock, Y. and Evans, D. (2001). Nursing management of chest drains. *Australian Critical Care*, **14**(4), 156–60.

Chaudhuri, N. and Page, R.D. (2005). Pneumothorax and insertion of a chest drain. *Surgery*, **23**(11), 417–18.

Cochran, J.B., Tecklenburg, F.W. and Turner, R.B. (2003). Intrapleural instillation of fibrinolytic agents for treatment of pleural empyema. *Paediatric Critical Care Medicine.* **4**(1), 39–43.

Davies, C.W.H., Traill, Z.C., Gleeson, F.V. and Davies, R.J.O. (1999). Intrapleural streptokinase in the management of malignant multilocated pleural effusions. *Chest*, **115**(3), 729–33.

Davies, C.W.H., Gleeson, F.V., Davies, R.J.O. and the BTS Pleural Disease Group (2003). BTS guidelines for the management of pleural infection. *Thorax*, **58**(Suppl.II), ii18–28.

Diacon, A.H., Theron, J., Schurmans, M.M., van de Wal, B.W. and Bolliger, C.T. (2004). Intrapleural streptokinase for empyema and complicated parapneumonic effusions. *American Journal of Respiratory and Critical Care Medicine*, **170**(1), 49–53.

Fox, V., Gould, D., Davies, N. and Owen, S. (1999). Patient's experiences of having an underwater seal chest drain: a replication study. *Journal of Clinical Nursing*, **8**(6), 684–92.

Gallon, A. (1998). Pneumothorax. *Nursing Standard*, **13**(10), 35–39.

Godden, J. and Hiley, C. (1998). Managing the patient with a chest drain: a review. *Nursing Standard*, **12**(32), 35–39.

Gray, E. (2001). Pain management for patients with chest drains. *Nursing Standard*, **14**(23), 40–44.

Gupta, N. (2001). Pneumothorax: Is chest tube clamp necessary before removal? *Chest*, **119**(4), 1292–93.

Hall, M. and Jones, A. (1997). Reducing morbidity from insertion of chest drains: clamping may be appropriate to prevent discomfort and reduce risk of oedema. *British Medical Journal*, **315**(7103), 313.

Henry, M., Arnold, T., Harvey, J. and the BTS Pleural Disease Group (2003). BTS guidelines for the management of spontaneous pneumothorax. *Thorax*, **58**(Suppl.ii), 39–52.

Hyde, J., Sykes, T. and Graham, T. (1997). Reducing morbidity from chest drains: knowledge of basic principles and use of appropriate equipment would help. *British Medical Journal*, **314**(7085), 914–15.

Jerjes-Sánchez, C., Ramirez-Rivera, A., Elizalde, J.J., *et al.* for the Collaborative Group Investigators of Intrapleural Fibrinolysis (1996). Intrapleural fibrinolysis with streptokinase as an adjunctive treatment in haemothorax and empyema. *Chest*, **109**(6), 1514–19.

Juneja, R., Kothari, S.S., Saxena, A., Sharma, R. and Joshi, A. (1999). Intrapericardial streptokinase in purulent pericarditis. *Archives of Diseases in Childhood*, **80**(3), 275–77.

Kam, A.C., O'Brien, M. and Kam, P.C.A. (1993). Pleural drainage systems. *Anaesthesia*, **48**(2), 154–61.

Laws, D., Neville, E., Duffy, J. and the BTS Pleural Disease Group (2003). BTS guidelines for the insertion of a chest drain. *Thorax*, **58**(Suppl.ii), 53–59.

Liu, C.-M., Hang, L.-W., Chen, W.-K., Hsia, T.-C. and Hsu, W.-H. (2003). Pigtail tube drainage in the treatment of spontaneous pneumothorax. *American Journal of Emergency Medicine*, **21**(3), 41–44.

Martinson, B.C., O'Connor, P.J. and Pronk, N.P. (2001). Physical inactivity and short-term all-cause mortality in adults with chronic disease. *Archives of Internal Medicine*, **161**(9), 1173–80.

Maskell, N.A., Davies, C.W.H., Nunn, A.J., *et al.* for the First Multicenter International Sepsis Trial (MISTI) Group (2005). UK controlled trial of intrapleural streptokinase for pleural infection. *New England Journal of Medicine*, **352**(9), 865–74.

Medford, A. and Maskell, N. (2005). Pleural effusion. *Postgraduate Medical Journal*, **81**(961), 702–10.

Miller, A. (1999). Pleural therapeutic procedures. *Medicine*, **27**(11), 174–76.

Miller, A.C. and Harvey, E. (1993). Guidelines for the management of spontaneous pneumothorax. *British Medical Journal*, **307**(6896), 114–16.

Norman, J. and Cook, A. (2000). Medical emergencies. In: M. Sheppard and M. Wright (eds) *High Dependency Nursing*. London, Baillière Tindall.

O'Hanlon-Nichols, T. (1996). Commonly asked questions about chest drains. *American Journal of Nursing*, **96**(5), 60–64.

Owens, S. and Gould, D. (1997). Underwater seal chest drains: the patient's experience. *Journal of Clinical Nursing*. **6**(3), 215–25.

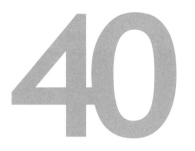

Radial artery puncture

Sally A. Smith

This chapter outlines the technique for obtaining an arterial blood sample from the radial artery. Radial artery samples are often required in ward areas when caring for acutely ill patients, and blood gases are like a window to a patient's body, informing the practitioner of key physiological changes.

A common reason for taking an arterial sample is to assess oxygenation, ventilation and the acid–base status during acute illness, for example in a patient who becomes acutely breathless or who was receiving non-invasive ventilation, or a diabetic in crisis.

Radial arteries are small but close to the skin's surface and can often be located quite easily. Before a sample is taken, collateral circulation must be checked using the Allen's test (Box **40.1**).

Box 40.1   Allen's test (based on Murray and White, 1999)

1. Ask the patient to clench his or her hand tightly for several seconds.
2. Compress the radial or ulnar artery and ask the patient to open the hand.
3. Colour should return quickly to the palm if the non-compressed artery is patent.
4. If colour does not return quickly, do not take arterial blood gases from this arm as circulation to the limb might be compromised.

The alveolar–arterial gradient will be raised by more than 2 kPa.

Equipment needed for taking the sample

- Cleaning agent.
- Gauze.
- Blood gas syringe.
- Dressing.

Local anaesthetic (EMLA cream or lidocaine) is optional – please follow your own hospital's procedures. Subcutaneous infiltration of the skin with lidocaine via a 23 G needle, and allowing time for it to work, is more comfortable patients. This is particularly so when repeated samples are required and finding the artery is difficult.

Procedure

This procedure is that given by Bucher (2001).

Step 1

Inform the patient of what you are about to do.

Step 2

Clean the site.

Step 3

Palpate the artery.

Step 4

With the bevel of the needle upward, insert the heparinised syringe (ideally a designated blood gas syringe) into the artery at an angle of 30–45 degrees.

Step 5

A pulsatile backflow of blood into the syringe indicates that the artery has been punctured.

Step 6

Stabilise the syringe and withdraw the sample.

Step 7

Remove, then apply pressure with sterile gauze to the puncture site for 5 minutes or until the puncture has stopped bleeding.

Ongoing care

Ensure that the site is checked for haematoma formation every 15 minutes for the first half hour, then every 30 minutes for 2 hours.

References and further reading

Bucher, L. (2001). Arterial puncture. In: D.J. Lynn-McHale and K.K. Carlson (eds) *AACN Procedure Manual for Critical Care*. Philadelphia, WB Saunders.

Murray, S.E. and White, B.S. (1999). *Critical Care Assessment Handbook*. Philadelphia, WB Saunders.

University of North Carolina Hospitals (2005). *Arterial Blood Sampling: Nursing Procedure Manual*. Available at: http//www.www.unchealthcare.net (last accessed September 2009).

41 Interpretation of arterial blood gases

Ann M. Price

The most important aspect of arterial blood gas (ABG) interpretation is being able to recognise normal ones and therefore to know when something is abnormal – identification of the specific abnormalities comes with practice. This easy guide aims to give you a logical format for identifying abnormal arterial blood gases based on Mays (1995) 'tic-tac-toe' method. When two of these three components (pH, CO_2 or HCO_3) fall into the same category you should be able to identify which type of condition the patient has.

By the end of this chapter you should:

- understand a normal arterial blood gas result
- understand how to interpret an arterial blood gas.

Normal values

The values of 'normal' arterial blood gases vary slightly depending which book you read – however, a fairly standard normal is stated by Woodrow (2000) as shown in Table 41.1.

Table 41.1 What is normal for arterial blood gases?	
Measurement	**Range**
pH	7.35–7.45
PaCO$_2$ (carbon dioxide)	4.5–6.0 kPa
PaO$_2$ (oxygen)	11.5–13.5 kPa
HCO$_3$ (bicarbonate)	22–28 mmol/L
BE (base excess)	−2 to +2
Saturation	> 95%

PaO_2 and $PaCO_2$ indicate the 'partial pressure' of oxygen (O_2) and carbon dioxide (CO_2) gases within the artery – thus it is always presented in this way. pH indicates the acidity or alkalinity of the blood. Blood is normally very slightly alkaline. Because the blood pH normally has such a tight range (just 0.10 of a difference), then slight changes towards acid or alkali have significant effects on the body. Most of the effects on blood gases are an attempt to bring the pH back to a normal range (Figure 41.1). The pH reflects the concentration of hydrogen ions (H^+) in the blood. High concentrations lead to *acidosis* (pH < 7.35) and low concentrations lead to *alkalosis* (pH > 7.45).

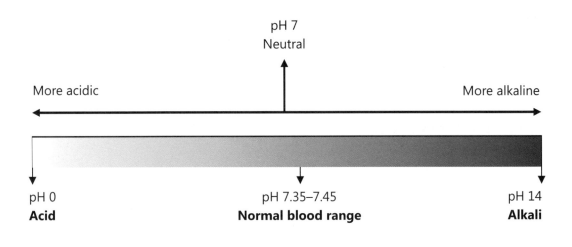

Figure 41.1 Acid and alkaline ranges.

The role of carbon dioxide

Hydrogen ions are formed when CO_2, a waste product of respiration, combines with water – thus CO_2 is considered to be an acid. In respiratory failure, CO_2 will increase and so lead to acid build up. In hyperventilation, it will drop and so lead to alkalosis.

Often respiratory acidosis will be accompanied by poor saturations and low oxygenation (PaO_2 < 11 kPa). However, there is no need to remove oxygen masks from patients with suspected respiratory failure to take an arterial blood gas, because their pH and CO_2 alone will indicate this.

Acidic	Normal	Alkaline
pH < 7.35	pH 7.35–7.45	pH > 7.45
$PaCO_2$ > 6.0 kPa	$PaCO_2$ 4.5–6 kPa	$PaCO_2$ < 4.5 kPa
Respiratory acidosis		Respiratory alkalosis

The role of bicarbonate

Bicarbonate (HCO_3) is the main alkaline substance in body fluids. It binds with excess hydrogen ions to reduce the concentration and maintain pH within normal limits.

When HCO_3 rises (such as in prolonged vomiting or Cushing's syndrome) a metabolic alkalosis will develop. In diarrhoea and renal failure, HCO_3 falls and a metabolic acidosis results.

Acidic	Normal	Alkaline
pH < 7.35	pH 7.35–7.45	pH > 7.45
HCO_3 < 22.0 mmol/L	HCO_3 22–28 mmol/L	HCO_3 > 28 mmol/L
Metabolic acidosis		Metabolic alkalosis

Compensation

The body quickly compensates pH for an acidosis and alkalosis to provide the best environment for cell function. Compensation is easy to recognise – if you have a normal pH (7.35–7.45) but CO_2 and HCO_3 are abnormal, you have a compensated arterial blood gas.

The nature of the compensation will depend on the original problem – for example, respiratory acidosis will be compensated by a rise in HCO_3.

A quick method for working out compensation is shown in Examples 1 and 2 below.

Example 1

Acidic	Normal	Alkaline
	pH 7.36	
$PaCO_2$ 7.0 kPa		HCO_3 34 mmol/L

When analysing compensation in an arterial blood gas, take the pH from the mid-point of the normal range (below 7.40 is acid and above 7.40 is alkaline).

Therefore this example of a compensated respiratory acidosis (shown in the acid column) becomes:

Acidic	Normal	Alkaline
pH < 7.40	pH 7.36	
$PaCO_2$ 7.0 kPa		HCO_3 34 mmol/L
Respiratory acidosis		Metabolic compensation

Example 2

Acidic	Normal	Alkaline
	pH 7.42	
PaCO$_2$ 7.0 kPa		HCO$_3$ 34.0 mmol/L

In this example, the CO$_2$ and HCO$_3$ are unchanged, but pH is above 7.40, thus this becomes:

Acidic	Normal	Alkaline
	pH 7.42	pH > 7.40
PaCO$_2$ 7.0 kPa		HCO$_3$ 34.0 mmol/L
Respiratory compensation		Metabolic alkalosis

Example 3

You can have *partial* compensation where the pH has not returned to normal but PaCO$_2$ and HCO$_3$ are abnormal. The two factors will be in one column and the compensation on its own in the opposing column, thus:

Acidic	Normal	Alkaline
		pH 7.47
PaCO$_2$ 7.0 kPa		HCO$_3$ 34 kPa
Partial respiratory compensation		Metabolic alkalosis

Combined metabolic and respiratory problems

Occasionally you will see a combination of metabolic and respiratory components – acidosis is most common often in a cardiac arrest situation. The patient has multiple problems to get a combination effect.

Example 4

Acidic	Normal	Alkaline
pH < 7.35		pH > 7.45
PaCO$_2$ > 6.0 kPa		PaCO$_2$ < 4.5 kPa
HCO$_3$ < 22 mmol/L		HCO$_3$ > 22 mmol/L
Combined respiratory and metabolic acidosis		Combined respiratory and metabolic alkalosis

Oxygen and saturation

If arterial oxygen levels (PaO_2) are below 11.5 kPa, the patient is described as 'hypoxic'. Thus a patient with a low pH, a high $PaCO_2$ and a low PaO_2 would be described as having 'a respiratory acidosis with hypoxaemia'. The PaO_2 is dependent on the inspired oxygen expressed as 'fraction of inspired oxygen' (FiO_2) with a value that has a decimal point (e.g. 0.21) or is a percentage (e.g. 21%). The inspired oxygen should always be presented with the PaO_2. Saturations should be greater than 95% in normal adults. Values of 90–95% indicate that the patient's respiratory state may worsen, even though they may have a normal PaO_2 level at that point. Saturations below 90% can indicate severe problems in the transportation of oxygen around the body – urgent treatment is needed in such cases.

Base excess

Base excess (BE) is displayed on arterial blood gas results and is an indication of the amount of compensation the body is having to make to maintain a normal pH. Thus, a base excess of –12 is a severe level of compensation; whereas values nearer to –2 to +2 (normal values) are less acute. For the purpose of working out acidosis and alkalosis, base excess is not needed.

Try working out the following examples (answers are given at the end of this chapter).

Scenario 1

This patient is in respiratory distress. Blood gases are pH 7.30, $PaCO_2$ 6.9 kPa, HCO_3 24 mmol/L and PaO_2 9.8 kPa. Fill in the columns below.

Acidic	Normal	Alkaline

Scenario 2

This patient is suspected of having renal failure. Blood gases are pH 7.30, $PaCO_2$ 5.2 kPa, HCO_3 18 mmol/L and PaO_2 11.8 kPa. Fill in the columns below.

Acidic	Normal	Alkaline

Scenario 3

This patient is admitted with a 4-day history of vomiting. Blood gases are pH 7.46, PaCO₂ 6.3 kPa, HCO₃ 34 mmol/L and PaO₂ 11.6 kPa. Fill in the columns below.

Acidic	Normal	Alkaline

Scenario 4

This man has just been put on a ventilator. Blood gases are pH 7.48, PaCO₂ 3.8 kPa and HCO₃ 24 mmol/L. Fill in the columns below.

Acidic	Normal	Alkaline

Scenario 5

This woman is admitted with chronic renal failure. Blood gases are pH 7.37, PaCO₂ 4.2 kPa and HCO₃ 19 mmol/L. Fill in the columns below.

Acidic	Normal	Alkaline

Scenario 6

This man with COPD for several years is admitted with acute-on-chronic respiratory failure due to pneumonia. Blood gases are pH 7.32, PaCO₂ 7.2 kPa, HCO₃ 33 mmol/L and PaO₂ 9.5 kPa.

Acidic	Normal	Alkaline

This patient is having a cardiac arrest. Blood gases are pH 7.29, PaCO$_2$ 7.1 kPa, HCO$_3$ 16 mmol/L and PaO$_2$ 22 kPa. Fill in the columns below.

Acidic	Normal	Alkaline

(Answers overpage.)

References and further reading

Mays, D. (1995). Turn ABGs into child's play. *Registered Nurse*, January, 36–39.

Woodrow, P. (2000). *Intensive Care Nursing: A Framework for Practice.* Routledge, London.

Answers (Scenarios 1-6)

Scenario 1. Respiratory acidosis with hypoxia.

Scenario 2. Metabolic acidosis.

Scenario 3. Metabolic alkalosis with some compensation because PCO_2 is slightly high.

Scenario 4. Respiratory alkalosis.

Scenario 5. Compensated metabolic acidosis.

Scenario 6. Respiratory acidosis with partial compensation and hypoxia.

Scenario 7. Combined metabolic and respiratory acidosis with too much oxygen being given.

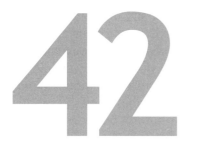

Pulse oximetry

Tim Collins

Hypoxaemia is common in critically ill patients and is a major cause of organ failure and death. A non-invasive method of assessing hypoxaemia is by pulse oximetry in addition to other methods of total patient assessment.

Pulse oximetry measures the amount of arterial oxygen that is combined with haemoglobin (Hb) and this is referred to as *oxygen saturations* (SpO_2) and recorded as a percentage. Pulse oximetry is simple to use, portable, non-invasive and frequently performed in all healthcare environments. The invention of pulse oximetry has been declared as the greatest advance in patient monitoring since electrocardiography (ECG) (Jevon and Ewens, 2002). However, all healthcare professionals need to be aware of the physiology behind and limitations of pulse oximetry in order to improve the care and outcome of their critically ill patients. A number of research studies have found that doctors and nurses have insufficient knowledge and understanding concerning the underlying physiology, clinical application and limitations of pulse oximetry (Kruger and Longden, 1999; Howell, 2002; Simon and Clark, 2002; Teoh *et al.*, 2003). The research highlights these deficits in knowledge among hospital staff, so this chapter will aim to address the following:

- the underlying physiology and mechanics of pulse oximetry
- the indications for monitoring oxygen saturations
- correct use of pulse oximetry
- the limitations of pulse oximetry in clinical practice.

Physiological basis of pulse oximetry

Haemoglobin is the oxygen-carrying component of the red blood cell. It is a compound consisting of iron and four polypeptide (globin) chains. Each globin chain is linked to one atom of iron (haem), each of which carries four molecules of oxygen (Woodrow, 1999). As each molecule of oxygen contains two atoms of oxygen (O_2), each molecule of haemoglobin can transport up to eight atoms of oxygen; 1 g of haemoglobin can carry the equivalent of 1.34 mL of oxygen (Woodrow, 1999).

Pulse oximetry records the percentage of haemoglobin that has been *fully* saturated with oxygen. Therefore, if all the body's haem molecules bind with an oxygen molecule, then all the body's haemoglobin is fully saturated, resulting in 100% oxygen saturations (Woodrow, 1999). When breathing room air (21% oxygen) it is rare for the body to be fully saturated, however with the high affinity of haem for oxygen, saturation levels are usually around 97% in healthy people.

Normal oxygen saturations should be around 95% and oxygen therapy should be instigated in patients to achieve oxygen saturations of 95% or above, otherwise hypoxaemia will develop. For patients who have chronic obstructive pulmonary disease (COPD), oxygen therapy should be given to maintain oxygen saturations of 90% (Smith, 2003). Pulse oximetry aids identification of hypoxaemia because cyanosis is a late sign of hypoxia that is only usually visible when saturations fall below 75%; but severe respiratory failure generally occurs with saturations between 90% and 85% although no visible cyanosis will be present (Woodrow, 1999; Casey, 2001).

Mechanics of pulse oximetry

A probe is placed over a pulsating arterial bed such as a finger or earlobe. The probe consists of two light-emitting diodes that transmit red and infrared light through the body tissue (the finger or earlobe) to a photodetector on the other side of the probe. The pulse oximeter then processes the absorption of red and infrared light and produces a display of the patient's oxygen saturation.

This process works on the principle of Beer's Law which states that the concentration of an unknown solute dissolved in a solvent can be determined by light absorption (Lynne *et al.*, 1990). Most of the light will be absorbed by the tissue between the probes, but the sensors detect the small amount of light that is not absorbed on the other side of the probe. It is this light that is not absorbed which allows the saturation of haemoglobin with oxygen to be calculated (Woodrow, 1999). Absorption of light varies between oxygen-rich and oxygen-poor haemoglobin. It is the difference of absorption between full capillaries at systole and empty ones at diastole that produces a measurable difference, enabling the microprocessor to calculate the oxygen saturation using a calibration curve obtained from experimental data (Woodrow, 1999; Jevon and Ewens, 2002). To accurately measure the difference between full and empty capillaries, the pulse oximeter needs to measure light absorption over a number of pulses (usually five) but some machines vary – and this is why there is a time delay before results are displayed (Harrahill, 1999; Woodrow, 1999).

Indications for pulse oximetry

Pulse oximetry machines are now very compact and portable which means they are frequently available in clinical environments. Just a decade ago they were mainly used within specialist areas such as intensive care or within operating theatres. Pulse oximetry has a pivotal role in any clinical situation where hypoxaemia may occur and should be monitored when managing all critically ill patients. Pulse oximetry should be monitored in the following situations:

- in all patients with (or suspected of) hypoxaemia
- during general anaesthesia and recovery
- during invasive or non-invasive ventilation
- during intravenous sedation or other procedures requiring continuous monitoring of oxygen status
- pre- and postoperative respiratory assessment

- for obtaining guidance regarding therapeutic oxygen and assessing its response
- when assessing severity of illness
- during intra- or inter-hospital transfer of potentially unstable patients
- to estimate oxygenation when arterial blood gas analysis cannot be performed.

Correct procedure for pulse oximetry

Step 1

Ensure the machine has been correctly calibrated (automatic on start-up) and serviced.

Step 2

Ensure the probe is clean.

Step 3

Wash and dry your hands (remember infection control measures are paramount if the pulse oximeter and yourself are going between patients).

Step 4

Select an adequate pulsating bed. If using a finger, assess the amplitude and strength of the radial pulse. Ear lobes and toes can be used instead of fingers but are less accurate (Jenson *et al.*, 1998; Hanning and Alexander-Williams, 1999).

Step 5

Avoid application of probe distal to blood pressure cuffs.

Step 6

Remove nail varnish or any blood or dirt from the patient's finger.

Step 7

Ensure the trace is reliable so that there is a strong plethysmographic waveform or visual light display, depending upon the machine.

Step 8

Ask yourself whether the patient has any conditions that may affect the accuracy of the readings. Always rely on clinical judgement rather than the SpO_2 reading in isolation (Teoh *et al.*, 2003). Decide whether the patient requires supplemental oxygen therapy or if an arterial blood gas needs to be taken.

Step 9

Record the oxygen saturation as well as the FiO_2 the patient is receiving on the observation chart.

Regularly monitor the probe site and alternate probe site every 4 hours to reduce the incidence of pressure sore development.

Limitations of pulse oximetry

In order for the pulse oximetry to be accurate, good peripheral perfusion to the fingers is essential. Depending upon the manufacturer of the pulse oximeter, the machine will either display an oximeter waveform or a digital light display which indicates the strength of the pulse reaching the probe.

Fig. 42.1 shows an accurate oximeter waveform. If the waveform is weak and displays a visual line consisting of limited positive upturns, the patient is in a low perfusion state, which makes it difficult for the probe to distinguish the pulsatile and baseline light absorptions – this results in falsely low readings. It may be particularly evident in clinical shock when a low perfusion state is likely to occur. It is beneficial to take an arterial blood gas if a patient is acutely unwell and possibly hypoxic.

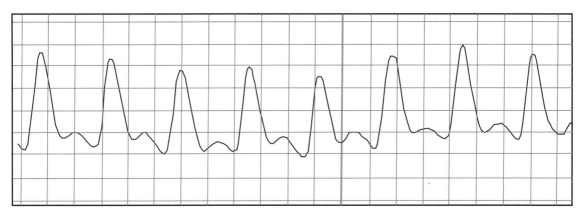

Figure 42.1   Oxygen saturation plethysmographic waveform.

There are a range of conditions that may affect the accuracy of the oxygen saturation recordings. Dysrhythmias may cause irregular perfusion and unreliably low readings (Woodrow, 1999; Smith, 2003). Shivering also causes problems with detecting saturations.

Bright external lighting such as overhead theatre lights interfere with the infrared absorption of the probe and may affect accuracy (Casey, 2001; Jevon and Ewens, 2002; Smith, 2003). Carbon monoxide poisoning causes falsely high readings due to the gas's greater affinity to combine with haemoglobin. When carboxyhaemoglobin is suspected, pulse oximetry should be avoided and arterial blood gases with carboxyhaemoglobin levels should be regularly obtained. Low-level accuracy of saturations occurs when the reading falls below 80% (Allen, 2004).

> **HOT TIPS**
>
> Errors also occur when anything interferes with light detection, such as dark nail varnish, dried blood, dark skin or intravenous dyes, which can also reduce the accuracy of the readings (Woodrow, 1999; Smith, 2003; Allen, 2004).

Pulse oximetry measures the oxygen saturation of haemoglobin but does not record carbon dioxide carriage. Therefore pulse oximetry gives an indication of oxygen transportation but it does not detect hypercapnia and acid–base balance disturbances caused by respiratory compromise. Haemoglobinopathies such as sickle cell disease sometimes alter the shape and properties of erythrocytes, causing over-readings or under-readings (Smith, 2003). Methaemoglobins that result in changes in the structure of iron in haemoglobin can inhibit oxygen release from the haemoglobin molecular, causing tissue hypoxia, which causes inaccurate readings (Jevon and Ewens, 2002).

> **HOT TIPS**
>
> Caution is necessary with anaemic patients. Pulse oximetry only records the available circulatory haemoglobin that has been saturated with oxygen – it cannot detect anaemia. Therefore patients may have oxygen saturations above 95% but have a low haemoglobin level (below 10 g/dL) which means that despite saturations being normal the oxygen reaching the cells via haemoglobin is reduced. This may result in hypoxia at a cellular level (Woodrow, 1999; Jevon and Ewens, 2002; Smith, 2003).

The probe should be alternated regularly between the fingers or toe digits, otherwise it may cause pressure sores to develop. Oxygen saturations should always be measured in conjunction with supplemental oxygen that the patient is receiving. Patients who are receiving oxygen may not have hypoxaemia detected early (Jevon and Ewens, 2002).

Conclusions

Pulse oximetry is a valuable and non-invasive method of assessing a critically ill patient's oxygen status. As it is routinely used to monitor patients in hospital, it is paramount that all healthcare staff are aware of the indications and limitations of its use. Remember that if a patient's saturations are low when observations are done, getting them to breathe deeply to get a better figure for recording is *not* helpful because the saturations will drop again for the next hour. Call for help for more effective long-term treatment such as repositioning the patient, physiotherapy or commencing oxygen therapy.

References and further reading

Allen, K. (2004). Principles and limitations of pulse oximetry in patient monitoring. *Nursing Times*, **41**, 34–37.

Casey, G. (2001). Oxygen transport and the use of pulse oximetry. *Nursing Standard*, **47**, 46–55.

Hanning, C. and Alexander-Williams, J. (1995). Pulse oximetry: a practical review. *British Medical Journal*, **311**, 367–370.

Harrahill, M. (1991). Pulse oximetry: Perils and pitfalls. *Journal of Emergency Nursing*, **6**, 437–439.

Howell, M. (2002). Pulse oximetry: An audit of nursing and medical staff understanding. *British Journal of Nursing*, **11**, 191–197.

Jenson, L., Onyskiw, J. and Prasad, N. (1998). Meta-analysis of arterial oxygenation saturation monitoring by pulse oximetry in adults. *Heart and Lung*, **6**, 387–408.

Jevon, P. and Ewens, B. (2002). *Monitoring the Critically Ill Patient*. London, Blackwell Science.

Kruger, P. and Longden, P. (1997). A study of hospital staff's knowledge of pulse oximetry. *Anaesthesia Intensive Care*, **25**, 38–41.

Lynne, M., Schnapp, M. and Neal, H. (1990). Pulse oximetry: Uses and abuses. *Chest*, **98**, 1244–1250.

Simon, S. and Clark, R. (2002). Using pulse oximetry: A review of pulse oximetry use in acute care medical wards. *Clinical Effectiveness in Nursing*, **6**, 106–110.

Smith, G. (2003). *ALERTTM: A Multiprofessional Course in Care of the Acutely Ill Patient*. Portsmouth, University of Portsmouth Learning Media Development.

Teoh, L., Epstein, A., Williamson, B., Morton, J., Papadopoulos, D. and Teng, A. (2003). Medical staff's knowledge of pulse oximetry: A prospective survey conducted in a tertiary children's hospital. *Journal of Paediatric Child Health*, **39**, 618–622.

Woodrow, P. (1999). Pulse oximetry. *Nursing Standard*, **13**, 42–46

43 Placement of a nasogastric tube

Catherine Plowright

Insertion of a nasogastric tube (NG) is relatively common among acutely unwell adult patients within a hospital environment. They are inserted for a variety of reasons, among which are to administer nutritional support and to aspirate gastrointestinal secretions. Staff who insert them should be aware of the complications associated with the procedure, such as accidental intubation of the respiratory tract and epistaxis. There are a number of contraindications to inserting nasogastric tubes: nasal injuries, basal skull fractures, and anatomical changes as a result of surgery or tumours. Care should also be taken in patients who have had recent upper gastrointestinal surgery.

Prior to inserting the tube

Before inserting a nasogastric tube, you must ensure that the patient requires the tube. Then decide on the most appropriate type of tube to use. This will depend on the reason why the tube is being inserted. The two main types of tube are:

- fine-bore tubes (for enteral feeding)
- wide-bore tubes (primarily for aspiration of gastric secretions, but can also be used for short-term feeding).

Different types of tubes are manufactured from different materials. The wide-bore tubes are made from polyvinylchloride (PVC) and the fine-bore ones from either PVC or polyurethane. Different hospitals will have local policies as to the size and type of fine-bore feeding tubes that are to be used. Rollins (1997) suggests that standard feeds can be administered through a size 6 Fr tube with ease, but that an 8 Fr tube may be required for patients receiving a fibre feed. Check with your local teams. Fine-bore PVC nasogastric tubes are only suitable for using for a maximum of 10 days; if used for longer than that, there is a risk to the patient of nasal ofoesophageal erosions (Best, 2005; 2007). Always check the manufacturer's instructions.

Nasogastric tubes that are inserted should be radio-opaque with clear markings on them to aid measurement and help guide the healthcare professional as to the position of the tube. Always gain verbal consent from the patient prior to attempting to insert a nasogastric tube. This ensures that the patient understands the planned procedure and gives a valid consent

(Nursing and Midwifery Council, 2008). The procedure for inserting differs slightly depending on the type of nasogastric tube being inserted. Before insertion, measure how far down the tube is to be inserted; note the distance from the patient's ear lobe to bridge of his or her nose, plus the distance to the bottom of xiphisternum (Best, 2007; see Fig. 43.1).

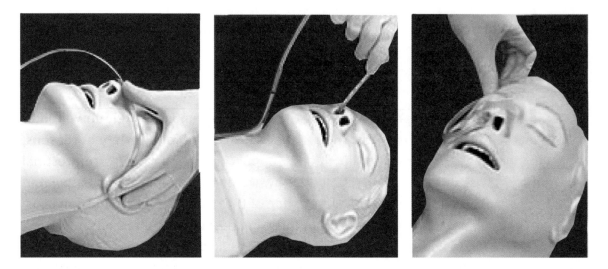

Figure 43.1   Nasogastric tube insertion. Measuring the length (*left*), passing the tube (*centre*) and securing the tube in place (*right*).

Equipment required for insertion

- Clean trolley.
- Non-sterile gloves and apron.
- Appropriate nasogastric tube.
- Sterile water.
- Syringe (10 mL for fine-bore tube; 50 mL for wide-bore tube).
- Receptacle to collect gastric aspirate.
- Lubricating jelly.
- Securing device/tape.
- Glass of water.
- pH indicator strips/paper.

(Best, 2005; Dougherty and Lister, 2008)

Procedure

Step 1

Prior to approaching patient, wash your hands and cleanse with bactericidal alcohol rub. Explain to the patient what is about to happen and discuss a signal that the patient can use to stop the procedure if wanted. Position the patient in a semi-upright position in a bed or on a chair and prepare all the equipment on the clean trolley. Open the nasogastric tube. Wash your hands and put on gloves and an apron, then measure the distance the nasogastric tube is to be inserted. Then, following the manufacturer's instructions, prepare the tube for insertion.

Step 2

Lubricate the end of the nasogastric tube with lubricating jelly.

Step 3

Inject water down the tube.

Step 4

Check that the patient's nostrils are clear. If necessary, ask him or her to blow their nose (or they can sniff with one nostril closed).

Step 5

Insert the rounded end of the tube into the nostril that is the clearest and slide it inwards and backwards following the floor of the nose towards the nasopharynx (Fig. 43.1 (centre)).

Step 6

If there is any obstruction or difficulty remove and try again. If necessary try the other nostril.

Step 7

As the tube passes into the nasopharynx, give the patient the glass of water and ask him or her to take and drink and swallow. As the patient swallows, advance the nasogastric tube. It will be necessary to let the patient take further sips of water. Advance the nasogastric tube until you have reached the mark that you previously measured.

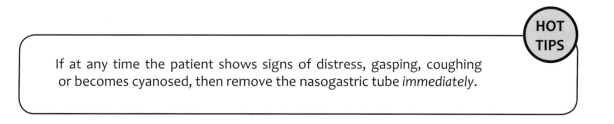

HOT TIPS

If at any time the patient shows signs of distress, gasping, coughing or becomes cyanosed, then remove the nasogastric tube *immediately*.

350   *PRACTICAL SKILLS*

If a fine-bore nasogastric tube has been used there will be a guide wire in situ. It is usual practice to leave this wire in until after an x-ray has been performed to check the position of the tube. After correct positioning of the tube is confirmed, then the wire must be removed. Secure the nasogastric tube using either a fixing device or tape (Fig. 43.1). Make a note of the position of the tube at the nostrils in the patient's records (Dougherty and Lister, 2004; Best, 2007).

HOT TIPS

No more than three attempts at inserting a nasogastric tube should be made by any one person. If unsuccessful, refer the patient to another healthcare professional for further advice (Best, 2007).

Checking the position of the nasogastric tube

The National Patient Safety Agency (2005a) recommends that only the following are attempted to establish the correct position of a nasogastric tubes. It is your responsibility as a healthcare professional to familiarise yourself with all the National Patient Safety Agency documents regarding nasogastric tubes (2005b).

1. Measure the pH of the aspirate using pH indicator strips or paper

- Aspirate about 2 mL of gastric secretions and test using pH indicator strip or paper.
- The pH should be below 5.5.

2. Radiography

- This is the method of choice in patients who are unconscious or who have no gag reflex.
- It should not be used routinely (National Patient Safety Agency, 2005a).
- It is highly recommended before nasogastric feeds are commenced to prevent iatrogenic instillation of feed into the lung.

After the procedure

Ensure that the patient is comfortable. Tidy up and dispose of or put away all the equipment used.

References and further reading

Best, C. (2005). Caring for the patient with a nasogastric tube. *Nursing Standard*, **20**(3), 59–65.

Best, C. (2007). Nasogastric tube insertion in adults who require enteral feeding. *Nursing Standard*, **21**(40), 39–43.

Dougherty, L. and Lister, S. (2008). *The Royal Marsden Hospital Manual of Clinical Nursing Procedures*, 7th edn. Oxford, Blackwell Publishing.

National Patient Safety Agency (2005a). *How to Confirm the Correct Position of Nasogastric Feeding Tubes in Infants, Children and Adults*. London, National Patient Safety Agency.

National Patient Safety Agency (2005b). *Reducing the Harm Caused by Misplaced Nasogastric Feeding Tubes Patient Safety Alert*. February 21. London, National Patient Safety Agency.

Nursing and Midwifery Council (2008). Advice Sheet Consent. Available at: http://www.nmc-uk.org/aDisplayDocument.aspx?documentID=4710 (last accessed November 2009).

Rollins, H. (1997). A nose for trouble. *Nursing Times*, **93** (49), 66–67.

Useful websites

British Association for Parental and Enteral Nutrition
www.bapen.org.uk

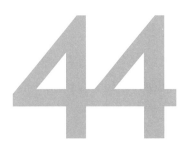

44 Meeting nutritional requirements

The Malnutrition Universal Screening Tool (MUST)

Ann M. Price

Nutrition in the critically ill patient is vital to aid healing, to hasten recovery and to improve prognosis. In the acute situation a patient's nutritional state is often forgotten, yet a poor nutritional state may have (at least in part) contributed to the patient's deterioration. Patients with a critical illness may be unable to eat, be nil by mouth, have restricted diets or poor appetites (Moore and Woodrow, 2004) which can lead to malnutrition and poor energy supply. Thus, nutritional assessment should be instigated as soon as is practical after the onset of critical illness – ideally, within the first 24–48 hours.

The Malnutrition Universal Screening Tool (MUST)

This tool is commonly used in acute hospitals to assess the nutritional needs of patients, but other tools are also available. The locally used tool should be employed to aid consistency of assessment and enable prompt referral to a dietician and other services when needed, according to local policy.

The MUST includes five steps for performing a full assessment. The full details are given on the website (see below).

Step 1

Measure the patient's height and weight and calculate their body mass index (BMI) using a table

- If 20 or below – score 1.
- If 18 or below – score 2.

If unable to do a BMI (or to estimate height) take a mid-upper arm circumference (MUAC) to estimate BMI.

Step 2

Note the amount of unplanned weight loss in the last 3–6 months and calculate the percentage (table available on the website).

- If below 5% – score 0.
- If 5–10% – score 1.
- If above 10% – score 2.

Ask the patient whether their clothes are loose, and about their appetite and food intake.

Step 3

Acute disease effect.

- Patient has not eaten or is unlikely to eat for 5 days or more – score 2.

Step 4

Add scores together from steps 1, 2 and 3.

- Total score of 0 – low risk.
- Total score of 1 – medium risk.
- Total score of 2 or more – high risk.

Step 5

Refer to hospital management guidelines (see below on meeting nutritional requirements).

- For 0 (low risk) – monitor weekly.
- For 1 (medium risk) – monitor food intake for 3 days and re-assess.
- For 2 or more (high risk) – refer to dietician and instigate nutrition support.

HOT TIPS

Record the presence of obesity but remember that a balanced nutritional intake is required in the acute situation and that obesity can be managed once the patient has recovered.

Also remember that critically ill patients can have large fluid shifts which make the patient heavier so that they may look more overweight than they really are. Weight loss is often increased in critical illness (due to catabolic state) so these patients can lose a lot of weight very rapidly.

Meeting nutritional requirements

Once the risk of malnutrition has been assessed it is important to implement strategies to improve nutritional intake. Consider the following strategies:

- Food daily intake record.
- Supplements.
- Referral to a dietician.
- Enteral feeding.
- Total parental nutrition.

Nutritional intake should be reviewed each day and feeding regimens commenced as required. Enteral and parental nutrition should ideally be commenced with a dietician's input but should not be delayed if this cannot take place (e.g. at a weekend).

If possible, medium-risk patients should be seen early by a dietician and a nutrition plan compiled so that appropriate nutritional regimens are in place if their nutritional intake does not improve.

References and further reading

Moore, T. and Woodrow, P. (2004). *High Dependency Nursing Care*. London, Routledge.

Woodrow, P. (2000). *Intensive Care Nursing*. London, Routledge.

Useful websites

British Association of Parental and Enteral Nutrition
www.bapen.org.uk

Malnutrition Universal Screening Tool (MUST; and related documents)
www.bapen.org.uk/must_tool.html/

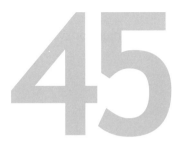

Undertaking a Glasgow Coma Score properly

Ann M. Price

There are three areas that need to be assessed in order to obtain a Glasgow Coma Score (GCS) score properly. These are: eye opening; best verbal response; and best motor response.

Section 1: Open Eyes (E)

Approach the patient

If the patient opens eyes spontaneously – **score 4**. The normal response is when the eyes open without speech or touch.

No response to approach

Try speaking to the patient. If the patient opens eyes – **score 3**. Take care not to approach, speak and touch all at the same time as you will not know which one caused the response. Also, consider hearing problems.

No response to speech

Try painful stimuli. If the patient opens eyes – **score 2**. Try touch or gentle shaking before using pain. Use the minimal level to elicit a response (a maximum of 30 seconds) and slowly increase the intensity of pain. Severe pain can make patients shut their eyes! Use the central pain method, not peripheral, at this point. See Box 45.1.

Box 45.1 Pain methods (Woodrow, 2006)

CENTRAL PAIN
Sub-orbital pressure: Place your thumb on the patient's eyebrow ridge and apply pressure.
Jaw pressure: Apply pressure to the angle of the jaw. This is unsuitable for patients with possible facial injuries or those with severe bruising.
Trapezium pinch: Squeeze the patient's trapezium muscle (on the top of the shoulder at the base of the neck) between your fingers and thumb. This has few side effects.
Sternal rub: Rub the centre of the chest on the sternum. This causes bruising if excessive pressure is used or there is a clotting disorder (not recommended).

PERIPHERAL PAIN
This includes pain on the side of a fingernail – *not* on the nailbed as this damages the nail. It is useful for assessing limb strength in deeply unconscious patients. It is *not* suitable for assessing GCS as it only elicits a local reflex response (Cree, 2003).

No response to pain

If the patient is deeply unconscious – score 1. If the eyes are closed due to injury or swelling – **record C** on the chart. Consider drug-induced unconsciousness.

Section 2: Best Verbal Response (V)

This is based on Waterhouse, 2005.

Orientated

If the patient knows where they are, who they are and why they are there, and talks in sentences and recognises people – **score 5**. Consider that patients lose track of time and date during a hospital stay; they should know the month and year. This is more difficult to assess in children.

Confused

If information is muddled and the patient is not sure of the above, but talks in sentences – **score 4**. Some patients seem to be talking sense and then make strange incorrect statements. Remember that some patients may not be able to express themselves but may be able to understand you.

Inappropriate words

If the patient uses recognisable words but incomplete sentences – **score 3**. The words may be swear words or odd and out of context.

Incomprehensible sounds

If the patient has no words, or grunts, moans and groans – **score 2**. Check that the sounds are not signs of airway obstruction (e.g. gurgling).

No response or tracheostomy

If there is no response – **score 1**. Consider injuries that may limit speech such as jaw fracture or tracheostomy or endotracheal tubes. Do not assume that a tracheostomy patient can speak. **Record T** on the chart.

Section 3: Best Motor Response (M)

Remember to record the 'best' response as limbs may differ.

Obeys commands

If patient follows commands (even if their limbs are weak) – **score 6**. Do not ask them to 'squeeze your hand' as this is a reflex response to touching the palm. Ask them to lift their arm or leg, or stick out their tongue. Remember to be specific!

Localises to pain

If the patient moves an arm or leg purposefully away from pain – **score 5**. The peripheral pain method is usually more useful because the central method gives a more generalised response.

Patients are localising if they try and pull at lines, endotracheal or nasogastric tubes or try to push you away.

Withdrawal from pain

If the patient moves an arm or leg away from pain but not purposefully – **score 4**. This differs from purposeful removal from pain because the patient may move all limbs away if they cannot distinguish where the pain is originating from.

Flexion to pain

If the patient demonstrates 'decorticate posturing' – **score 3**. The arms will bend at the elbows and the wrists will flex. This response is slower than withdrawal to pain.

Extension to pain

If the patient demonstrates 'decerebrate posturing' – **score 2**. The arms and legs straighten, and there is internal rotation of the shoulder and wrist. This is a very abnormal response.

None

If there is no response – **score 1**. Consider other causes, such as paralysing agents or spinal injury.

Now add up the scores according to Box 45.2.

Box 45.1   Producing the Glasgow Coma Score

Record the E, V and M scores separately and add them together.

— A total score of 8 and below is considered as coma.
— Deterioration of 2 or more points is considered significant (Waterhouse, 2005).
— The lowest score possible is 3 (completely unresponsive).
— The highest possible score is 15 (normal).

Record GCS half-hourly until the patient is stable – the frequency depends on the individual patient's needs.

Limb response

Assess differences in limb strength and type of movement. Record the left and right separately. For GCS, record the best limb response (Waterhouse, 2005).

To assess arm and leg strength, ask the patient to lift the limb and hold it off the bed. Observe for weakness or drifting down of the limb.

For patients who are unable to respond to a command or who do not move their limb you will need to assess their response to pain (Waterhouse, 2005).

Pupil response

Pupil reaction is not part of the score but provides important additional information. Open both eyes and examine whether the pupils are equal to begin with. Then shine a bright light from the side into one eye at a time and assess the response. The pupils should constrict swiftly and both evenly. Any differences in size or response should be reported. Consider eye injuries and cataracts (Cree, 2003).

Cardiovascular state

Blood pressure, pulse, respiration rate and temperature should be recorded. Changes in the cardiovascular state can be linked to changes in the GCS score and may be significant (Cree, 2003), for example the following is usually true:

- **Early** signs of deterioration
  — *Hypo*-tension
  — *Tachy*-cardia.

- **Late** signs of deterioration
  — *Hyper*-tension
  — *Brady*-cardia.

References and further reading

Cree, C. (2003). Acquired brain injury: Acute management. *Nursing Standard*, **18**(11), 45–56.

Waterhouse, C. (2005). The Glasgow Coma Score and other neurological observations. *Nursing Standard*, **19**(33), 56–64.

Woodrow, P. (2006). *Intensive Care Nursing: A Framework for Practice*, 2nd edn. London, Routledge.

46 Examination of the sick ward patient

Alistair Challiner

This chapter assumes that the patient has already been admitted and fully clerked with a full history and that examination has already taken place. Assume this is an unwell patient who has deteriorated. A basic examination system is described here that will quickly help you ascertain the salient points of why the patient is deteriorating and what you need to do to manage the situation straight away.

First of all, assess for life-threatening problems by assessing and treating (using ABCDE) as already described in initial assessment and a review of the notes. An effective assessment of *Breathing* and *Circulation* requires examination skills.

Medically qualified staff are trained in clinical examination. Nursing staff do not have this full training during their qualifying training but the skills can be learned and are particularly relevant initially in detecting any abnormality. There are many texts on the technique of clinical examination, which should also be consulted, but the best way is through observation of an expert and through practice. The key points covered in this chapter are how to determine whether something has changed from the normal or from how it was before.

Always follow the order:

1. Inspection.
2. Palpation.
3. Percussion.
4. Auscultation.

Examine from the patient's right and ideally have him or her sitting up at a 30° angle.

Examination of the respiratory system

Look for the following key things during examination of the respiratory system.

1. Inspection

Initially look at the colour of the patient, particularly looking for cyanosis, pallor or mottling. Also look for recent or old scars that imply previous surgery; cardiac surgery if the scar is down the middle of the sternum, or lung surgery if it is running between the ribs. Check the sputum pot or ask either the nurses or the patient what their sputum is like. Is it clear, thick, yellowy brown or is there any blood in it?

Stand at the foot of the bed and observe the patient's chest movements. You may find that one side of the chest does not move as much as the other (as in pneumothorax). Movement of the chest may be very shallow if there is an underlying chest infection, or if the patient is exhausted or has muscular weakness.

Check also for an abnormal rate of breathing. This is covered in the initial assessment. You may observe increased work of breathing, or usage of accessory muscles in the neck from working hard to breathe. This can be due to obstruction in the upper or lower airways or because the patient is getting tired out from prolonged difficulty in breathing (as in pneumonia, pulmonary oedema or respiratory compensation in acidosis).

2. Palpation

Decreased chest movement on one side or both sides can be checked for by placing the hands flat on each side of the chest with the thumbs meeting in the middle. Check the position of the trachea. It should be in the middle. If it is deviated to one side it is abnormal.

- *Lung collapse* pulls the trachea towards the affected side. This occurs when there is an obstruction to one of the lung airways (such as a mucous plug).
- *Tension pneumothorax* pushes the trachea towards the non-affected side.

3. Percussion

The technique of percussion is done using both hands. The left hand is placed flat over the chest with the fingers apart. With the right hand, tap over one of your left fingers with the tip of your right middle finger. Do this as if tapping out morse code, extending your right wrist fully and then flexing it quickly. The aim is to detect whether the space under the body wall is hollow or solid (it is like tapping on a wall to find a door that has been wall-papered over).

Percussing over the rib cage should produce a hollow sound if there is lung underneath. Compare both sides. It should sound dull over the heart if you tap over the lower sternum and dull over the lower right chest where there is liver under the ribs. The upper part of the rib cage on each side should sound resonant (hollow). If there is *consolidation* of the lung (as in a lobar pneumonia) it should sound dull. If there is an *effusion* then the dullness is pronounced and termed 'stony' dull. A *pneumothorax* should sound more resonant than on the opposite side of the chest.

HOT TIPS

This technique should be demonstrated by a doctor and practiced. It will help to determine effusions and consolidation if dullness is where it should not be, and a pneumothorax if it is more resonant.

4. Auscultation

Listen over all areas of the chest at the front and the back using the diaphragm of the stethoscope. Normally you will hear quiet sounds of air moving in and out; these are termed vesicular. Listen over each zone, comparing the right with the left. If breath sounds are absent then the underlying lung is not being ventilated (as in collapse, consolidation or a large effusion). A pneumothorax may be quiet or may sound like quiet or distant breath sounds.

At the edge of a consolidated area there may be loud hissing-like sounds called bronchial breathing; these help the diagnosis.

Listen for added sounds. Wheezing, particularly on expiration, means lower respiratory obstruction (as in asthma). Louder added sounds on inspiration are usually caused by upper airway obstruction. Expiratory wheeze can be caused by bronchospasm, as in asthma, chronic obstructive pulmonary disorder and anaphylaxis. It can also be caused by left ventricular failure.

Crackles in the chest can be caused by pneumonia due to increased secretions. Also classic of pulmonary oedema are crackles in both lung bases when listening to the lower part of the back over the lower ribs. Ask the patient to cough: if the crackles clear then they were due to secretions; otherwise they are likely to be caused by left ventricular failure. There is often confusion between chest infection or left ventricular failure, especially in elderly patients who often have difficult-to-determine signs. Look for other signs of chest infection (temperature, sputum, white cell count) and history of pre-existing lung disease. For left ventricular failure, ask if this is sudden onset and whether there are cardiovascular signs, ECG abnormalities or a history of poor cardiac function. If it is still unclear, obtain senior medical help because the treatments are completely different.

HOT TIPS

> The key point of the examination is to determine whether something has *changed*. Patients should be examined every day and the results recorded in their notes. This provides a baseline for determining an acute change.

Examination of the cardiovascular system

The same systematic method is used to examine the cardiovascular system in a patient who is deteriorating.

1. Inspection

Look at the colour of the patient as you did in the respiratory examination. Look at the patient's observations, and particularly check the blood pressure, pulse rate and ECG monitor, if present.

Ask for a recent 12-lead ECG to look at. Look at the patient's neck. Can the pulse be seen over the carotid or the jugular vein? Are the veins in the neck distended, showing either a well-filled patient or raised pressure in the thorax (as in severe asthma or tension pneumothorax)?

Assess the jugular venous pulse (JVP). Ensure that the patient is positioned on their back at an angle of 45 degrees, with his or her head resting on a pillow and the neck relaxed. Ask them to turn their head just a little left of centre. By looking across the neck, identify the pulsation of the internal jugular vein – it is normally visible just above the level of the clavicle (remember, patients who are breathless may find it difficult to lie in this position).

Estimate the height of the JVP using the sternal angle as 0 cm; the height of the top of the pulsation is the JVP. It should not be higher than 4 cm above the sternal angle. Remember that the respiratory and cardiac systems are very closely related.

HOT TIPS

The *internal jugular vein* is seen to pulsate twice for every one heart beat (except when there is atrial fibrillation) and this is one way of distinguishing it from the carotid pulse – the other is that venous pulsations are impalpable.

The *sternal angle* is found by running the fingers along one of the clavicles to the midline. This point is the sternal notch. Run your fingers down the sternum at this point for a few centimetres – the palpable 'lump' is the sternal angle.

Check for oedema. The ankles are usually swollen in right heart failure but may not be obvious in bed-bound patients (check the sacral area instead). The oedema is typically pitting, meaning that direct thumb pressure will cause a dent (like that in uncooked pastry).

Remember other causes of oedema such as fluid overload and low serum proteins in debilitated patients.

2. Palpation

Feel the pulse at the radius. Is it strong or weak? Is it regular, irregular or irregularly irregular as in atrial fibrillation? Also feel the character of the pulse to determine whether it is weak but slowly rising, or bounding. If the pulse is weak, how does it compare with the carotid? The radial pulse is very difficult to feel if the blood pressure is around 80 mmHg or less.

Check the blood pressure. If the diastolic pressure is low, it may be due to vasodilation (as in early sepsis). A high blood pressure may be due to pain or stress. Compare the blood pressure with that obtained earlier on admission and with those recorded on the observation charts.

Other peripheral pulses may be useful to check, particularly in vascular patients, such as the femoral and dorsalis pedis on the top of the foot between the first and second metatarsals.

Palpation over the heart is useful for feeling the apex beat which can be displaced further left with an enlarged heart.

> **HOT TIPS**
>
> It is *essential* that blood pressures are recorded in the notes!
>
> Knowing the patient's normal blood pressure is necessary in order to determine whether it is currently abnormal.
>
> A blood pressure of 111/65 mmHg may be good for most people, but if the patient's normal is 170/94 then this may indicate shock and be the reason for a poor urine output.

3. Auscultation

Listen over the heart. The apex is the easiest to listen to. Practise listening to the sounds made by a normal heart. Most people can hear two sounds of *lub* (systolic) and *dub* (diastolic). The initial *lub* is the atrioventricular valves closing, and the *dub* is the pulmonary and aortic valves closing. Hearing other specific sounds takes lots of practice and practical teaching, but most people are able to hear murmurs. Some murmurs are not harmful, but some can be serious.

Murmurs due to *congenital heart disease* will have been present for life and the patient may well be aware and have to take antibiotics for dental work or surgery to prevent endocarditis. Serious valve disorders produce murmurs, for example the systolic murmur of aortic stenosis. If severe, the patient may have a slow rising pulse and a low blood pressure.

Remember that the patient will already have been clerked. Has the murmur been recorded in the notes? If not, check with the doctor. It may have been missed or something may have changed. In endocarditis, a changing murmur is significant and *must* be reported to the medical team. A sudden-onset murmur in a post-myocardial infarction patient could be due to papillary muscle rupture and onset of a valve regurgitation. In most other cases murmurs do not change. The lung fields need to be checked (as above) to determine signs of pulmonary oedema.

Abdominal examination

The patient may become unwell if there is an acute abdominal problem. Therefore a basic knowledge of examination is required.

1. Inspection

Examine the patient lying flat, with his or her arms by their side and relaxed. If there are any dressings over the abdomen due to recent surgery, the abdomen will be tender and difficult to examine.

Look at the patient's colour, particularly for jaundice or pallor (as in anaemia). Are there old scars? Find out by asking the patient what they were or check the notes. Is there a colostomy or ileostomy? Does it work? If it has recently been formed, does it look healthy and pink? If it looks dusky or black, get the surgical team to check it. This does not necessarily mean it has failed – but it could do.

Does the abdomen look distended? This could be due to fat or pregnancy. Otherwise it could be due to gaseous distension from obstruction, ascites or blood. Blood lying free in the abdomen could be due to catastrophic haemorrhage (several litres may show no signs except for severe hypovolaemic shock and possibly pain). Measuring girth circumferences is pointless in this case. Are there signs of bruising? If along the posterior of the abdomen and back (Gray–Turner's sign), they may be due to pancreatitis or extraperitoneal bleeding. Bruising around the umbilicus (Cullen's sign) is another possibility with pancreatitis.

2. Palpation

Ask the patient if there is any pain before touching them and ask where it is. Initially gently palpate over the whole abdomen, watching the patient's face. The point is to detect tenderness – not to hurt them. If tenderness is found, isolate where it is worse or if it is generalised. This could be peritonitis. Typically there may be 'guarding' whereby the patient tenses their abdominal muscles and looks very anxious because the pain is severe. Talk to them to distract their attention – is there still guarding? Severe peritonitis presents as a board-rigid abdomen that is very tender. Confirm this by eliciting release tenderness (sometimes called *rebound*). Warn the patient and then press *slowly* over the site of tenderness. Then suddenly lift your hand. If this causes a sudden worsening of the pain, then peritonitis is likely.

HOT TIPS

At this point call for medical help or a surgeon to confirm peritonitis. Do not examine the abdomen further. Make sure bloods have been recently taken for full blood count, white cells, urea and electrolytes, liver function tests and amylase (test for pancreatitis).

Keep the patient 'nil by mouth' until seen by the specialist team.

If there are no signs of peritonitis further examination may not be necessary. A full abdominal examination requires a detailed knowledge of the underlying anatomy. At initial clerking, an enlarged liver should have been detected.

- *Pancreatitis* causes an acute abdomen with pain radiating through to the back, also there may be signs of septic shock and the amylase may be raised.
- *Acute ruptured aortic aneurysm* presents with abdominal pain and shock. Usually the aneurysm has already been found.
- *Acute appendicitis* usually presents with nausea and vomiting. The patient will be off food and have acute abdominal pain starting in the middle, over the umbilicus, and moving to the right iliac fossa. There is usually guarding and release tenderness. Similar pain on the left side is usually due to a gynaecological condition.

- *Generalised peritonitis* can be caused by perforations of the bowel (such as diverticular abscess or tumour). Upper abdominal pain may be from a perforated gastric ulcer or duodenal ulcer. Perforations cause gas under the diaphragm which shows up on an erect chest x-ray.

Remember any of these conditions can occur with an adult inpatient admitted for any other reason.

3. Percussion

This is especially useful for detecting ascites, where there is increased dullness in the flanks. It can also be used to detect an enlarged liver or spleen. Usually the front and middle of the abdomen are resonant due to an air-filled gut.

4. Auscultation

Bowel sounds are normally heard as occasional gurgling sounds when listening over the abdomen. No sound at all is usually caused by a paralytic ileus, which means there is no peristalsis in the gut. This is common after abdominal surgery and can delay feeding as the stomach may not empty. It usually resolves with time. Loud tinkling sounds may be caused by obstruction of the bowel. The classic signs of obstruction with loud tinkling sounds are vomiting, distension of the abdomen and constipation with an empty rectum. If this is a new finding, call for medical or surgical help to confirm this.

Neurological examination

The importance of this is to determine acute changes and call for medical help. Assessment of the level of consciousness is vital, as well as pupil signs as described elsewhere (see Chapter 45 on how to determine a Glasgow Coma Score). What is important is to determine whether anything has changed due to an acute stroke so that it can be dealt with urgently.

Loss of motor function down one side of the body needs to be elicited. The simplest way of doing this is to look at the patient and see if there are any differences on either side (such as drooping of one eye or one side of the mouth) or if the limbs look different.

- Ask the patient to smile. Is it even?
- Ask the patient to stick their tongue out. Does it deviate?
- Get the patient to lift their arms up. Do they move evenly?
- Check their grip simultaneously.

As a further check, test their strength. Get them to bend and straighten their arms as you resist them. Compare on both sides and record the strength on a scale of 0 to 5 thus:

- No movement – **score 0.**
- Flicker of muscle movement – **score 1.**

- Moves sideways but cannot lift against gravity – **score 2.**
- Can lift against gravity but not against gentle downward pressure – **score 3.**
- Weak against your resistance – **score 4.**
- Normal power – **score 5.**

Ask the patient to flex their legs at the hip, bringing the knee up against you as you push down. Also check the foot bending up and down. Run your nail firmly along the sole of the foot from the heel to the ball. Do not cause scratch marks. This looks for the Babinski sign. Normally the big toe will bend. The result is considered abnormal (indicating a possible stroke) when the big toe extends.

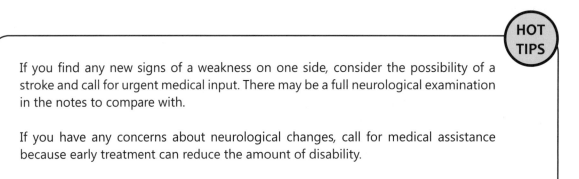

HOT TIPS

If you find any new signs of a weakness on one side, consider the possibility of a stroke and call for urgent medical input. There may be a full neurological examination in the notes to compare with.

If you have any concerns about neurological changes, call for medical assistance because early treatment can reduce the amount of disability.

Conclusions

With all examinations and assessments, record your findings. If the patient was normal this morning and there is something different now, then that is significant. If you think there is a problem with the patient, call a member of the outreach team and/or the medical team. See if they agree with you, watch what they do, ask questions. If they find something different to your findings, ask them why and get them to show you – after all, that's how they learned.

References and further reading

Cox, C. (1994). *Physical Examination for Nurses*. Oxford, Blackwell Publishing.

Jarvis, C. (2000). *Physical Examination and Health Assessment*, 3rd edn. London, WB Saunders.

Epstein, O., Perkin, G.D., Cookson, J. and de Bono, D.P. (2003). *Clinical Examination*, 3rd edn. Edinburgh, Mosby.

MacLeod, J., Munro, F. and Campbell, I.W. (eds) (2000). *Clinical Examination*, 3rd edn. Edinburgh, Churchill Livingston.